RB Acc N° 1601

Please return to:

PHARMA
R & D LIBRARY

Johnson/Lloyd-Jones

Drug Delivery Systems

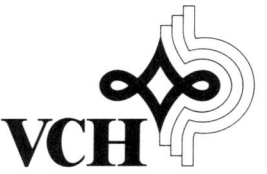 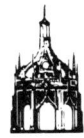

Ellis Horwood Series in Biomedicine

Series Editor: Dr. Alan Wiseman, Department of Biochemistry, University of Surrey

The Blood-Brain Barrier: Drug and Therapeutic Aspects J. P. Bates and N. G. Burnet

Cholecystokinin (CCK) in the Nervous System: Current Developments in Neuropeptide Research J. de Belleroche and G. J. Dockray (Eds.)

Chemiluminescence: Principles and Applications in Biology and Medicine A. K. Campbell

Steroid Hormone Receptors: Their Intracellular Localisation C. R. Clark (Ed.)

Brain 5-HT$_{1A}$ Receptors: Behavioural and Neurochemical Pharmacology C.T. Dourish, S. Ahlenius and P.H. Hutson **(Eds.)**

Cellular and Molecular Basis of Cholinergic Function
M. J. Dowdall and J. N. Hawthorne (Eds.)

Peptidergic Mechanisms in the Cerebral Circulation L. Edvinsson and J. McCulloch (Eds.)

Neuropharmacology and Pesticide Action M. G. Ford, G. G. Lunt, R. C. Reay and P.N. R. Usherwood (Eds.)

Combating Resistance to Xenobiotics: Biological and Chemical Approaches M. G. Ford, D.W. Holloman, B. P.S. Khambay and R. M. Sawicki (Eds.)

Fibrinogen, Fibrin Stabilisation and Fibrinolysis J. L. Francis (Ed.)

Drug Delivery to the Respiratory Tract D. Ganderton and T. Jones (Eds.)

Biological Oxidation of Nitrogen in Organic Molecules J. W. Gorrod and L. A. Damani (Eds.)

Development of Drugs and Modern Medicines: A Conference to Honour Professor Arnold H. Beckett J.W. Gorrod, G. G. Gibson and M. Mitchard (Eds.)

Clinical Pharmacy: Pathology and Therapeutics R. J. Greene and N. D. Harris

Affinity Labelling in Steroid and Thyroid Hormone Research: Techniques, Biological Application and Cloning H. Gronemeyer (Ed.)

Drug Delivery Systems: Fundamentals and Techniques P. Johnson and G. Lloyd-Jones (Eds.)

Monitoring Neurotransmitter Release During Behaviour M. H. Joseph, M. Fillenz, I. A. Macdonald and C. A. Marsden (Eds.)

Blood Substitutes: Physiology and Medical Applications K. C. Lowe **(Ed.)**

Handbook of Cardiac Glycosides: Chemistry, Pharmacology and Toxicology of Nonrenal Digitalis Substances N. Rietbrock and B. G. Woodcock

The Modification of Primary Translation Products by Glycosylation and Acylation
M. F. G. Schmidt and R.T. Schwarz

Interaction of Steroid Hormone Receptors with DNA M. Sluyser (Ed.)

Growth Factors and Oncogenes in Breast Cancer M. Sluyser (Ed.)

Extending Drug Uses: Postmarketing Development of Medicines E. Snell (Ed.)

The Molecular Biology of Receptors: Techniques and Applications of Receptor Research
A. D. Strosberg (Ed.)

The Blood-Brain Barrier in Health and Disease A. J. Suckling, M. G. Rumsby and M.W. Bradbury (Eds.)

Neuropeptides and their Peptidases A. J. Turner (Ed.)

Critical Factors in Haemostasis: Evaluation and Development C. E.Williams, P. E. Short, A. J. George and M. P. B. Entwistle

Drug Delivery Systems

Fundamentals and Techniques

Edited by
P. Johnson and J. G. Lloyd-Jones

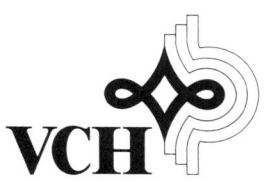

VCH

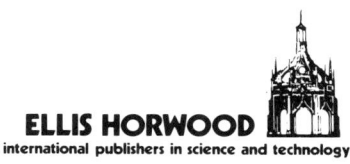

ELLIS HORWOOD
international publishers in science and technology

Editors:
Dr. J. G. Lloyd-Jones
Reckitt and Colman
Pharmaceutical Division
Dansom Lane
Hull, UK

Dr. P. Johnson
Smith Kline and French Research Ltd.
Welwyn
Hertshire, UK

Series Adviser in Pharmaceutical Sciences:
Prof. J. W. Gorrod
Chelsea Department of Pharmacy
University of London
London, UK

Published for the Society for Drug Research
London, UK

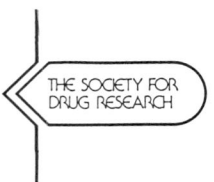

THE SOCIETY FOR
DRUG RESEARCH

Deutsche Bibliothek Cataloguing-in-Publication Data

Drug delivery systems : fundamentals and techniques
/ ed. by P. Johnson and J. G. Lloyd-Jones. –
Weinheim ; New York : VCH ; Chichester : Horwood,
   (Ellis Horwood series in biomedicine)
   ISBN 3-527-26558-9

NE: Johnson, P. [Hrsg.]

ISSN 0930-3367

British Library Cataloguing in Publication Data

Drug delivery systems: fundamentals and techniques. —
(Ellis Horwood series in biomedicine, ISSN 0930–3367).
1. Delayed-action preparations
I. Johnson, P. (Peter)   II. Lloyd-Jones, J.G.
615'.6   RS201.C64

Library of Congress CIP data available

Published jointly in 1987 by
Ellis Horwood Ltd., Chichester, England
and VCH Verlagsgesellschaft mbH, Weinheim, Federal Republic of Germany

Distribution:

Great Britain and Ireland: VCH Publishers (UK) Ltd., 8 Wellington Court, Wellington Street,
   Cambridge CB1 1HW (Great Britain)

USA and Canada: VCH Publishers, Suite 909, 220 East 23rd Street, New York,
   NY 10010-4606 (USA)

Switzerland: VCH Verlags-AG, P.O. Box, CH-4020 Basel (Switzerland)

All other countries: VCH Verlagsgesellschaft, P.O. Box 1260/1280, D-6940 Weinheim
   (Federal Republic of Germany)

ISBN 3-527-26558-9 (VCH Verlagsgesellschaft)   ISBN 0-89573-580-6 (VCH Publishers)

Printed in Great Britain by Unwin   Bros. of Woking

Table of contents

Preface 7

1 **Drug delivery — where now?** 11
   C. R. Gardiner

2 **Biological opportunities for site-specific drug delivery using particulate carriers** 32
   E. Tomlinson

3 **Therapeutic utility of liposomes** .66
   F. H. Roerdink, T. Daemen, I. A. J. M. Bakker-Woudenberg, G. Storm,
   D. J. A. Crommelin and G. L. Scherphof

4 **Monoclonal antibodies as carriers for drug delivery** 81
   G. F. Rowland

5 **Soluble polymers as targetable drug carriers** 95
   J. B. Lloyd

6 **Design of biodegradable polymers for controlled release** 106
   F. G. Hutchinson and B. J. A. Furr

7 **Implantable osmotically powered drug delivery systems** 120
   N. Ray and F. Theeuwes

8 **Implantable pumps for insulin delivery: current clinical status** 139
   P. J. Blackshear

9 **Technological advances in oral drug delivery** 150
   D. Ganderton

**10   Evaluation of the gastrointestinal transit and release characteristics of
     drugs** 164
     S. S. Davis

11   Mucoadhesive polymers in drug delivery systems 180
     G. Hunt, P. Kearney and I. W. Kellaway

12   Transdermal drug delivery 200
     B. W. Barry

13   Recent advances in intranasal drug delivery systems 224
     K. S. E. Su, H. C. Wilson and K. M. Campanale

14   New systems for the ocular delivery of drugs 243
     J. W. Shell

15   Drug delivery: advances and retreats 266
     A. T. Florence

Index 277

Preface

Over the past 25 years, drug delivery technology has made significant advances. This has been spurred on by two major factors: (a) the substantial decline in recent years in the rate of appearance to the medical profession of new drug entities — this being principally attributed to the increased safety requirements associated with drug registration in all major countries — and (b), the advances in precise analytical techniques which have allowed the growth of the science of pharmacokinetics. Drug delivery has increasingly come to be recognized as offering a means of optimizing therapy with established drugs through a better understanding of factors affecting drug absorption, drug release kinetics, drug distribution, pharmacokinetics, bioavailability and toxicity.

Through the rapid advances of recent years, the field of drug delivery has become a multidisciplinary science which for this book has been divided into the following discrete areas of research:

(1) Site-specific drug delivery systems
(2) Implantable drug delivery systems
(3) Oral drug delivery systems
(4) Other non-invasive delivery systems

Site-specific drug delivery systems utilizing various carrier systems such as colloidal and non-colloidal particles, liposomes, monoclonal antibodies and soluble polymers have been developed over the years. Chapters on each of these provide a balanced view of the potential and limitations of each delivery system. Although many unsolved problems remain in these areas, there is every indication that interesting developments can be expected from this technology in the next decade, which may well find major therapeutic uses by the turn of the century.

Implantable drug delivery systems offer an alternative to conventional controlled-release systems, particularly where variable-rate delivery is demanded.

These systems, surgically implanted under the skin, can be driven by osmotic action, by direct mechanical activation or when a continuous controlled flow is required by biodegradation of the implanted polymer matrix. In this section, the authors describe in detail the systems available and their potential for use in both animal toxicology and human studies. From these accounts, it is clear that implantable delivery vehicles currently pioneered with insulin in the treatment of diabetes hold significant opportunities for new and improved therapeutic application of many marketed drugs.

Oral controlled-release systems, although having been intensely researched over the years, will continue to offer new opportunities. The appearance of novel systems like the 'hydrodynamically balanced system', polymer-coated drug/ion-exchange resin complex, mucoadhesive coating, 'Oros' osmotic pump and coated particulate systems offers new approaches to this conventional route of drug administration. The need to fully understand the physiological and physicochemical factors dictating drug release in the gastrointestinal tract is strongly emphasized and needs to be continued through the use of both *in vitro* and *in vivo* techniques. Approaches to these are discussed.

Other routes of drug delivery have gained prominence over the years, particularly directed at improving the therapeutic utility of drugs with comprised systemic availability or where a particular local action is desired. Transdermal, nasal and ocular are among the principal routes considered to offer positive benefits over conventional oral systems.

Transdermal absorption of drugs is a particularly complex process. The development of appropriate systems has been pioneered with scopolamine and nitroglycerin, and the stage is now set for these to be followed by transdermal devices for the treatment of many other disease states. The factors affecting transdermal absorption have been addressed, along with the difficulties associated with interpretation of data.

Increased research effort has been directed towards the development of the nasal route of delivery. This route, having potential for allowing absorption of both polar and non-polar molecules, is of particular interest to peptide- and protein-based drugs. The potential of this route in achieving both rapid and sustained-release absorption is discussed through reference to data derived for a number of drugs. Although, as yet, this remains essentially an under-exploited route, it has potential for providing therapeutic opportunities for the 1990s.

Occular administration of drugs is principally associated with the need to treat ophthalmic diseases and is not regarded as a route for gaining systemic drug action. Although a readily accessible body site, the introduction to the eye of clinically acceptable controlled-release systems has not been without problems. The types of systems available are reviewed and their potential for future use in treatment of various ophthalmic diseases is discussed. Some of these are considered to hold significant promise, particularly in the treatment of disorders prevalent in the Third World, provided the difficulties associated with the development of an eye-drop system with controlled-release properties can be overcome.

It is impossible in a single volume to encompass every area of drug delivery research. However, the topics covered here have the advantage of being based on up-to-date information and in several cases form comprehensive reviews of current progress in the field with appropriate glimpses into the future. Although great challenges lie ahead in designing drug delivery systems for products of biotechnology, the marriage of drug delivery technology with the advancing techniques of molecular biology and genetic engineering holds particular promise.

ACKNOWLEDGEMENTS

The Society for Drug Research, founded in 1966, has been instrumental in providing common ground for those interested in all aspects of drug research. The contributions for this book are derived from the Society's residential meeting 'Advances in Drug Delivery' held at Cambridge in July 1986. The publication of this book has particular significance since it records the papers presented at a meeting held in the year of the Society's 20th anniversary.

We are grateful to the Society for Drug Research for providing the initial forum through which the various contributors were contacted and for making many other arrangements.

Our thanks go to the authors for the time and effort they have spent in providing us with the manuscripts and we acknowledge the invaluable secretarial help of Miss Sue Ibbotson.

P. Johnson
J. G. Lloyd-Jones

1

Drug delivery — where now?

Colin R. Gardner, Merck Sharp & Dohme Research Laboratories, West Point, PA 19486, USA

1. INTRODUCTION

The task of predicting the future is fraught with danger and, at best, can only be as effective as the data set upon which the predictions are based. This presentation can be described as a highly personal, subjective and perhaps controversial view of the current status and future directions of the area we have come to call drug delivery. No doubt many of my colleagues will disagree with my analyses, but through their scientific endeavours they will have ample opportunity to prove me right or wrong.

Let us start with an overview of drug discovery, for I believe that it is in the context of this process that we must see the future of drug delivery research. The pharmaceutical industry of the 1980s no longer relies on blind, mass screening of thousands of compounds in a battery of 'animal models' of human disease. Rather it has chosen a rational approach to drug design where various macromolecular structures (receptors, enzymes) are recognized as potential targets for activation, deactivation or modification as a means of allaying the principal symptoms of a disease, or better still, attacking its root cause. In many cases there is sufficient information on the nature of the endogenous 'substrates' for the macromolecular complexes to permit rational design of agonists, inhibitors, etc. In other cases the leads have come from screening synthetic or natural products in appropriate test systems. What distinguishes this approach from the classical or traditional drug discovery process is that the screening systems are much more selective, involving the use of *in vitro* receptor binding techniques and enzyme inhibition assays. The throughput in such screens is much greater and the responses more specific than in whole animal screening, thereby permitting more effective identification of compounds active at the target site. However, a potential liability of this approach is that active compounds may be selected without indication of their bioavailability, i.e. their ability to transport across biological membranes and their resistance to metabolic inactivation. We shall return to these issues later.

While these changes in the drug discovery process have been occurring over the last 20 years, there has been a corresponding period of change in the area of physical pharmacy and pharmaceutical research and development. There have been advances in assay techniques, formulation stability, sustained-release dosage forms and our understanding of pharmacokinetics and metabolism of drug molecules. This has led to the development of the field of drug delivery which I define as a strategy using processes or devices designed to enhance (ideally optimize) the efficiency of therapeutic agents. It may result in one of a number of consequences:

(1) Enhanced bioavailability
(2) Enhanced therapeutic index
(3) Reduced side-effects
(4) Improved patient acceptance or compliance.

It might be instructive at this point to review the current technology available to achieve these goals, to review how successful we have been and to determine where the future needs lie.

2.   CURRENT TECHNOLOGY

Examples of some drug approaches and drugs which have been incorporated into them are shown in Table 1. It is clear that there is a wide range of technology available for pharmaceutical development, yet only a few products using this technology have reached or survived in the market place.

Why? To respond we need to examine the problems associated with the use of these approaches and to define the information required to devise successful dosage forms (Table 2). It is convenient to use delivery route as a means of subclassifying drug delivery issues.

2.1   Ocular delivery

There are a number of problems associated with delivery of ophthalmic drugs. These depend on a number of factors:

(1) Is there a need for ocular penetration, e.g. topical infection versus glaucoma?.
(2) Drug residence time at the target site — local, intraocular.
(3) Potential for systemic side-effects from nasolacrymal absorption.

In many cases patient compliance and drug efficacy could be improved by the existance of an easily applied, long-lasting delivery system. Despite considerable effort in this field, there is as yet no well-tolerated system available. The Ocusert® (Alza Corporation) [1] is a very sophisticated and effective delivery system which has been used with pilocarpine to treat glaucoma. Despite the elegance of the device it has not proven to be a great commercial success probably for two reasons:

(1) Patients (particularly elderly ones) find it difficult to put a solid insert into the eye, and some find it uncomfortable, giving a foreign body sensation. There is also concern for loss of the device from the eye particularly during sleep.

Table 1 — Examples of drug delivery systems

Route	System	Marketed drug
Ocular	Lacrisert	None
	Ocusert	Policarpine
	Thermogel	None
Transdermal	Skin control	Nitroglycerin
	Device control	Scopolamine
	Enhanced flux	Estradiol
Oral	Polymer-coated pellets	Indomethacin
	Oros	Phenylpropanolamine
	MODS	
	MODAS	
	Pennkinetic	
	Hydrodynamically	Valium
	Balanced capsule	
Rumenal	Rumisert	
Implants	Silicone	Levo-norgestrel
	Poly lactide/glycolide	
	Poly (ortho ester(s))	
Prodrugs	Ophthalmic	Dipivaloyl epinephrine
	Oral	Clinoril
	Oral	L-dopa
	Oral	Aldomet

(2) The second reason is due to a major change in the available therapy for glaucoma. Around the time that Alza was developing the pilocarpine Ocusert there was a movement to beta-blockers as the primary therapy for this disease. Beta-blockers have longer-lasting effects than pilocarpine and do not need such frequent dosing schedules. Thus, the need for an insert may not be so great.

Since many patients seem to object to inserting solid devices, a number of investigators have developed gels and viscous fluids as drug carriers [2,3]. Although residence times are longer than for simple solutions, the major problem again appears to be patient acceptance, since crusting of the gels on the eyelids is an unacceptable occurrence.

More recently there has been interest in the use of liposomes and other emulsions [4,5] for ocular drugs. As yet the evidence for their success is not compelling. Even if they were to show improved efficacy, the stability issues associated with their manufacture, storage and use are not insignificant. As will be reiterated several times in this presentation, I believe that each drug needs to be looked at as a separate entity and its local and systemic pharmacokinetics examined carefully to determine the optimum delivery pattern to achieve satisfactory therapeutic efficacy with acceptable

Table 2 — Problems and needs for current delivery systems

	Problem concern	Need
Ocular	Patient acceptability — Foreign body sensation — Stickiness of 'gels'	Easily applied long-lasting system
Transdermal	Transport rate Irritation Wearability Depot effects Tachyphylaxis	Understand transport processes; enhancers
Oral	Absorption does not necessarily parallel release rate	GI transit control
Implants	Erodibility Reproducibility of erosion and release rates	Chemical and biological information on implant erosion and rate and compatibility

dosing frequency. Methods of achieving this delivery pattern must then be found. Perhaps there needs to be a considerable effort to educate ophthalmologists and patients in the use of novel delivery devices. After all, a whole generation has come to accept contact lenses: why can we not develop a similar acceptance for drug delivery systems? — perhaps our vanity exceeds our desire for effective health care.

2.2 Transdermal delivery
Over the last 5 years there has been a dramatic surge in interest in drug delivery through the skin to produce systemic, as opposed to local, effects associated with topical drug application. The concept of using the skin as a delivery route came largely from developments at the Alza Corporation in the early 1970s [6]. The initial commercial success of the nitroglycerin patches [7] was a further impetus to invest in this approach. It also evoked a number of predictions (or fantasies) regarding the future of this delivery route, with estimates as high as 70% of all new drugs being delivered transdermally by the end of the century. Much of this is hyperbole and does not deserve to be discussed in a scientific forum — rather we should look critically and realistically at the pros and cons of transdermal delivery and decide its value on its scientific merits and true commercial potential. There are now four drugs available in transdermal patch systems:

(1) Scopolamine for motion sickness [8]
(2) Nitroglycerin for angina pectoris [7]
(3) Clonidine for hypertension [9]
(4) Estradiol for post-menopausal hormone replacement [10].

It is, as yet, too early to assess the success of the estradiol system. Of the others, scopolamine has a limited market and clonidine has not achieved any significant market penetration. On the other hand the organo-nitrates have clearly been remarkably successful, although there have been a number of concerns about the possibility of tachyphylaxis possibly due to depletion of an endogenous factor necessary for nitrate activation [11].

The criteria for choosing transdermal drug candidates have been widely discussed [6]. The principle restrictions appear to be:

(1) Is the transport rate fast enough to permit manufacture of an acceptably sized patch to give optimal therapeutic response?
(2) Is the drug non-irritating to the skin, or at least is the irritation acceptable?
(3) Can patches be fabricated which will permit wearing times that are convenient for the patient without being unacceptable aesthetically and functionally (e.g. peeling)?
(4) Does constant input rate give rise to tolerance to the drug effect (e.g. some organo-nitrates)?
(5) Is it possible to use enhancers of dermal penetration which will be safe and effective and can only be incorporated into transdermal delivery systems?
(6) What are suitable models (*in vitro* and *in vivo*) on which to base development of these patches?

Clearly, there are still many scientific issues to be addressed. In addition, the commercial success of these systems will depend on patient acceptance. Where once-a-day oral therapy in available, a 1-day patch is unlikely to be marketable. Thus the need to address extended-wear systems is critical. It will be interesting to observe this market segment over the next 10 years. My prediction is that we shall see transdermal products for carefully chosen, very potent, short half-life drugs, but that transdermal delivery will never be the major route of drug administration.

2.3   Implants

If one traces the interest in controlled drug delivery back to its origins, one finds a paper by Folkman and Long [12] on the use of silicone implants to prolong a drug effect. Despite much activity in the years since 1964 (particularly related to delivery of contraceptive steroids), the progress to a safe, effective and acceptable implant system(s) has been slow. In recent years two implant systems have been approved for human use:

(1) A silicone-based device releasing levo-norgestrel over a 5-year period (Norplant [13]).
(2) More recently, a system based on lactide/glycolide polymers to release a luteinizing hormone-releasing hormone (LHRH) agonist for treatment of male reproductive tract tumors. (See later chapter in this volume.)

This approach to drug delivery is very appealing for a number of classes of drugs, particularly those which cannot be given via the oral route. The major issue is: can we make implants sufficiently reliable in the biologial milieu to deliver potent drugs at a well-defined rate and with a duration of release which will permit a frequency of administration acceptable to the patient? The evidence from two products suggests that this goal can be achieved. We must work to see how these successes can be built on for other compounds. We shall return to this subject later in the discussion.

2.4 Oral route

Despite the interest in other routes of administration (transdermal, implants, etc.) the oral route is, and will continue to be, the primary means of drug administration. There is a vast array of technology available for oral drug delivery, ranging from liquids, capsules and tablets through various sustained-release systems to highly sophisticated osmotic devices. The major question is how to apply this wealth of technology to the solution of a particular problem. To design or select an effective system we must have a full understanding of the biological parameters: how the body treats the drug delivery device and the drug released from this system; and how it responds to the drug and its input rate (see Table 3).

Table 3 — To take advantage of current technology a fuller understanding of the biological parameters is required

GI transit
GI absorption — site and rate
Presystemic metabolism
Drug pharmacokinetics
Effect of constant input rate on biological response

It is only in the last 5 years that the pharmaceutical community has really embraced the importance of gastrointestinal (GI) transit as it relates to drug dosage forms, due largely to two reasons:

(1) A fuller understanding of the physiological factors controlling gastric emptying and the effect of food on the size selectivity of the pylorus.
(2) The availability of safe, non-invasive techniques which permit visualization of dosage forms in the GI tract of animals and humans (e.g. gamma-scintigraphy).

It is beyond the scope of this review to discuss all aspects of gastric emptying and GI transit. (The reader is referred to an excellent review of GI physiology [14], and to chapters in this volume.) Briefly, there are two patterns of gastric emptying. In the fed state, the food is retained in the stomach and subjected to mechanical grinding and enzymatic digestion to reduce the particle size so that effective digestion to molecular constituents can occur in the small intestine prior to absorption.

Older studies using sizing of intestinal contents suggest that the fed stomach retains particles greater than a few mm in diameter. More recent information in dogs [15] would suggest that larger particles can still empty from the stomach during the digestion period, but, in general, as particle size increases, the likelihood of emptying decreases, so that particles >7 mm are essentially retained. After a meal has been digested, the stomach moves into a pattern of mobility controlled by the interdigestive migratory myo-electric complex (IMMC, 'housekeeper wave') which repeats on an approximate 2 h cycle. During the third phase of this cycle there are string contractions of the stomach muscles which expel the entire contents of the stomach (including any undigested material) through the fully open pylorus into the intestines.

The effect of feeding pattern and the digestive cycles on gastric residence time of a non-disintegrating capsule (simulating a controlled-release dosage form) has been determined in a number of human studies using Heidelberg capsules [16] and gamma-scintigraphy [17]. The data from one of these studies are shown in Fig. 1.

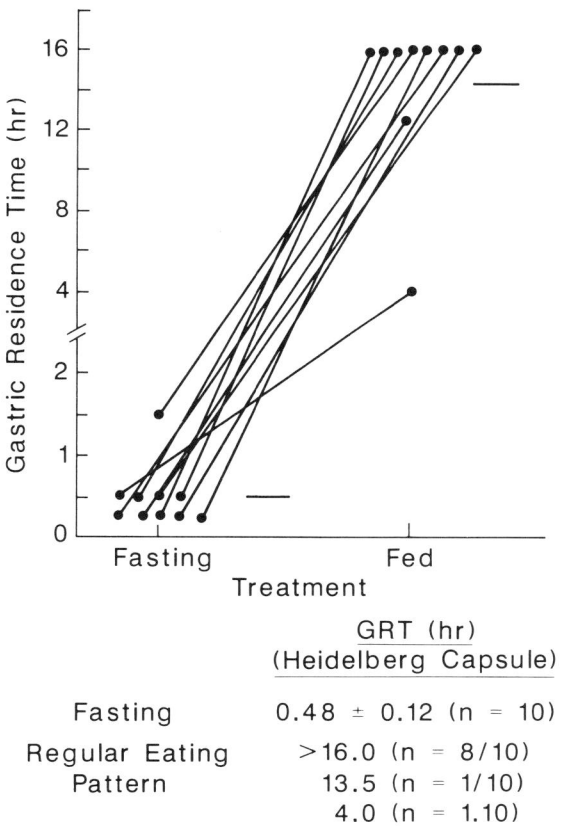

| | GRT (hr) |
	(Heidelberg Capsule)
Fasting	0.48 ± 0.12 (n = 10)
Regular Eating Pattern	>16.0 (n = 8/10)
	13.5 (n = 1/10)
	4.0 (n = 1.10)

Fig. 1 — Gastric residence time of a Heidelberg capsule in ten volunteers in the fasting state and during a regular eating pattern.

Given in a fasting state the capsule was retained in the stomach for less than 1 h, when the subjects took the capsule after breakfast and ate regularly during the day the capsule was retained in eight of ten cases for >16 h but emptied from the stomach during the night, probably as a consequence of an IMMC after digestion of the food was complete. The significance of such information for dosage forms is shown in Fig. 2 where the effect of food on delivery of aspirin from an enteric-coated product is

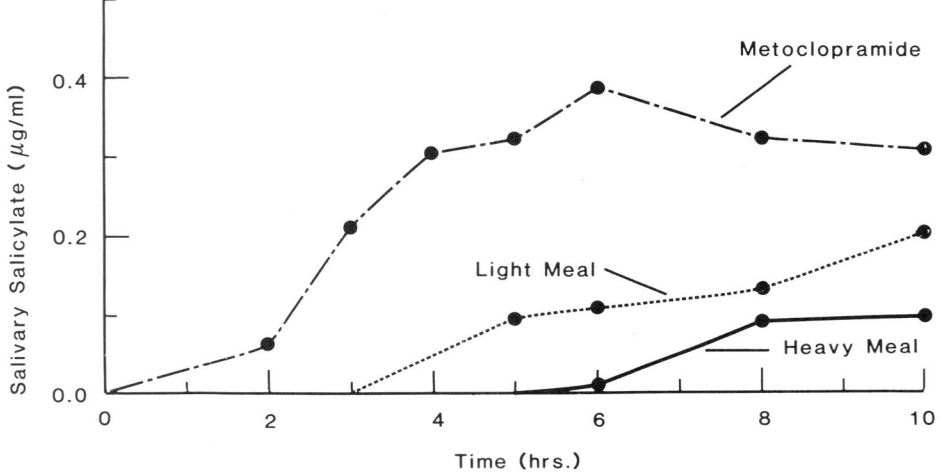

Fig. 2 — Time course of salivary salicylate levels after administration of enteric-coated aspirin with a light meal (dotted line), a heavy meal (solid line) or with metocioptamide (dashed and dotted line), which accelerates gastric emptying. Data replotted from Bogentoft *et al.* [18].

plotted. A reasonable interpretation of these data would suggest that rapid gastric emptying (i.e. with metoclopramide) results in rapid release and absorption of aspirin in the small intestine. On the other hand, in the presence of food, the enteric-coated tablet was retained in the stomach and was ineffective in delivering drug until the food had been digested, the tablet had emptied from the stomach during a 'housekeeper' and the coating had dissolved in the intestine.

A second aspect of the GI tract which affects delivery device performance is the drug absorption site. From the data obtained with a controlled-release device (Oros) delivering an ester of alpha-methyldopa (AMD; Aldomet) in the fasted state, the drug was shown to be effectively absorbed for a period of approximately 4 h. When the device was given to the same subjects in the fed state (feeding pattern as in [16] and Fig. 1 above), the drug was shown to be effectively absorbed for a period of 8.5 h (Table 4). A reasonable interpretation would be that the ester is only well absorbed in the small intestine and that when the device reaches the ileo-cecal junction (~4 h in the fasted state [17]), absorption is no longer effective. Given with food the device was retained in the stomach and the release drug absorbed as it 'trickled' down the

Table 4 — Bioavailability of α-methyldopa — POE ester

	Oros® Fasted	Oros® Fed
Bioavailability	26.5%	36.3%
Absorption rate/ duration	12 mg eg/h 4 h	1.4 mg eg/h 8.5 h

Data from Dobrinska *et al.* [19].

entire length of the small intestine. Clearly the efficacy of such treatment would depend critically on the timing of the dose relative to the eating pattern of the patient.

Another important factor is the concentration dependence of the rate of absorption and presystemic metabolism of a drug. For a drug which is absorbed via a 'carrier' system (e.g. amino acid analogs), the uptake process is saturable and thus more efficient at low drug concentrations. On the other hand, for drugs which are subject to saturable presystemic metabolism in the gut wall or liver, maintaining the drug concentration as high as possible may permit a fraction of the drug to avoid degradation and reach the systemic circulation intact. When both of these effects occur with the same drug, the delivery rate of the drug may be critical in determining its oral bioavailability. Based on *in vitro* [20] and *in vivo* studies in rats we believed that such a situation would pertain to AMD (Aldomet). Since the AMD uptake process resembles that of large neutral amino acids, the uptake from the large intestine is unlikely to be effective. Thus a sustained-release formulation of AMD will only deliver drug effectively while it is in the stomach or small intestine. Given in the fasted state this would limit the delivery period to approximately 4–6 h. On the other hand, if the dosage form were given with a meal, gastric residence time would be extended and the duration of delivery to the small intestine prolonged. However, if food interferes with the absorption or metabolism of AMD, the bioavailability of drug given under these conditions might be affected adversely.

In order to determine if an effective sustained-delivery system for AMD could be developed, we designed the protocol shown in Table 5 to compare the absorption rate, metabolism and total oral bioavailability of AMD under conditions of slow delivery rate in the presence and absence of food compared to bolus administration under the same eating conditions. A summary of the results (which will be presented elsewhere) is shown in Table 6. It is clear that slow infusion of AMD in the fed state results in dramatically reduced bioavailability of AMD and that a sustained-release formulation of AMD would not be effective. These predictions were later confirmed by experimental studies with a controlled-release device.

These results indicate the desirability of obtaining a drug delivery system which will have a slow GI transit. This might be achieved either by retaining the device in the stomach even in the fasting state or by increasing the transit time in the small intestine. So far no effective solution to this problem has been identified.

A summary of what we have learned from past drug delivery experiences is given in Table 7. It is clear that optimizing drug delivery is not a matter of putting a drug in

Table 5 — Protocol for determining feasibility of a sustained-release formulation of α-methyldopa (AMD)

Five-way cross-over in ten healthy male volunteers age 21–40 years	
A: Oral bolus/fasted	400 mg
B: Oral bolus/fed[†]	400 mg
C: Slow nasogastric infusion/ fasted	400 mg (50 mg/h)
D: Slow nasogastric infusion/fed*	400 mg (50 mg/h)
E: IV/fasted	225 mg/15 min

[†]Breakfast, lunch, dinner.
  Plasma and unrine samples were assayed for AMD and metabolites.

Table 6 — Comparative bioavailability of α-methyldopa (AMD) delivered by oral bolus or gastric flow infusion in the fed and fasting states

Delivery pattern	Bioavailability of AMD ($n = 10$) (% of IV AUC)
Oral bolus/fasted	25.5 ± 16.4 (S.D.)
Oral bolus/fed	21.7 ± 6.9
Slow gastric infusion/fasted	24.9 ± 7.7
Slow gastric infusion/fed	12.0 ± 3.1

Table 7 — Drug delivery — where are we now?

Physical and chemical systems available
Requires appropriate choice of drug
No generic approach — each compound has to be researched thoroughly
Needs multidisciplinary effort
Should start early in development of research program

any available drug delivery system. The absorption site and rate and presystemic metabolism have to be considered carefully in assessing whether the drug is a candidate for oral controlled release and in deciding on the design crtieria for an effective dosage form. This strategy will require a multidisciplinary approach which ought to start early in the development of a potential new therapeutic agent.

3. THE FUTURE

The previous sections argued that although much technology exists, the application to effective drug delivery optmization has been slow and in many cases driven by purely commercial rather than a combination of scientific and commercial criteria. It is now time to take a look into the future and attempt to predict where fruitful directions may lie. Table 8 lists six areas which I believe are worthy of investigation

Table 8 — Potential areas of future drug delivery interest

Pulsatile systems
Feedback control
Implants
Drug targeting
Selective drug delivery to the CNS
Delivery of peptide and protein drugs

---

and where breakthroughs could have significant therapeutic and commercial impact.

3.1 Pulsatile delivery

There is good evidence from many systems (neurotransmitters, peptide hormones, etc.) that continuous receptor stimulation can lead to reduced response (tachyphylaxis), while continuous receptor blockade can lead to supersensitivity. This has many profound implications for the use of sustained-released dosage forms. (I have already discussed a similar situation with transdermal nitroglycerin patches.) Thus, for animal and human health products we have to consider the possibility of using systems which will permit delivery or release of drug in a pulsatile fashion; either predetermined or controlled by the patients themselves. Because of the GI transit time considerations discussed earlier, it is unlikely that human oral controlled-delivery systems will be required to deliver in a pulsatile fashion; however, the use of such devices is being studied in cattle where residence time can be many months.

Thus, pulsatile delivery is more likely to be used in controlled-release devices designed to function over several days to months, such as transdermal patches or implantable or injectable depots.

The control of pulses can be either chemical or electronic. For example, controlled erosion of a bioerodible polymer could be used to trigger the release mechanisms. Despite considerable efforts in the area of erodible systems there is still a lot to be learned, and achieved in this area, particularly where precise control is essential (see later). The other possibility is through microchip technology. In this case the timer will be electronic and the driving force for drug release could be via one of many mechanisms — mechanical, electrical, magnetic or chemical. For an implant the device will have to be surgically inserted and removed when the drug load is depleted, or the device will have to be capable of being refilled via an external septum. Clearly the severity or inconvenience of the disease will have to be sufficient to warrant such heroic measures on the part of the patient. A transdermal delivery system would obviate some of these problems, but, as we discussed in an earlier section, the criteria for drugs suitable for this route of administration are strict and may exclude many of the candidates likely to require pulsatile delivery (e.g. peptides; see later discussion).

3.2 Feedback systems
In all living systems there exists a multitude of feedback mechanisms, many of them redundant, which control and fine-tune the responses critical to the well-being of the organism. If we are to be able to attempt to mimic the performance of many biological mediators we need to understand fully the minimum control required for each modulator and have some mechanism to monitor the appropriate parameters and modify the drug release rate. This type of control is well known to chemical engineers and the technology exists to employ it on a large scale. The problems we face are to miniaturize the components and to guarantee their reliability and precision over long periods of time in a biological environment. Given the current state of our technology, this type of approach has to be very long range and to be considered only for a small group of potential users.

3.3 Implants
I have already reviewed the current status of drug implants in an earlier section. Suffice it to say, that while this is a very appealing idea for many therapeutic uses, the success rate to date has been remarkably poor. The critical factors which need to be addressed are listed in Table 9. While it is possible to surgically implant and remove

Table 9 — Critical questions for implant research

Erodibility
Reproducibility
Lack of irritation/carcinogenicity
Lack of dose dumping
Duration (days, months, years?)
Pulses?

drug-containing devices or polymeric matrices, the requirement for such intervention could have a significant negative impact on the acceptability of a product candidate. Two avenues seem possible. The first is the use of implanted mechanically or electrically driven pumps which can be refilled by simple injection of drug through a septum into the pump reservoir. The advantage of such systems is that the pumping rate can be under microprocessor control. It can be reliably programmed and altered via radio signals. The major disadvantages are the size of the devices, the need for surgical implantation and the possibility of infection and reduction at the implant and refilling sites. The use of these types of device is reviewed elsewhere in this volume.

The second approach is the use of erodible implants. Here the requirements are for a system which will be safe and whose erosion rate can be sufficiently well controlled to give a reproducible and precise drug release rate over the entire lifetime of the implant. While, in theory, this does not seem to be unobtainable, the success to date has been remarkably limited. The desire to build in precise zero-order surface erosion of polymers without alteration of the structural integrity of the inner structures has been difficult to meet. Thus, although surface erosion can account for a significant portion of the release process (particularly if the device lifetime is relatively short), diffusion of drug out of device or water into the polymer ultimately contributes to the drug release process and causes unpredictable changes in release rate, some of which may be catastrophic. A discussion of how some of these problems have been addressed is contained in another chapter in this volume.

Clearly the future use of polymeric systems as implants requires greater input from polymer chemists and materials who have learned to understand the nature and properties of the biological milieu. The nature of the drug and its required release characteristics are also critical. It would seem prudent to start efforts with candidates whose therapeutic index is relatively large, whose delivery rate is not narrowly defined and where continuous release is unlikely to lead to tolerance and lack of response (unless this is the therapeutic goal!)

Despite the difficulties inherent in the development of safe, effective and manufacturable implant systems, the potential usefulness of such devices in human and animal health care is enormous and is well worth pursuing. As with all drug delivery areas, success will only be achieved by use of appropriate multidisciplinary teams dedicated to choosing problems capable of solution and to persevering with efforts to overcome the difficulties.

3.4 Drug targeting

The term drug targeting is one which evokes different types of concepts in our minds depending on the discipline from which we come or which we represent. However, it usually conjures up thoughts of directing therapeutic agents specifically to their desired site of action without permitting them to interact with non-tissue. I have discussed previously [21] three ways in which this might be achieved:

(1) Using the selectivity of the biological receptors and finding agents which act only at this site. This latter approach will work only if the receptor subtype is responsible for a single pharmacological response.
(2) Having the drug in an active form which is converted to active drug only at the required site of action
(3) Directing the drug selectively to the target tissue while preventing it from 'seeing' other tissues.

The first approach is the realm of the medicinal chemists and many of our currently available drugs owe their efficiency and safety to the remarkable ingenuity of this group of scientists who have subdivided adrenergic receptors into alphas and betas and further subdivided them into α_1, α_2, etc. and β_1, β_2, etc. However, despite this capability there are still many situations where selectivity at receptor subtypes is not enough, where no such subtypes are yet known to exist or where the target disease stems from some biological response whose dependence on receptors is as yet unclear.

The second approach has been practised by chemists and pharmaceutical scientists alike. The prodrug approach, as it is called, has a number of successes in improving transport across biological barriers and a few successes in achieving selectivity, if not specificity, of action at a particular organ [22]. Perhaps the most classically well known of these is the use of L-dopa as a precursor of dopamine to treat Parkinson's disease. By the administration of peripherally acting inhibitors or aromatic L-amino acid decarboxylase (AADC) it has proved possible to remarkably reduce the peripheral side-effects of L-dopa therapy while retaining the therapeutic response to the enhanced central nervous system (CNS) levels of dopamine. However, even this achievement is not absolute and centrally mediated responses to poorly controlled brain dopamine levels can still result in undesirable side-effects.

Until recently the third approach has involved mainly pharmaceutical agents such as the use of microcapsules, emulsions, liposomes or other microparticulates. Although, in the past, there have been efforts to use 'biomolecules' to direct drugs or drug-containing vehicles to specific targets, it is only recently, with the development of monoclonal antibodies, that renewed interest has appeared in this approach to targeting.

The disease targets have been different for each type of approach. With the microparticulate and/or antibody direction, the major interest has been in the field of cancer treatment. There has been a great deal of endeavor in this area by some skilled (and some not so skilled) contributors. However, despite these efforts, success has been conspicuous by its absence. Much of the early lack of success was due to failure to understand the nature of the problem. There were many reports of enhanced uptake of drugs by tumor cells in the culture dish and even some cases of claimed success with treatment of peritoneal ascites tumors. In neither situation does this build a case for effective systemic therapy. In the first case the cells have unlimited access to the drug/vehicle particles, and the use of the peritoneal cavity as a model has been criticized by George Poste as use of an *in vivo* test tube where again the drug particles have access to the tumor cells without having to escape the reticuloendothelial system (RES) or pass across capillary endothelial barriers to reach the target site. In retrospect, but perhaps it should have been with foresight, many of these approaches were naive and ill-conceived [21,23]. It is remarkable that many investigators still continue to plod along this well-worn path with apparent disregard of the fate of their own or others' efforts. A true success in this area might come from an understanding of the nature of the surface chemistry involved in particular recognition by the RES. However noble this goal, its conversion to effective commercial products still seems to be well in the future.

Likewise, there is now reason to believe that the antibody approach is less attractive than was at first perceived. The goal here seems to be treatment of metastatic cancer, hitting particularly microscopic tumor foci undetectable by standard procedures. The problem seems to be in the nature and heterogeneity of the tumor surface antigens and the ability of secondary tumors to display epitopes different from those on the surface of the primary tumor. This is clearly a very serious barrier to this approach. Work is still progressing in this area, but it seems unlikely that a breakthrough is just around the corner, as a number of investigators would have us believe. In terms of cancer treatment, the breakthrough seems more likely to come from a better understanding of the molecular biology associated with the disease process. This will ultimately lead to new, better-defined and more specific targets than have existed with previous therapeutic modalities which have tended to attack cells on the basis of properties common to many normal as well as malignant cells. Success in these endeavors once again will result in providing the medicinal chemist with a challenge to make agonists or antagonists which are selective for the particular receptor. This time, however, the targets may be more complex since peptides and nucleic acids may be the endogenous ligands for these recognition sites.

The prodrug approach is still a viable one [22]. It has a track record of successful agents and an understanding of the limitations of this approach [24,25] will certainly help to define targets which are likely to be amenable to solution. It must be clearly borne in mind that, getting the drug to the target site without it being exposed to other interactive sites, is only part of the task. Once there it must be retained preferentially or, if released, its half-life in the external environment must be short. Failure to apply these principles will result in systemic drug concentrations not significantly different from those achieved by giving the parent drug, and all 'targeting' effect will be lost [24].

A somewhat easier, though by no means simple task, is the use of targeting to identify the existence and site of tumors, particularly metastatic neoplasms. Here, one does not need to obtain very high concentrations of the targeting 'vehicle' at the target site and the distribution to other sites such as the RES may be tolerated provided the tumor remains 'visible' for a sufficiently long term to permit the body background to decay to a low level. This goal may best be achieved by use of gamma-emitting labels attached to targeting vehicles. Whole body scans using gamma-scintigraphy can then be used to try to localize secondary tumors. This type of research is still in its infancy. If antibodies are to be used as the targeting vehicle, the question of antigenic multiplicity and evolution remains a major concern.

Since the RES remains the major obstacle to delivery of particulate material from the vascular system, the idea of targeting to the RES has been addressed. There are a number of diseases where parasitic infections of the RES are particularly difficult to treat due to poor penetration of active chemotherapeutic agents. The use of particulates or colloids to enhance uptake by the reticuloendothial cells in which the parasites are residing may be the most effective use of the targeting research which has been conducted over the last 20 years.

3.5 Central nervous system selectivity

One area where selective site distribution would clearly be advantageous is in the treatment of CNS disorders [26]. Frequently the CNS receptors or enzymes which are targets for intervention are indistinguishable from corresponding receptors or enzymes in the periphery. In some instances it is possible by careful dosing to interact sufficiently at CNS sites without inducing side-effects to such a degree as to be intolerable (e.g. Aldomet, clonidine). However, in other situations, notably the cholinergic system, the potential for serious peripheral side-efects severely limits what might otherwise be potential therapeutic successes.

To date the use of inhibitors of AADC such as carbidopa or benserazide have proved to be the most effective means of achieving central selectivity. The situation with L-dopa treatment of Parkinson's disease has already been discussed. A more recent application of this approach lies in confining to the CNS activation of a prodrug of a potent manoamine oxidase inhibitor (MDL 72394). This concept has proved useful in animal studies [27] and awaits demonstration of activity in the clinical setting.

3.6 Peptides and proteins as drugs

The very significant advances in synthetic chemistry of peptides and recombinant DNA technology for production of proteins have created a vast potential for novel types of drug therapy. While the means of production and the mechanisms for testing efficacy *in vitro* and *in vivo* are in place, the limiting factor in making drugs out of these interesting research leads lies in the lack of effective means of delivering them to the patient population in an acceptable manner. The magnitude of this problem depends on the nature of the disease being tested. For example, patients suffering from life-threatening diseases such as cancer, diabetes, and severe cardiovascular occlusions will, in most cases, be willing to accept parenteral administration of useful or potentially useful drugs, such as peptides or proteins. However, if the disease is not immediately life threatening, regardless of the potential long-term threat, the majority of the patient population is unlikely to accept frequent injections.

Thus, there are two major areas of interest in delivery of peptides and proteins. The first is finding adequate ways to prepare stable, effective formulations for parenteral administration. This raises a number of potential problems including:

(1) Stability of the protein (in storage; during use)
 — chemical
 — conformational
(2) Solubility
(3) Adsorption to surfaces.

The nature and severity of these problems will depend on the particular protein. However, these should be amenable to solution in most cases using the multidisciplinary efforts of biochemists and pharmaceutical chemists. The second type of problem is much more difficult to overcome; that is, to find a more acceptable method of delivering peptide and protein drugs. It is highly unlikely that we shall be able to achieve oral absorption of intact proteins in a reliable and predictable manner. Claims in the literature of GI absorption of insulin (a large peptide rather than a protein) usually prove to be optimistic and close examination of the data reveals that only 1% or, at most, 2% was bioavailable. Thus, the problem for larger proteins does not seem to be solvable.

We know very little about the oral absorption of small peptides. There are a number of marketed drugs which are peptides and some of these are orally bioavailable. One of these is the dipeptide angiotensin-converting enzyme (ACE) inhibitor enalapril (MK-421). This compound is a prodrug in which an ester function is cleaved following absorption, releasing the active enzyme inhibitor enalaprilat (MK-422). The oral bioavailability of enalapril is at least an order of magnitude better than that of enalaprilat in a number of species (rat, dog, human). The absorption of enalapril is rapid and extensive with peak plasma levels appearing within 1 h of dosing. On the other hand, lisinopril, an analog of enalapril which has the alanine replaced by lysine, shows lower oral bioavailability with absorption occurring over a more extended period [26]. The exact mechanism whereby these compounds are absorbed has not yet been determined, although some data on the pH dependence of enalapril absorption have suggested that it may be absorbed via a passive mechanism high in the small intestine [27].

The oral absorption of a number of other peptide drugs has been examined. Cyclic hecapeptide somatostatin analogs have shown poor oral bioavailability while cyclosporin A (a cyclic undecapeptide) shows fairly respectable absorption. This latter phenomenon has been reported to be critically dependent on the formulation of the compound (Table 10). Exactly how the oil-based formulation assists the

Table 10 — Biopharmaceutical properties of cyclosporin A

Oral doses (human)	~12.5 mg/kg/day
Average oral absorption	37%
First-pass metabolism (lipid vehicle)	25%
Oral bioavailability (dependent on formulation)	27%
Biliary excretion (rat)	>50% after IV
Recovery of intact compound in urine	0.1%
Urinary recovery of radioactivity	6%
Metabolites contain intact ring system	

Information extracted Borel [30].

absorption is not fully understood, although there is a requirement for intact bile flow to achieve good absorption [31,32]. Given what we thought we knew about the relationship between molecular weight and absorption, it is somewhat surprising to find that a molecule like cyclosporin A (1200 daltons) is so well taken up. Cyclosporin A has a very unusual structure with no free functional groups on its surface. It would be interesting to know how important its structural features are in promoting good absorption.

Other routes of administration have been used or proposed for peptides. In particular, nasal delivery is the route by which oxytocin and vasopressin and their analogs are administered. The bioavailability of these agents is fairly low and there has been considerable research effort in recent years to pursue the nasal route. A number of absorption-promoting agents have been tried. Bile salts are reported to signficantly enhance nasal absorption of insulin [33] but irritation and mucosal cell damage seem to be a major concern [34]. Recently some investigators have reported the use of polyacrylic acid gels to enhance nasal absorption. They have claimed significantly enhanced bioavailability of insulin and calcitonin [35]. Further safety and clinical studies will be required to demonstrate the efficacy or acceptability of such dosage forms.

Absorption enhancers have also been applied to the GI tract. The literature abounds with references to compounds which promote rectal absorption of drugs [36]. Without a clear idea of the mechanism of such events it is difficult to assess the safety or toxic potential of this approach. Perhaps the need to find alternative, non-parenteral delivery of the peptide and protein products of recombinant DNA technology will stimulate the answering of these critical questions.

The other method of delivery of peptides and proteins is via implants which have already been discussed at length earlier in this text. Again the impetus of overcoming delivery problems for these agents may be the stimulus to improve the chemistry and biology of implant technology.

Another important aspect affecting the potential of peptides and proteins as drugs is the ability of the liver to extract many of these compounds very efficiently. The mechanisms of this extraction and the relationship between extraction efficiency and structure are poorly understood. A clear understanding of the process would be extremely useful in helping to design molecules with longer half-lives, hence, reducing the frequency of dosing or the dose burden imposed on a long-term delivery system.

4. CONCLUSION

This presentation has listed some of the topics which I believe should be the top priorities for drug delivery in the last decade of this century. There are no magic solutions to improving the adminsitration of a new or old drug entity. Only a full understanding of the problem, a clear definition of the goals and a multidisciplinary effort is likely to succeed (Fig. 3). Even then there will be some problems which are not amenable to solutions with today's knowledge and technology. They are best left alone.

My final plea is that we let good science and not entrepreneurial zeal be the guide in determining the future directions of drug delivery. Failure to do so can only result in disillusionment and a sullied reputation for the pharmaceutical research area.

REFERENCES

[1] Chandrasekaran, S. K., Benson, H. & Urquhart, J. (1978) Methods to achieve controlled drug delivery. In: Robinson, J. R. (ed.) *Sustained and Controlled Drug Delivery Systems*, Marcel Dekker, New York, p. 557.

[2] Haslam, J., Higuchi, T. & Mlodozeniec, A. *Ophthalmic Drug Delivery System Utilizing Thermal Setting Gels*, U.S. Patent No. 4 474 751.

[3] Hui, H.-W. & Robinson, J. R. (1985). Ocular delivery of progesterone using a bioadhesive polymer. *Int. J. Pharmaceut.* **26** 203.

DRUG DISCOVERY

RATIONAL DRUG DESIGN PROCESS

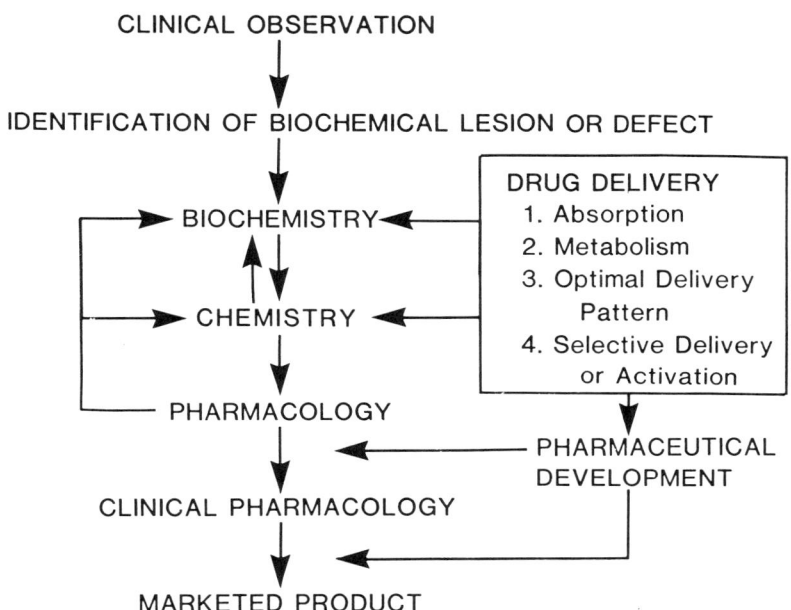

Fig. 3 — Multidisciplinary approach to rational drug design. Incorporation of drug delivery
consideration into the design and development cycles. Reproduced from Gardner [21].

[4] Lee, V. H. L. (1985) Topical ocular drug delivery: recent advances and future perspectives. *Pharmacy Int.* **135**.

[5] Robinson, J. R. & Li, V. H. K. (1984) Ocular disposition and bioavailability of pilocarpine from Piloplex and other sustained release drug delivery systems. In: Ticho, U. & David, R. (eds), *Recent Advances in Glaucoma*, Elsevier, Amsterdam, p. 231.

[6] Zaffaroni, A. (1982) Industrial development of transdermal therapeutic systems. In: Brandan, R. & Lippold, B. H. (eds). *Dermal and Transdermal Absorption*, Wissenschaftliche Verlagsgesellchaft, Stuttgart, p. 188.

[7] Abrams, J. (1984). Nitrate delivery systems in perspective; a decade of progress. *Am. J. Med.* **76**, 38.

[8] Chandrasekran, S. K. & Shaw, J. E. (1977) Design of transdermal therapeutic systems. In: Pearce, E. M. & Schafgen, J. R. (eds) *Contemporary Topics in Polymer Science*, Vol. 2, Plenum, New York, p. 291.

[9] Weber, M. A. & Drayer, J. I. M. (1984) Clinical experience with rate-controlled delviery of anithypertensive therapy by a transdermal system. *Am. Heart J.* **108**, 231.

[10] Chetowski, R. J., Meldrum, D. R., Steingold, K. A., Randle, D., Lu, J. K., Eggena, P., Hershman, J. M., Alkjaersig, N. K., Fletcher, A. P. & Judd, H. L. (1986). Biological effects of transdermal estradiol. *New England J. Med.* **314**, 1615.

[11] Fung, H.-L. (1985) Nitrate formulations and drug delivery systems — an overview. *Z. Kardiol.* **74**, (Suppl. 4) 4.

[12] Folkman, J. & Long, D. M. (1964) The use of silicone rubber as a carrier for prolonged drug therapy. *J. Surg. Res.* **4** 139.

[13] Sivin, I. (1983) Clinical effects of Norplant® subdermal implants for concentration. In: Mishell, D. R. (ed.) *Long-Acting Steroid Contraception*, Raven Press, New York, p. 89.

[14] Kelly, K. A. (1981). Motility of the stomach and gastroduodenal junction. In: Johnson, L. B. (ed.) *Physiology of the Gastrointestinal Tract*, Raven Press, New York, p. 393.

[15] Itoh, T., Higuchi, T., Gardner, C. R. & Caldwell, L. (1986) Effect of particle size and food on gastric residence time on non-disintegrating solids in beagle dogs. *J. Pharm. Pharmcol.* **38**, 801.

[16] Mojaverian, P., Ferguson, R. K., Vlasses, P. H., Rocci, M. L., Oven, A., Fix, J. A., Caldwell, L. J. & Gardner, C. R. (1985). Estimation of gastic residence time of the Heidelberg capsule in humans: effect of varying of food composition. *Gastroenterology* **89** 392.

[17] Davis, S. S., Hardy, J. G., Taylor, M. J., Whalley, D. R. & Wilson, C. G. (1984). The effect of food on the gastrointestinal transit of pellets and an osmotic device (Osmet). *Int. J. Pharmaceut.* **21** 331.

[18] Bogentoft, C., Carlsson, I., Ekenued, G. & Magnusson, A. (1978). Influence of food on the absorption of acetyl salicylic acid from enteric-coated dosage forms. *Eur. J. Clin. Pharmacol.* **14** 351.

[19] Dobrinska, M. R., Titus, D. C., Harris, K. E., Walkow, J. C. Fara, J. W., Kulaga, S. F., McWilliams, E. J. & McMahon, F. G. (1985) Effect of Food/Transit Time on Bioavailability of Methyldopa from a Controlled-release Formulation, A.Ph.A. Annual Meeting Abstracts, Minneapolis.

[20] Osiecka, I., Cortese, M., Porter, P. A., Borchardt, R. T., Fix, J. A. & Gardner, C. R. (1987) Intestinal absorption of alpha-methyldopa: in-vitro mechanistic studies in rat small intestinal segments, *J. Pharmac. Exp. Therap.* (in press).

[21] Gardner, C. R. (1985). Potential and limitations of drug targeting: an overview. *Biomaterials* **6** 153.

[22] Gardner, C. R. & Alexander, J. (1985) Pro-drug approaches to drug targeting: past accomplishments and future potential. In: Buri, P. & Gumma, A. (eds) *Drug Targeting*. Elsevier, Amsterdam, p. 145.

[23] Poste, G., & Kirsch, R. (1983) Site-specific (targeted) drug delivery in cancer therapy. *Biotech.* **1** 869.

[24] Stella, V. J. & Himmelstein, K. L. (1980) Prodrugs and site specific delivery. *J. Med. Chem.* **23**, 1275.

[25] Stella, V. J. & Himmelstein, K. J. (1985). Prodrugs: a chemical approach to targeted drug delivery. In: Borchardt, R. T., Repta, A. J. & Steel, V. J. (eds)

Directed Drug Delivery, The Humana Press, Clifron, NJ, p. 247.

[26] Gardner, C. R. (1985). Chemical approaches to drug delivery to the central nervous system. *Psychopharmacol. Bull.* **21** 657.

[27] Palfreyman, M. G., McDonald, I. A., Fozard, J. R., Mely, Y., Sleight, A. J., Zreika, M., Wagner, J., Bey, P. & Lewis, P. J. (1985) Inhibition of monoamine oxidase selectivity in brain monoamine nerves using the bioprecursor (E)-β-fluormethylene-m-tyrosine (MDL 72394), a substrate for aromatic L-amino acid decarboxylase. *J. Neurochem.* **45** 1850.

[28] Ulm, E. H., Hitchins, M., Gomez, H. J., Till, A. E., Hand, E., Vassil, T. C., Biollay, J., Brunner, H. R. & Schelling, J. L. (1982). Enalapril maleate and a lysine analogue (MK-521): disposition in man. *Br. J. Clin. Pharmac.* **14** 357.

[29] Gardner, C. R. (1985). Gastrointestinal barrier to oral drug delivery. In: Borchardt, R. T., Repta, A. J. & Stella, V. J. (eds) *Directed Drug Delivery*, The Humana Press, Clifton, NJ, p. 61.

[30] Borel, J. (1981). The history of cyclosporin A and its significance. In: White, D. J. G. (ed.) *Cyclosporin A*, Elsevier Biomedical Press, Amsterdam, p. 5.

[31] Zaghloul, I., Takaya, S., Noguchi, T., Ohmori, Y., Iwatsuki, S., Burchardt, J. G., Ptachcinski, R. J. & Venkataramanan, R. (1985). *Effect of Bile Duct Ligation on Cyclosporin Pharmacokinetics*, A.Ph.A. Annual Meeting Abstracts, Minneapolis, Abstract No. 131, p. 169.

[32] Menta, M. U., Venkataramanan, R., Gray, J. A., Ptachcinski, R. J., Burchardt, J. G., Starzl, T. E., VanThiel, D. H., Iwatsuki, S., Staschak, S. & Shaw, B. W. (1985). *Effect of Bile on Cyclosporin Absorption in Humans*, A.Ph.A. Annual Meeting Abstracts, Minneapolis, Abstract No. 130, p. 169.

[33] Moses, A. C., Gordon, G. S., Carey, M. C. & Carey, M. C. & Flier, J. S. (1983) Insulin administered intranasally as an insulin-bile salt aerosol. Effectiveness and reproducibility in normal diabetic subjects. *Diabetes* **32** 1040.

[34] Salzman, R., Manson, J. E., Griffing, G. T., Kimmerle, R., Ruderman, N., McCall, A., Stoltz, E. I., Mullen, C., Small, D., Armstrong, J. & Melby, J. C. (1985). Intranasal aerosoluized insulin. Mixed-meal studies and long-term use in type I diabetes. *New England J. Med.* **312** 1078.

[35] Morimoto, K., Morisaka, K., & Kamada, A. (1985). Enhancement of nasal absorption of insulin and calcitonin using polyacrylic acid gel. *J. Pharm. Pharmacol.* **37** 134.

[36] Fix, J. A. & Gardner, C. R. (1987) Rectal drug delivery — a viable alternative? *Pharmacy Int.* **7** 272.

2

Biological opportunities for site-specific drug delivery using particulate carriers

E. Tomlinson, Advanced Drug Delivery Research, Ciba-Geigy Pharmaceuticals, Horsham, RH12 4AB, UK.

1. INTRODUCTION

Recent and continued advances in cell and molecular biology are helping to further our understanding of both normal and pathological physiology. It is believed that such new knowledge will result in both a clearer definition of disease states, as well as their management via (bio)chemical intervention. Additionally, improved control of gene expression in eukaryotes and prokaryotes is leading to the production of new homologous and heterologous peptidergic mediators of high specificity and complexity.

Drug administration has come of age during the past decade with many interesting devices and approaches utilized for achieving a controlled input of drug into the blood pool. Unfortunately, often the pharmacological parameters used to determine such levels are derived from simple bolus or infusion dosing approaches, which can lead to a less than clear appreciation of the clinical management of the steady-state pharmacology of many of the drugs being administered using controlled-release systems. Although this will change, it is also apparent that drug use currently relies on two processes to ensure efficiency and safety, i.e. first, that after passively reaching its site of action(s) a drug is able to interact specifically with its pharmacological receptor, and second, that the body's capacity to detoxify and eliminate the unwanted drug is such that untoward effects do not arise. In hundreds of thousands of documented instances, putative drugs fail to reach clinical use because *in vivo* either of these two processes are not favourable. Witness for example the difficulty with cytotoxic agents, or agents such as the corticosteroids in inflammation. Also, the use of paracrine- and endocrine-like peptidergic mediators, when administered as drugs by conventional dosing regimes, can be described as inefficient, often due to their widespread disposition and placement, rapid inactivation (catabolism and liver extraction), and variable and inefficient extravasation, as well as possessing unduly high toxicities because of the high circulating levels they require to reach their site(s) of action. Although it is traditional to deal with these issues by a process of molecular roulette (and its bioengineering equivalent — gene jockeying), it is clear that achievement of site-specific delivery of drug molecules would be a clear advantage, particularly if this could occur in an exclusive manner such that prior to interaction with the pharmacological receptor protection of the drug from the body (and vice versa) occurred (Table 1).

Table 1 — Rationale for site-specific drug delivery

Exclusive delivery to specific compartments (and/or diseases)

Access to previously inaccessible sites (e.g. intracellular infections)

Protection of drug and body from unwanted deposition which could lead to untoward reactions and metabolism, etc

Controlled rate and modality of delivery to pharmacological receptor

Reduction in the amount of active principle employed

Tomlinson [1].

We have argued [1] that for site-specific drug delivery to occur, therapeutic systems have to be designed such that they have the functions of site access, and retention, and that the issue of timing of release may be critical to successful drug use. Approaches to site-specific delivery include either the *de novo* synthesis of constructs (using synthetic and bioengineering approaches) and/or the use of carrier systems.

Drug targeting is a much worked term, though it is only in very recent years that the biological opportunities which exist for site-specific delivery have come to be elucidated. This has followed from an understanding of both anatomical and (patho)physiological opportunities and constraints, as well as from a proper consideration of the nature of the drug's interaction with the disease, including, for example with peptidergic mediators, target cell responses, unique dose–response relationships and the influence of time effects on these, the intravascular to extravascular localization required, potential side-effects, and clinical use of developed therapeutic systems.

Two types of system can be considered as drug carriers, i.e. particulates and soluble (bio)(macro)molecules. In this present contribution the use of colloidal and non-colloidal particles for site-specific drug delivery will be described in terms of the biological opportunities which exist for their use. Particulate carriers of sizes 20 nm to up to 200 microns have been proposed because of (a) the presumably high payload of drug that could be released in a controlled and sustained fashion, and (b) the unique biological pathways that such materials can have. Reference will be centred around the features of access, retention, and timing. Particles can be monolithic or capsular, and include such constructs as lipid and protein nanoparticles and liposomes, etc. However, it is argued from the outset that current knowledge gives that because of their general inability to leave the general circulation, particulate carriers will only have a use that is restricted to either biochemical or cellular targets within the vasculature, to discrete anatomical compartments or to extravascular targets at highly specialized areas or where the pathological state permits it.

Table 2 gives the properties that appear to be needed for site-specific carriers [1].

Table 2 — Idealized characteristics of a site-specific drug delivery system

---

Biological factors
    Vascular carriage to site of action
    Placement at site (via active or passive means)
    Epi- and/or endothelial passage
    Restricted drug distribution to target site
    Drug and host protected from one another
    Release controlled by biological processes
    Release related to the responsiveness of the target

Drug-related factors
    Controlled modality and frequency of release
    No premature drug release during transit
    Adequate levels of drug carried

Carrier-related factors
    Biologically compatible
    Biodegradable/excreted
    No carrier modulation of the disease
    Convenient and cost-effective to prepare and to formulate
    System chemically and physically stable in its dosage form

---

Tomlinson [1].

2. ANATOMICAL AND PHYSIOLOGICAL CONSIDERATIONS

Two features of intact particles largely determine their biological localization, i.e. size and surface character. Site-specific delivery with particles relies on a combination of anatomical and (patho)physiological events/constraints/opportunities, involving anatomically accessible and non-accessible compartments, as well as normal and dysfunctioning cellular processes of both a passive and an active type [1].

These *biological opportunities* will be examined in turn, with exemplification of some of the potential therapeutic possibilities which could arise.

3. DISCRETE ANATOMICAL COMPARTMENTS

Several anatomical compartments exist where direct introduction of particulates will lead to their retention due to the physics of the space. This opportunity has been used for the treatment of diseases which require a persistent and sustained presentation of the drug at that site. Such compartments include the eye, joints, vagina, anal vault and the respiratory tract. Usefully, although small particles of less than 5 microns can be taken up by phagocytic tissue histiocytes, this can lead to their retention at these sites of administration.

With intra-articular injection in the treatment of both cancer and chronic inflammation, both liposomes and monolithic particles have been examined, as have simple colloid aggregates of drug and/or radiocolloids. The persistence of such materials at these sites is of obvious importance, and Noble *et al.* [2] have shown this to be related to the size of the particles, with larger particles (7 to 15 microns diameter) being retained for longer periods. It is unclear how particles are retained within joints, though some groups have suggested that this is due to uptake by fixed macrophage cells present within the synovium [3]. The host compatibility of monolithic particulate carriers is most important with, for example, gelatin and albumin being better tolerated than polylactic acid and polybutylcyanoacrylates. What has been established is that the intra-articular administration of liposome particles containing cortisol palmitate does lead to a successful treatment of experimental arthritis in the knee joints of rabbits, using relatively low doses of steroid [4, 5]. Preliminary studies in humans have given similar results. Issues such as cost and suitability of alternative colloidal systems (including phospholipid emulsions), have reduced the potential use of this carrier system here. Interesting further developments have been to use liposomes of unique composition that can release their drugs at the higher temperatures found at sites of inflammation [6].

The use of particles for the controlled release of drugs in the lungs have often been proposed. Recent patents have indicated that liposomal sustained-release aerosol delivery systems are technically possible [7].

The accepted model for respiratory tract desposition patterns for man (international Commission on Radiological Protection, 1966) predicts a low probability for disposition in the pulmonary region of inhaled particles larger than 5 microns real size. The dynamics of airflow within the lungs, and the physical sizes of the bronchioles, coupled with the ability for particles to be removed from the lungs via the mucociliary escalator, coupled with the problems of administration to the lungs in an efficient manner, suggest that only particles having an aerodynamic diameter of less than 2 microns could be of use. Recent work has shown that instilled microspheres of size larger than 7 μm are strongly retained in the pulmonary region, and that small percentages of particles of 3 μm and 7 μm administered by instillation into the lungs of beagle dogs can translocate to the tracheobronchial lymph nodes (though this does not occur above 7 μm) [8]. These data give that approximately 2–3% of the dose clears the lungs after a few days (via the mucociliary escalator); thereafter the 3 μm microspheres clear the lungs with a biological retention half-time of 850 days, and the larger particles in excess of several thousand days. Translocation of particles from the alveoli to the tracheobronchial lymph nodes appears to lead largely to their *extracellular* accumulation, though the dynamics of this are only just beginning to be elucidated [9]. Clearly, opportunities for controlled administration and delivery to the lungs exist here. Other studies on particle retention have shown that drug carrier systems can be retained successfully in the respiratory tract [10, 11]. Small liposomes of 50 nm are retained for many hours, though as with all particles, those depositing in the tracheal bronchial regions are cleared under normal conditions within 6 h. Although mucociliary clearance is impaired in chronic respiratory disease [10], it has been shown that liposomal formulations can be effective (in guinea pigs) in providing a sustained drug input to the lung at the tissue level, leading to both an increase in drug efficacy and a decrease in drug toxicity [12].

Other compartments for the constrained retention of particulate carriers include the eyes and the nasal cavity. Size is most important for retention. The ocular irritancy which exists with most grains could well be obviated by making them hydrophilic, coupled with their clearance after release of drug. Recent studies have shown that *in situ* gel-forming systems of nanoparticles can be used to give a prolonged ocular therapeutic effect, combined with ease of application and good tolerance [13]. These systems work by using a latex of approximately 300 nm diameter (e.g. cellulose acetate hydrogen phthalate), onto which is adsorbed drug, and which (in the example cited) has a low enough buffer capacity to gel effectively in the cul-de-sac of the eye. After administration, the latex formulated at a stable pH of 4.4 coagulates within a few seconds when placed into the pH 7.2 environment within the cul-de-sac. The almost instantaneous change from a highly fluid polymeric particle dispersion to a viscous gel ensures retention of the dosage form at the site of action.

The eye contains some highly phagocytosing cells able to take up particulate materials. For example, it has been shown recently that polystyrene latex particles are taken up (presumed to be via phagocytosis) by the rabbit corneal endothelium [14]. However, it is disturbing to note that when carbon microparticles (210–70 nm diameter) are injected intravitreally in monkeys, stimulation of phagocytic cells appears to induce cell proliferation, manifesting itself as neovascularization and retinal detachment [15].

One of the most ambitious studies here has been that of Klipstein *et al.* [16], who showed that oral immunization could be achieved with heat-labile enterotoxin encapsulated in orally administered and pH-dependent (albumin) microspheres. Here the microspheres act as both a protectant against acid as well as an adjuvant, giving rise to a strong serum and mucosal antitoxin response. Diseases of the gastrointestinal tract which could be suggested for access via this route include both colon carcinoma and Crohn's disease.

4.   EPITHELIAL PASSAGE

The epithelial membrane of the gastrointestinal tract comprises an anatomically continuous barrier of cells which permit the passage of low molecular weight material by simple diffusion and various (nutrient) carrier processes. Additionally, low molecular weight polar materials are able to diffuse through the tight junctions of epithelial cells (the paracellular route), and macromolecules may be absorbed from the lumen by cellular vesicular processes by either fluid-phase pinocytosis or specialized (receptor-mediated) endocytosis. This may result in direct transport of material through the epithelial membrane. Particles can pass through this membrane, but only in specialized cases where either the barrier has been disrupted by chemical means, or where it is incomplete. For example, spheres of 20 nm diameter given orally to suckling mice pass through the epithelium of the intestinal lumen and become localized in the omentum, the Kupffer cells of the liver (probably via hematogenous translocation), the mesenteric lymph nodes and the thymic cortex [17]. With mature epithelia there is little evidence of transport *through* the barrier [18].

Claims have frequently been made that drugs given orally in liposomes have an enhanced intestinal absorption. Evidence suggests that if so, this is due to either a protection effect or an enhanced availability of drug at the mucosal surface, rather than a direct transfer of the liposome (e.g. [19, 20]). Also, a recent study with radiolabelled polymethyl methacrylate nanoparticles (mean size 130 nm) shows that after oral administration to bile cannulated rats, 10–15% of the dose found in bile and urine is undoubtedly due to the uptake not of intact particles, but of low molecular weight polymers arising from the particles [21].

Specialized cells within the gastrointestinal tract can take up particles. Thus, it has been demonstrated that the M cells lining the intestine can absorb indigenous bacteria (*Vibrio cholera*), and transport these through into Peyer's patches [22]. Mucosal immune responses are initiated within this lymphoidal tissue, and one can postulate that a drug carrier system sampled through the M cell could be used to bring an appropriate immunomodulator to the attention of the mucosal system. M cells are specialized absorptive cells that overlay both Peyer's patches and other mucosal lymphoid follicles, and are known to transport macromolecules such as ferritin and horseradish peroxidase [23], viruses [24] and even carbon particles [25], from the lumen of the intestine to submucosal *lymphoid* tissue. Further translocation to the systemic system through lymph fluid and via recruitment of lymphocytes does appear possible. The crucial question is: does this system provide an opportunity for the uptake of particulate carriers? Present evidence is ambivalent, and indicates that capacity and onward translocation are limiting features, though work on the utility of M cell extraction related to specificity, abundance and capacity to handle particulate (and macromolecular) material does appear warranted.

Certainly living virus particles can enter the general circulation through the nasal or intestinal mucosa, but whether their passage through to the circulation is as an intact species or is effected though replication is uncertain.

In conclusion, it must be currently regarded that colloidal particles are not able to traverse the epithelia of the gastrointestinal tract intact and in a manner significant for drug use, except under exceptional and unusual circumstances.

5.   INTERSTITIAL ADMINISTRATION

The administration of particles into the interstitium provides an opportunity for either uptake by the lymphatic system or as a local depot of drug.

Administration of carrier systems to the lymphatic system is one which has received scant though important consideration. Clearance of materials from interstitial sites depends upon a number of factors, including size and surface character of particle, formulation medium, administration point with respect to lymphatic anatomy, the composition and pH of tissue interstitial fluid, hydrostatic pressure differences, intrinsic smooth muscle action and extrinsic muscle action, as well as disease within the interstitium. Two prime routes of administration have been considered for colloidal carrier systems, namely into the peritoneal cavity (for delivery of cytostatics to the lymph nodes of the thorax, and subcutaneous administration for targeting of regional nodes [26]. This is based on the fact that small molecules of up to 1000 daltons, when administered either peritoneally or interstitially, pass directly into the bloodstream, whereas macromolecules and colloids enter the lymphatic system through clefts in the terminal vessels [27]. Leak has shown recently [28] that access of colloids and macromolecules may be related to the presence of high density anionic sites within the intercellular clefts of mesothelial and lymphatic endothelial cells, such that these clefts can provide channels between endothelial cells which permit movement of macromolecules and colloids. A further suggestion is that particles can also enter the lymphatic system by being transported in pinocytotic vesicles through the cells [29]. The dynamics of macromolecule exchange across lymphatic capillaries has been well studied by Taylor and Granger [30]. In contrast to endothelia lining the cardiovascular system, the terminal lymphatics do not possess as developed a continuous and uninterrupted subendothelial basement membrane. If present, this tends to be variable in extent, and indeed is often absent — the lining endothelium being the only cell membrane present [31]. Also, adjacent endothelial cells may have gaps of between 20 nm to more than 100 nm, which are known to be extremely enlarged at sites of both inflammation and extensive tissue movement [32]. Hence in some cases, access into the lymphatics is possible with large particles of up to perhaps 1 micron diameter. However, the terminal lymphatics drain into larger vessels (the collecting lymphatics), which have an endothelium possessing an extensive basement membrane and with few endothelial gaps.

These physiological opportunities have long been exploited diagnostically for examining both lymphatic drainage and malignant lymph nodes. The size dependency for interstitial particle uptake has been determined for both small animals and humans, and in lymphoscintigraphy, a wide variety of inert colloids in the 40–100 nm range have been successfully used to outline the lymphatic system (see references in [29]).

Once within the lymphatic system, particles may be phagocytosed, though this is a saturable process. Lymph node status is important in the staging of many malignancies; however, as recently pointed out by Weinstein *et al.* [33], the scope for tumour therapy via the lympatics is more limited than it is for diagnosis. In the case of breast cancer, for example, regional nodes are currently considered to be an indicator of metastatic spread, rather than a site at which spread can be arrested. Local control may be useful in other malignancies such as Hodgkin's, which disseminate early via the lymphatic chains. The subcutaneous or intramuscular administration of cytostatics entrapped in liposome particles can result in an improved access to the lymph nodes and in suppression of tumour metastases within the lymphatics (see references in [34]). Recent work has shown that coating liposomes with a non-specific immunoglobulin can result in these particles becoming accumulated in lymph nodes [35].

Formulation of particles appears to affect their lymphatic uptake. For example, Hashida and Sezaki [36] have developed a lymphotropic system based on either lipid-based particles or particles administered in an oil, both approaches which appear to facilitate uptake into the lymphatic system.

Numerous groups have shown that particles injected intraperitoneally into rodents can pass through the lymphatics and enter the cardiovascular circulation intact [37, 38]. Hirano *et al.* [34] give that for approximately 200 nm diameter liposomes, composition does affect the absorption rate of these colloids into the lymphatic system, but that it is unclear whether this then affects their passage through the lymph capillaries — though there is little doubt that surface character will affect phagocytosis. It is technically difficult to determine lymph node retentions, but this group has pointed to a trend which gives that surface charge affects rate of absorption into the lymphatic system from the peritoneal cavity, with the apparent half-life for absorption of positive liposomes (i.e. the least absorbed) being 9.7 h (assuming a first-order process), whilst that for negative liposomes was 5.1 h. The anionic binding sites present on the lymphatic endothelial surface may be the cause of this retention at the endothelial surface, which manifests itself as a slower absorption. These data suggest that inclusion of a charged lipid into a liposome can reduce its systemic availability, while neutral particles can rapidly pass through the lymphatics to the bloodstream. The corollary to this is that charged particles will probably be better retained at the nodes. Results do show a wide interanimal variation, which could be due to differences in the lymphatic systems combined with differences in their physiologic status. It may be that these latter differences will limit the number of cases where lymphatic carriers can be used.

Particles of 50 microns and above will be retained in the interstitial tissue after subcutaneous and intramuscular administration, and can act as a sustained-release depot. This has been used for the controlled release of a variety of peptidergic mediators, as well as for potentiating and providing a sustained-release formulation for prolonged local anaesthesia. In the latter case, drug release is dependent upon both drug amount in the particle and particle surface area (see references in [39]). An interesting feature here is the relative biodegradation of different particles given either intraperitoneally or subcutaneously, with poly(ethylene carbonate) particles being degraded relatively much faster after administration by the former route.

6.   INTRALESIONAL/INTRATISSUE ADMINISTRATION

The parenteral administration of materials into discrete compartments can also include tumour areas. It has been suggested [40] that the most efficacious means of administration of cytotoxic and immunostimulant agents could be by localized intratumour injection. Retention of both solid particles and even water-in-oil emulsions containing drugs seems possible. For example, water-in-oil emulsions of bleomycin injected directly into carcinomas and adenocarcinomas in humans have longer drug retention times compared to when given as aqueous solutions. However many questions arise with such an administration route, including the potential for inflammatory responses, dangers of inducing metastatic cell loss and local immune responses. Intratumour administration does seem to be an extremely limited case for the use of colloidal carriers, with less prosaic questions such as needle size, injection volume, duration of leakage from the injection site, etc., being complicating factors.

7.   PARENTERAL ADMINSTRATION

7.1   General considerations

When introduced into the vasculature, particles can either access targets within the circulation, or, upon leaving the vasculature, can access other targets. However, as subsequent discussion will show, the opportunities for the latter are extremely limited. Extravasation in normal endothelia is possible via either specialized endothelial gaps, or vesicular processes of either a fluid phase and a constitutive and/or a non-constitutive receptor-mediated nature, or when carried within extravasating cells.

Table 3 gives the anatomical features of capillary endothelia. It is seen that

Table 3 — Anatomical features of endothelial barriers

Type/characteristics	Tissue
Continuous Tight junctions Vesicular trafficking Continuous basement membrane	Skeletal, smooth, cardiac muscles; connective tissue; central nervous system; pancreas; gonads; lung
Discontinuous *Fenestrated* Interruptions 20–80 nm Thin membrane 4–6 nm thick Continuous basement membrane	Exocrine and endocrine glands; gastrointestinal tract; renal glomeruli; peritubular capillaries; choroid plexus

Sinusoidal
 Gaps about 150 nm
 Basement membrane absent in
    liver, interrupted in spleen
    bone marrow
	Liver; spleen; bone marrow

capillaries with continuous endothelia and an uninterrupted basement membrane are the most widely distributed and although small molecular weight solutes and a large number of macromolecules are able to pass through this barrier [30], generally, particles of greater than approximately 40 nm diameter will not. On the other hand, capillaries with fenestrated endothelia and a basement membrane which are usually found in organs whose functions require high rates of fluid exchange, have pores which are able to permit very small particles of less than 40 nm to pass, and capillaries having a discontinuous endothelia and no basement membrane have relatively large and abundant pores. For example, electron microscope studies show pores of up to 150 nm in the liver sinusoids.

7.2 Intravascular targets

7.2.1 Capillary filtration

Particles of sizes larger than the narrowest capillary beds will become filtered by these. This phenomenon has been exploited for various disease states including cancer, emphysema and thrombus formation. The rationale is that within a diseased organ, at the point of filtration there will be a high concentration of drug for an extended period of time, leading to an increased availability of drug for either direct action or absorption through endothelia. The hypothesis is unproven but a number of groups have worked on this approach with some degree of success.

All such particles injected intravenously (apart from into the portal vein) will become entrapped in the capillaries of the lungs. Indeed, this is the basis of the use of human serum albumin particles radiolabelled for the scintigraphic examination of various masses within the lungs. Interestingly, although the supply to the lungs is arterial in origin, tumour masses are indicated as cold spots, i.e. the particles go to everywhere within the lungs except the tumour mass.

The studies by Martodam *et al.* [41] clearly show that particles of 15 μm diameter are blocked in the lungs of emphysemic rats after IV administration. Attachment of human leucocyte elastase inhibitor resulted in the alleviation of the symptoms of emphysema.

To overcome filtration by the lung, attempts have been made to administer particulates intra-arterially for both diagnostic and therapeutic purposes. To illustrate the potential that this has, the injection of particles greater than 15 μm into, for example, the mesenteric artery, portal vein or renal artery, leads to their complete entrapment in the gut, liver or kidneys, respectively. This approach has been exploited by Torchilin [42], who used microgranules of Sephadex, to which were bound different thrombolytic enzymes including fibrinolysin, streptokinase and urokinase. Approximately 10–60 mg of enzyme can be bound to one gram of this carrier. The immobilized enzymes were shown to be highly effective in the treatment of thromboses and thromboemboli of vessels that were accessible via catheterization. This was demonstrated by the successful lysis of an experimental thrombus in a dog femoral artery by means of catheterization of the artery and administration of a dose of immobilized enzyme (fibrinolysin) 100 times lower than that required with normal IV injection of the enzyme. Sephadex is completely degraded within about an hour, although it does not lend itself to use as a carrier because to link drugs chemically is a somewhat difficult procedure, and long-term release *in vivo* (i.e. grater than 15 days) does not appear possible.

Intra-arterial delivery to cancerous sites by filtration uses one of two approaches either where drug is incorporated into the particles [43], or where the presence of a coadministered particle increases the dwell time within the particular capillary of a solution of drug [44]. Intra-arterial administration of a bolus of particles of size greater than 15 μm in rabbits bearing intrahepatic V2 carcinomas, results in particles distributing to tumour capillaries, in preference to the surrounding (normal) capillaries by a factor of four [45]. This effect is probably due to a quantitative difference in capillary networks of the tumour compared to those of the host organ [46].

7.2.2   *Mononuclear phagocyte system (MPS)*

Particles that are able to move freely through the cardiovascular system are generally cleared within minutes from the circulation by the MPS. Particle clearance has been shown to be related to a large number of factors including size, dose, surface charge, nature of the particle matrix, particle stability, and physiological state of the species (e.g. [47]). The MPS can be regarded as either a constraint to site-specific delivery, or as both an opportunity for targeting and as a disease target.

The MPS is a connective tissue system of cells distributed throughout the body. Cells of the reticuloendothelial system (RES) do include cells of the MPS; however, other RES cells do not phagocytose, including the endothelial cells of the liver which take part in the clearance of foreign particles by endocytic (though non-phagocytic) processes. In addition, Langerhans cells and related cells can be potent accessory cells but are often non-phagocytic and may lack Fc and C_3 receptors [48]. The main functions of the MPS include the clearance of a large variety of potentially harmful substances from plasma, catabolism of ingested macromolecules, participation in the immune response and the synthesis and secretion of various effector molecules. These effects can sometimes be age-related. Materials cleared include effete red blood cells, circulating tumour cells, inert colloids, autologous tissue debris, immune complexes, denatured proteins, specific glycoproteins, bacterial endotoxins, steroids and lipoproteins. Macrophages and other phagocytic cells synthesize and excrete monokines, including enzymes such as collagenase, as well as several effectors such as pyrogens, prostaglandins, procoagulants, colony-stimulating factor(s), interferons and tumouricidal factors (reviewed in [49]). The cells of the MPS are mesenchymal in origin and include the phagocytically active reticulum cells of the reticular connective tissue, the Kupffer stellate cells lining the wall of the hepatic sinusoids, the Hortega cells (microglia) of the central nervous system, the histiocytes (i.e. tissue macrophages) and the blood macrophages or monocytes (see Bradfield [50] for a more complete description). Phagocytosis is a potential route for uptake of colloidal drug delivery systems, and it is of interest to note that such cells include platelets, which take up latex particles of (87 nm diameter) in their open-channel system, followed by their location in platelet vacuoles, with phagocytosis being chronologically similar to that given for polymorphonuclear leukocytes [51].

When foreign particles are introduced intravenously, about 90% are extracted by the Kupffer cells, 5% by the spleen and a few per cent enter the bone marrow. There is considerable species variation observed, with the rabbit in particular exhibiting much greater bone marrow uptake than other observed species [52]. The dominance of the liver does not reflect the concentration of macrophages in the body, rather their accessibility. After 100% transit through the lungs, about 28% of the blood from the heart goes through the liver and then through the spleen and intestine, with less than 10% going through the skeleton.

Macrophages are able to bind and to engulf a variety of particles through both a specific process involving specifically adsorbed opsonins, as well as through non-specific processes [53]. In addition, macrophages present on their surface membrane receptors for the Fc part of the immunoglobulin molecule and for the C3b component of the complement sequence. They also characteristically express Ia antigens. Serum factors which promote phagocytosis are called opsonins (a term coined by Wright in 1902 from the Greek *opsono*, meaning, 'I prepare a meal for thou'). Opsonins may be divided into immune and non-immune components, though both mediate the onset of phagocytosis through their bifunctional binding to the target and the receptors on phagocytes. The recognition of foreign particles depends upon opsonin selectivity and perhaps specificity for surface structures [54]. Czop *et al.* [55] have demonstrated a further type of recognition mechanism in human monocytes which does not require exogenous opsonin but involves the human complement system. The immune components include immunoglobulin G and complement C3b, though each appear to have a somewhat different subsequent mode of clearance by macrophages and can operate independently of one another. The processes are complicated, for example, C3b-mediated adherence to macrophages may involve cleavage of this component on the surface so that it now becomes coated with C3d and is released back into the blood for prolonged circulation. Fibronectin may also be involved in these processes as well as fibrinogen.

Interaction of particles with cells takes the form of opsonization followed by adherance and engulfment and then attempts at digestion. For non-drug-bearing particles it is of interest to note that ingestion can lead to stimulation of the glycolytic and arachidonic acid pathways and the hexose monophosphate shunt; also, lysosomal enzymes are released within the cell and interleukin-1 is secreted. Interference with the phagocytic process is possible by hindering both adsorption (of opsonins) and perhaps particle cell adherance. Various surface manipulations of particles will lead to qualitative and quantitative alterations in opsonization and macrophage uptake. Bradfield [50] has noted some of the differences found. For example, gentle treatment of a person's own red blood cells with N-ethylmaleimide results in splenic extraction after reinjection, but more severe treatment leads to hepatic uptake. Such procedures cause complement C3b to become opsonized, whereas red blood cells treated with glutaraldehyde are opsonized by IgG — which leads to Fc-mediated adherance. Also, gelatin-coated particles are opsonized by fibronectin. Related to these findings are those which show that when autologous red cells are coated with low concentrations of non-complement-fixing IgG, the main site of clearance is the spleen, whereas coating with complement-fixing IgM causes liver sequestration — which is in contrast to the removal of *soluble* immune complexes by an Fc-mediated, complement-independent process. In humans the removal of sialic acid from red blood cells exposes terminal galactosyl residues, resulting in their hepatic uptake, whereas the further (and sequential) removal of the surface galactose residues results in N-acetylglucosamine or mannose being revealed. This leads to their uptake by Kupffer cells.

A number of factors can affect the interaction of particles with macrophages apart from the presence of specific surface ligands such as mannose and galactose. Studies by Schwendener *et al.* [56] have shown that with sterylamine incorporated (at 15%) into the surface of egg phosphatidyl:cholesterol liposomes, the number of larger vesicles (100 nm and 160 nm dimater) associated with rat peritoneal macrophages *in vitro* was 100-fold less than that found for smaller vesicles of 25 nm. Interestingly for drug delivery, the total entrapped aqueous volume introduced into the macrophages by large vesicles was an order of magnitude greater than with small vesicles. Increasing the sterylamine content, i.e. increasing the net surface positive charge on the particles, increased their interaction with peritoneal macrophages. In contrast, work with crystalline metal sulphide particles gives that *in vitro*, negatively charged particles are far better phagocytosed by cultured mammalian cells [57]. This is somewhat peculiar since macrophages themselves exhibit an overall negative charge, but is in accord with the reported phagocytosis of other negatively charged particles such as quartz, and certain bacteria [58]. Other factors influencing clearance of blood-borne particles *in vivo* include therapeutic levels of ultrasound [59]. The mechanisms for this are unclear but may involve either mechanical or biochemical effects.

7.2.2.1 *Diseases of the MPS*

Many diseases either reside within the cells of the MPS, or may be fought by marshalling the MPS to effect various events. The selective delivery of drugs encapsulated in liposome particles for targeting to various disease states of the MPS have been given by Schroit *et al.* [60] (Table 4). The MPS has an important role in

Table 4 — Macrophage-associated disease amenable to treatment with particulate drug delivery systems

Disease	Drug
Intracellular parasites	
Leishmania	Antimony drugs
Histoplasmosis	Amphotericin B
Leprosy	Sulphones
Neoplasms	
Histiocytosis	Doxorubicin
Enzyme storage disease	
Gaucher's disease	Glucocerebrosides

resistance to many infectious diseases. In numerous instances facultative parasites are able to survive and proliferate within the cytoplasm of these cells [61]. Also, the chronic persistence of parasites stimulates the infiltration of more macrophages resulting in severe granulatomous lesions. In addition, neoplasms of the histiocytes and monocytes (including histiocytic medullar reticulosis, monocytic leukaemia, hairy cell leukaemias and certain forms of Hodgkin's disease), would appear to be amenable to an approach of using phagocytosed particulate carriers containing cytotoxic drugs. Although access is assured, persistence of drug and/or carrier to give a therapeutically significant effect is still an open question.

Clinical success has been gained in this field of passive targeting to fungally infected cells of the MPS. Systemic mycoses caused by *Candida albicans, Aspergillus* sp., and *Mucor* sp. are mainly intracellular fungal infections which are difficult to treat due to problems of selective drug access. It has been demonstrated both *in vitro* and *in vivo* in animals and in humans, that there is a marked improvement in the selective toxicity of liposomal polyene antibiotics (e.g. amphotericin B) when administered systematically as the liposomal preparation [62]. *in vivo* this results in an improved drug therapeutic index due to normal mammalian tissue/cells becoming protected. It has been argued that polyenes transfer effectively from lipsomes to fungal cells but not to mammalian cells [63]. The successful access to the diseased cells, plus the almost complete abolishment of nephrotoxic effects, mean that this delivery approach is indicated in the therapy of systemic fungal infections in both cancer patients and in other immunodebilitated persons.

Further successful uses of liposomal anti-infective drugs have been reported, [26], as has the use of cytotoxic agents and organic antimonial drugs for the treatment of parasites living within the endocytic vacuoles of mononuclear phagocytes (see Poznansky and Juliano [64]).

The use of particulate systems for treating viral diseases has been examined recently. This can be considered in two ways, either by treating a virally infected macrophage or by providing a vechicle for drugs which are able to stimulate macrophages to effect cytostasis or cytolysis of other (virally infected) cells. Fidler [66] has shown that an important aspect in the treatment of viral infections is the ability to selectively deliver antiviral agents to the sites of virus replication. Several groups of viruses infect cells of the MPS, and hence naturally targeted particles can be used to direct antiviral drugs to infected phagocytic cells, though it is not yet possible to ascertain how this could be made exclusive for the population of infected cells. Viral infections usually manifest themselves by inflammation, including perivascular infiltration by mononuclear phagocytes.

The body rids itself of unwanted substrates by degrading those within the lysosomes of various cells, including cells which are phagocytic. Abnormalities in this process, often due to the absence of the cellular machinery for the enzyme to enter the cell and to be routed to the lysosome can manifest themselves as a number of storage diseases, including adult Gaucher's disease and mucoliposes types II and III. Direct enzyme supplementation/replacement is seemingly inappropriate due to enzyme breakdown and immune responses. However, knowledge of the lysosomal processing of enzymes and the mechanisms and routes of endocytosis, has caused several groups to suggest various carriers for enzymes which would be able both to *protect* the enzyme and the body from one another, as well as to exploit phagocytic processes of cells to effect deposition of the enzyme(s) within the cellular lysosomes. The use of microspheres, low density lipoproteins, fibroblasts and leucocytes and encapsulated cells as both lysosomally directed particulate carriers and as circulating enzyme depots has been reviewed by Poznansky and Juliano [64], and is exemplified by the study of Umezawa *et al.* [66] on direct enzyme replacement using liposomes containing beta-galactosidase in (murine) globoid cell leukodystrophy.

There are many othe dysfunctions of marcophages. For example in rheumatoid arthritis, phagocytic cells may overproduce collagenase and secrete prostaglandins, which can be responsible for much of the pathology associated with this disease.

(Protection of healthy tissues from deleterious drug effects is central to the use of carrier systems, and examples exist where drugs are not necessarily targeted to their site of action, but still are diverted from unwanted sites of disposition. For example, the use of doxorubicin in lipsomes enables the cardiomyelopathy seen with anthracyclines to be greatly reduced.)

Types of particles which are indicated for targeting to macrophages are the lipid-like, those which are hydrophobic or which can be readily opsonized, and even altered erythrocytes [67].

7.2.2.2 *Modulation of MPS action*

Two of the most important aspects of cancer chemotherapy that relate to site-specific delivery are tumour cell heterogeneity and the extravascular positions of tumour cell masses. Phagocytosis of particles by the cells of the MPS can be turned to advantage in the treatment of low tumour burden. That is, mononuclear phagocytes may become activated by effector molecules to acquire the ability to destroy neoplastic cells. This process may also be considered for treating facultative and obligate intracellular parasites.

Antigen- and mitogen-stimulated T-lymphocytes release lymphokines which interact in a highly specific manner with target cells bearing appropriate receptors. Activation can be caused by numerous molecules, and appears to include an initial priming step that can be induced by lymphokines and a second triggering step. It is clear that lymphokines can also act as this second trigger, though other molecules may be more effective [68]. In addition, secretory products of the macrophages themselves regulate macrophage activation by both a positive and a negative feedback control.

Much attention has been given to the question of macrophage activation by bacterial cell wall components and their synthetic analogues. Such molecules (e.g. muramyl dipeptides) and lymphokines (e.g. MIF, MAF, gamma-inteferon and TNF) tend to have poor disposition to macrophages and are rapidly excreted and catabolized by the liver. For this reason attempts have been made to deliver these molecules to mononuclear phagocytes using colloids. Lymphokines and muramyl peptides encapsulated within liposomes are highly effective in activating macrophages both *in vitro* and *in vivo* (reviewed by Poste and Kirsch [69] and Fidler [65]). Recent work [65] gives that drugs do not necessarily have to leave their carrier to be effective, so long as they are available to activate the macrophage. Evidence also suggests that once activated, macrophages are able to extravasate and seek out their target cells, though which macrophages do this and why, are still unknowns.

Fidler [65] has proposed that liposomal drugs could be used to activate macrophages to treat viral infections. This is based on the finding that activated human monocytes or mouse macrophages are able to distinguish between normal and HSV-2-infected cells. (One further issue here reviewed [65] is that some viruses have been shown to be able to replicate with a greater efficiency within activated macrophages, and hence this should be taken into account in developing clinical modalities involving macrophage activation.) Impaired MPS function occurs during the pathogenesis of numerous diseases including diabetes, liver disease, chronic heart failure, and malnutrition, and these may complicate the treatment of diseases of the MPS or the exploitation of phagocytosis to activate macrophages. In addition, MPS function changes with age. For example, Brouwer and Knook [49] have found that the clearance capacity of macrophages shows a moderate age-related decrease, which probably correlates with a decreased endocytic capacity of Kupffer cells.

For clinical use, the relationships between particle size, matrix composition, dose, composition, colloidal stability, surface character, particle degradability, and macrophage responsiveness and the synergistic use of multiple activators are still large uncertainties.

7.2.2.3 *Avoiding the MPS*

Access of particles to other vascular or extravascular targets is initially largely dependent upon an avoidance of interaction with the phagocytosing cells of the MPS. Various successful attempts have been made to achieve this (Table 5). Immediately upon entry into biological fluids, colloids have adsorbed to them flexible and globular (glyco)proteins. Some of these will be opsonins of the type discussed previously.

Table 5 — Suggested approaches for avoiding uptake of particulate carriers by the mononuclear phagocyte system

Process	Example
Alteration of particle surface	
Charge	Charged liposomes
Hydrophilic	Albumin nanoparticles
Hydrophilic and sterically stabilized	Poloxamer/poloxamine copolymers adsorbed to hydrophobic surfaces; polyethylene glycols
Mimics of natural particles	Erythrocytes
Blockade of MPS	
By saturation	Dextrans; empty mannosylated liposomes
By receptor-block	Anti-Fc receptor antibodies

Opsonization can be avoided or altered in such a way that particles either adhere to other surfaces or take advantage of passive and receptor-mediated processes to access other compartments.

Most of the approaches appear to be limited for clinical use. For example the practicalities of producing natural particles such as red blood cells on a large scale appear formidable, although study of why these avoid uptake could be invaluable in designing MPS-avoiding particles.

(a) Saturation of MPS capacity Attempts have been made to temporarily block the functioning of the MPS by using materials-inert colloids such as carbon, methyl palmitate, latex beads, dextran sulphate, and empty lipsomes and nanoparticles. Gregoriadis *et al.* [70] attempted to alter liposome distribution by prior blockade of the MPS with empty liposomes, and although their goal of thence increasing uptake of drug-bearing liposomes by tumour tissue was not achieved, MPS function was depressed. Proffitt *et al.* [71] have successfully imaged tumours with labelled neutral liposomes by prior blockade of the MPS with small unilamellar vesicles that incorporated a 6-aminomannose derivative of cholesterol into the liposome bilayer (this was based on the finding that phagocytosis of aminomannose-modified vesicles proceeds *in vitro* at a high rate). Suppression often leads to the redirection of particles to the lungs and to other blood cells and to the lungs [50].

Clinically, this approach does not seem viable. Although it is possible to reversibly block the MPS, repeated intravenous injections of liposomes are accompanied by long-term paralysis of the MPS [72]. It is interesting to look at the mechanism of blockade. Lehnert and Tech [53] have shown that a reduction in phagocytosis after preloading macrophages with particles is due to a loss in surface sites required for particle recognition and binding, and not to limitations in the phagocytic capacity or particle loading of macrophages *per se.*

Hopkins [73] recently discussed a novel approach to blockade, using pretreatment with monoclonal antibodies to the low affinity Fc receptors of macrophages.

An example quoted gives, for the chimpanzee, that an injection of 1 mg kg^{-1} antibody prolongs the half-life of immune-coated red cells from 50 min to 23.5 h.

(b) Altering opsonization. As discussed above, phagocytosis is generally preceded by opsonization, adherence to cells and then ingestion after engulfment and vesicularization of the phagocytosing cell membrane. Both processes of opsonization and adherence can be diminished if the attractive forces between the interacting particles, surfaces and macromolecules are diminished. Adsorption and adhesion effects are complex phenomena, and are controlled by electrostatic, dispersion and steric forces, by hydration, and by other short-range interactions [74]. Interfacial adsorption is dependent upon a balance between these forces. Colloidal particles will attract each other through van der Waals interactions (short range), and repel each other through longer range, repulsive (e.g. Coulombic) forces. As particles approach one another there is a net attraction, with a potential energy barrier to interaction at closer proximities, and with strong interaction at very short ranges. For avoidance of opsonization one wishes to avoid interactions. This can be achieved by creating a high potential energy barrier.

It has been shown that particles coated with either negative or positive macromolecules can have altered organ uptakes [75]. As described by Napper and Netschey [76], a high potential energy barrier can be formed by creating a sterically stablized surface by introducing a hydrated (i.e. hydrophilic) polymer at the surface. This results in a surface which is both hydrophilic and stabilized. The hydration effect is enthalpic in origin, and the stabilization effect is manifested by both osmotic effects and chain entanglements, both of which are entropic in origin [77]. The size of this repulsive barrier should be determined by both the thickness of the polymer layer and its density, as well as by polymer–polymer interactions caused by specific interactions along the polymer chain.

The use of sterically stabilized coats for reducing opsonization and eventual (liver) clearance has been tried for both soluble marcomolecules such as enzymes [78], and monolithic particles. Tightly adsorbed block copolymers have been studied (in which a hydrophobic portion of the ABA copolymer is adsorbed to the surface of a hydrophobic particle), e.g. using poloxamers of different hydrophilicity/hydrophobicity, as has chemical grafting in order to covalently attach hydrophilic macromolecules to the surface of particles. The former approach has been used to reduce the liver upake of emulsion droplets [79, 80, 81] and monolithic particles [82, 83, 84]. The effect of adsorbing different poloxamers is not only to reduce liver uptake (by Kupffer cells), but also to divert non-extravasating particles to other vascular target cells, including monocytes and bone marrow cells [85]. Other materials considered for this effect include poloxamines and natural xanthans [85].

(c) Mimics of natural particles. It is probable that steric stabilization is akin to the mechanism whereby blood cells and various bacteria and parasites escape detection by the MPS [5]. Some groups have attempted to exploit the behaviour of natural particles such as erythrocytes [68] and bacteria to increase the circulation times of particles. For example Utsumi *et al.* [86] have demonstrated that incorporating the sialoglycoprotein of human erythrocytes into liposomes of 0.2 to 1.0 μm diameter causes a marked suppression in their clearance by the liver.

7.2.3   Circulating systems/other intravascular targets

To remain in the blood pool is attractive as particles could act as long-term storage depots for the release of, for example, anti-infectives, cytostatics and fibrinolytics. Numerous systems, other than sterically stabilized synthetic particles, have been proposed. For example, erythrocytes have been studied as depots for asparaginase in the treatment of cancer [87].

Blood cells are now defined in terms of subsets having differentiation markers, and detailed classifications are becoming possible. These subsets represent defined intravascular targets which may be recognized by various ligands including antibodies, hormones, and simple sugars, etc. Microparticles linked to such ligands have been successfully targeted to blood cells both *in vitro* [88] as well as *in vivo*. For example, Singhal and Gupta [89] have shown that the covalent attachment of anti-rat erythrocyte F(ab')$_2$ antibody to liposomes both enhanced their binding to rat erythrocytes *in vivo*, as well as reducing vesicle uptake by the liver. The contents of the liposomes were also delivered to the cells to which they were bound. Similarly, a recent study by Laakso *et al.* [90] to enhance the cell elimination has mirrored this finding. Although such approaches appear attractive, the *internalization* of particles by blood subsets differs [91] and this needs further consideration.

Further, recent work has shown that by constructing transferrin-coated liposomes these can be used *in vivo* to transport exogenous DNA to bone marrow erythroblasts in anaemic rabbits. Such cells have many transferrin receptors on their surfaces [92].

7.2.4   Normal and abnormal endothelia, and endothelia-related targets

Organ-specific antigens exist on capillary endothelial cells [93], as do disease-related markers. For example, recent work has shown the presence of a unique endothelial marker on endothelia derived from an AIDS-associated Kaposi's sarcoma [94]. Targeting with a ligand able to recognize and attach to such markers has been often mooted, but little study has been performed. Undoubtedly, certain of these endothelial markers can be imaged by scintigraphy, but whether this is of significance for chemotherapy is uncertain. Although most imaging studies have been carried out with soluble conjugates, particulate carriers have been successfully directed to endothelial targets where a pathological condition exists. For example there are a number of diseased states of the cardiovascular system where subendothelial structures that are normally thrombogenic come into contact with blood. This is the case in transluminal angioplasty of stenotic vessels, which causes the exposure of intimal and often medial vascular wall structures. The work of Smirnov *et al.* [95] gives that by binding either anti-collagen type I antibodies, or human fibronectin to cholesterol oleate-containing liposomes in perfused *in situ* arteries, partially denuded to expose underlying basement membrane structures, such constructs are selectively bound by endothelia-free zones of arterial segments. This finding is suggested for use in preventing platelet aggregation and thrombus formation of fissures of atherosclerotic caps, as well as for local delivery of anti-platelet drugs, which, in some cases, need to be present at the moment of plaque rupture. Other suggested targets for local delivery by this method include exposed antigens of activated and spread platelets, newly formed fibrin and other specific antigens of the plaque surface. The delivery to these lesions of drugs able to both inhibit further platelet aggregation over the plaque surface and to lyse the formed clot was also proposed. Previously studies by the same group have given that in myocardial infarct, the exposure of cardiac myosin enables anti-myosin antibodies linked to liposomes to accumulate at these sites [42].

7.3 Extravascular targets

As discussed above, endothelial membranes can provide either a continuous or a discontinuous barrier to the passage of particulates. Membrane permeability is altered by some diseases.

7.3.1 Disease-related particle extravasation

7.3.1.1 Inflammation

Endothelial hyperpermeability at various sites of inflammation is well established. This is of potential use for access of anti-inflammatory drugs to inflamed extravascular regions. For example, in areas of inflammation induced by carrageenin, the accumulation of lipid microspheres of approximately 200 nm diameter around endothelial cells of blood vessels, and the penetration of these to the outer layer of blood vessels, have been reported [96]. however, other groups have shown that in other models of inflammation, such extravasation does not occur [97]. An enhanced anti-inflammatory response has been demonstrated with cortisol palmitate in liposomes after intravenous administration in rat models of inflammation [98]. What this means in terms of the pathogenesis of the underlying disease and the retention of the carrier is unknown, particularly when one appreciates that inflamed sites often contain phagocytic cells. Interestingly, intravenously administered radiolabelled 'small' liposome particles can be used to image joints of patients affected by rheumatoid disease [99], though when the disease is in remission, with no active synovitis, then accumulation of the radiolabel does not occur. This group has suggested that accumulation is due to phagocytic activity.

7.3.1.2 Ischaemia/hypertensive vascular lesions

An increased permeability in the endothelia is seen as an important factor in the pathogenesis of hypertensive lesions leading to infiltration and accumulation of plasma material. For example, in experimental malignant hypertension, colloidal iron and carbon particles of between 5 and 50 μm diameter are able to extravasate [100]. In addition, capillaries have been shown to be permeable at sites of tissue ischaemia, both in the mesenteric artery [101] and myocardium [102], though whether these are opportunities for drug use is unclear. However, this is not the case for other hypertensive states. In spontaneously hypertensive rats the endothelial wall, although exhibiting various severe types of damage, does not have an altered permeability for colloidal carbon.

7.3.1.3 Tumour endothelia

Poste [97] has described as a 'fading prospect' the possibility of an increased permeability of tumour endothelia enabling access of colloidal particles. Although it is true that the permeability of the microcirculation in tumours is often higher than that found for normal tissues, it is highly variable and, as Poste points out, is an unpredictable component of tumour physiology. For inorganic colloids only limited access has been shown, and then when particles are as small as 30 nm in diameter. Knowledge on the vasculature of tumours is scanty. In some models of cancer, endothelial cells can be seen which are leaky (e.g. Lewis lung carcinoma), but due to a build-up of necrotic tissue, areas of damage are poorly perfused with only limited access possible. Unfortunately, in the studies performed to date, particles targeted to tumour masses have had to *compete* with the MPS cell pool, and although 'fading', the prospects for accumulation of small drug-bearing particles may be brighter if this competing pool was negated by, for example, using sterically stabilized particles. Poste [97] gives a detailed discussion on tumour endothelia and its role as a barrier to colloidal particle passive extravasation, and shows that in contradistinction to arterial endothelia, changes in venous structures are quite common — malignant tumours, for example, generally invade veins.

For active targeting to tumours, irrespective of the serious challenge that tumour cell heterogeneity and extravasation poses, during endothelial proliferation in, for example, tumour angiogenesis, high levels of receptors may be expressed which are normally present at low levels.

A further hope for particulate carriers has been the use of particles containing magnetic material. Here, drug-bearing particles can be directed into the tumour mass using two-dimensional magnetic fields. This approach has been used for solid monolithic particles [103] and for oil-in-water emulsions [104], and is a further means of avoiding the competing MPS cell pool [105]. The approach relies on knowledge of the position of the tumour mass, and although it is unlikely to have any great applicability in cancer chemotherapy, its use in treating, for example, diseases of the joints could be considered.

7.3.2 Passage through normal endothelia

Passage of soluble and particulate macromolecules through normal capillary endothelia is possible under certain circumstances.

7.3.2.1 *Continuous endothelia*

Capillary wall permeability for soluble macromolecules is well documented [30]. Soluble materials of less than 80 nm diameter are able to permeate through continuous endothelia, which is in contrast to liposome particles of 30–80 nm diameter, which are not able to pass the (alveolar) endothelia [97].

Endothelial cells process soluble and particulate materials via pathways which include a vesicularization step. Considerable evidence exists to show that endothelia undergo endocytosis of both the fluid phase, and the constitutive and the non-constitutive receptor-mediated types [73]. The size of vesicle (20–100 nm) is of importance when considering if particulate carriers could use this route to either enter cells (i.e. endocytose), or even pass through them (i.e. transcytose). Some evidence exists with *in vitro* sytems to suggest that *particulates* of less than 40 nm are able to enter such pathways, in particular when receptor-mediated events are involved. Similar studies are beginning with whole organs. For example, Ghitescu *et al.* [106] have perfused homologous and heterologous albumin–gold particle complexes (AGC) into continuous endothelial capillaries of mice *in situ*. Using gold particles of mean diameter 5 nm they have been able to show that for the endothelia examined (i.e. in lung, heart and diaphragm), AGC is first absorbed onto specific binding sites and then transported in transcytotic vesicles across the endothelium by receptor-mediated transcytosis and, to a lesser extent, by a fluid-phase process. Although no binding could be found when the complex was injected *in vivo* (even with the portal vein and hepatic artery ligated to minimize liver uptake), these workers have suggested that the existence of albumin receptors on such continuous endothelia may provide a specific mechanism for the transport of albumin, and hence conversely, for adducted particles. It is unclear whether this provides a biological opportunity for access through endothelia with particulates, particularly when tissue specificity of the receptor, and the capacity of the pathway, are considered.

7.3.2.2   *Discontinuous endothelia*

Discontinuous endothelia exist at different tissue regions. Passage of particles of approximately 100 nm diameter and below through such discontinuous endothelia, with onward transport to underlying tissues, be they basement membranes, or, as is the case in the liver, underlying parenchymal cells, is possible. For example, low density lipoprotein (LDL), the carrier for cholesterol ester, which is monolithic and has a diamter of about 22 nm, is able to pass through liver sinusoids, enter the Space of Disse and then interact with liver hepatocytes. Interaction is due to the apolipo-protein ligands on the surface of LDL interacting with specific receptors on the surface of the hepatocytes.

Interestingly, manipulation of the surface of LDL by acetylation causes it to be recognized and be taken up via an endocytic pathway by liver *endothelial* cells rather than the parenchymal cells [107]. Numerous other studies exist which show that not only can particles interact with underlying parenchymal cells in the liver, but that this can be modified by altering the particle surface with ligands specific for the plasma membranes of various liver cells — leading to their redistribution within the liver, as well as to other organs such as the spleen [108]. Such ligands are often simple carbohydrates and this redistribution reflects the diverse carbohydrate recognition assemblies present throughout both of these organs.

These data reflect the principle that particles of the correct size may have their surface altered to enable them to be taken up not only by specific organs but by specific cell types within that organ, and that endothelial uptake and passage of particles are also possible. This, of course, has been employed by virus particles, whose tissue and cell tropisms are becoming increasingly well documented [1].

Low density lipoprotein itself has been examined as a carrier of drugs and radiolabels because of its unique deposition, and has been studied for the imaging of injured and healing arterial walls and the adrenal cortex [109], and for targeting to cancerous cells [110].

7.4 Extravascular, extracellular targets

Extracellular matrix components present as the basement membrane have a number of important physiological roles, including cellular translocation and chemotaxis. Recent studies using polystyrene latex as probes of these events show that such particles can be translocated from extracellular matrices lacking in fibronectin to areas containing it [111]. Although such studies are in their early stages, they do point to a further possible unique behaviour that a colloidal particulate delivery system would have once it gained access to such regions, particularly as (cell) translocations are important in some types of tissue reorganization such as those which occur in inflammation, would healing and tumour invasion.

8. POTENTIAL TOXICITIES OF PARTICULATE CARRIERS

The potential toxic effects that could arise due to the use of carriers are given in Table 6. Many of these are based on experiences with liposomes.

Table 6 — Potential toxicities of particulate carriers

MPS Depression, exhaustion
Propensity to bacterial and viral infection
Immunological depression
Haemorrhagic and endotoxin shock
Altered drug deposition/metabolism (uptake by specilized immune
    compartments (e.g. in skin and gut))
Altered responses to drugs

Low level activation of MPS
Production of interleukin-1
Amyloidosis
Hyperplastic liver foci
Altered bone marrow stem cell kinetics

Carrier material toxicity

Adapted from Poste [31, 98].

The major concern is with potential immune responses and alteration (either poisoning or by activation) of the functioning of the MPS. Also, as for any novel administration or delivery mode, the potential toxic effects that new patterns of tissue exposure bring will need to be determined. Studies relating to these issues can be found in the following references [31, 63, 72, 97, 98, 112].

9. SYSTEM DESIGN

Apart from the properties of size and surface character, little attention is paid in this present contribution to the design of systems in terms of the matrix material, drug loading or whether systems need to be capsular etc. Table 7 lists some of the more

Table 7 — Types of particulate carrier

Type	Material (and examples)
Lipid carriers	Liposomes; low density lipoproteins; chylomicrons; lipid emulsions; waxes
Polymeric carriers	Polyalkylcyanoacrylate; polylactides; polyamides
Proteinaceous carriers	Albumin; gelatin
Carbohydrate carriers	Starch; dextran (celulose, agarose)
Natural particles	Erythrocytes

important matrix materials that have been studied.

Biological opportunities do exist for effecting the release of drugs. Apart from simple diffusion and carrier breakdown, the influence of hydrogen ion concentration and heat on drug release has been considered. A particularly interesting approach has been the use of pH-sensitive liposomes to greatly enhance the cytoplasmic delivery of encapsulated macromolecues (e.g. [113, 114]). The latter *in vitro* studies give that negatively charged lipsomes are endocytosed and accumulate in endosomes of pH 4.5 to 5.5 before fusion with lysosomes. By producing oleic acid/phosphatidy-lethanolamine (as opposed to using serine or choline lipids), liposomes are formed which are unstable below pH 7. The system has great potential, though again *in vivo* access to the cell is needed. Other novel *in vivo* approaches to release include the warming of (liposome) particles above their transition temperature — when flux from the delivery system is greater (e.g. [115, 116]), and the use of microwaves [117].

(Tables 8 and 9 give the types of release possible from particular carriers and the factors which can affect these.)

10. PROSPECTS

Prospects for the limited use of particles as site-specific delivery systems are clearly good so long as they are not regarded as a panacea for access problems. For clinical purposes they must be considered alongside other similar approaches (i.e. using carriers), as well as other therapeutic strategies not necessarily involving targeting.

Table 10 gives some of the areas where useful progress is being made in exploiting the various anatomical, physiological and pathological opportunities for particle use. Passive targeting to cells of the MPS is now possible for both direct therapy and also for modulating the behaviour of MPS cells. In addition, use of ligand receptor-mediated processes to target particles containing high payloads of drugs to cells within the vasculature, the lympathic system, the bone marrow, and even in some

Table 8 — Types of release from particle carriers

Control of membrane permeability
    pH
    heat
    microwave
    magnetic

Diffusion

Ion exchange
    particle diffusion and leaching

Surface erosion

Total sphere disintegration
    enzyme attack

Adapted from Tomlinson [118].

Table 9 — Factors affecting the release of drugs from particle carriers

Drug	
	— position in the particle
	— molecular weight
	— physicochemistry
	— concentration
	— drug/carrier interactions
Particle	
	— type and amount of matrix material
	— size and density of the particle
	— extent and nature of any cross-linking, denaturation, or polymerization
	— presence of adjuvants
Environment	
	— hydrogen ion concentration
	— polarity
	— ionic strength
	— presence of enzymes
	— temperature

Adapted from Tomlinson [118].

Table 10 — Accessible biological targets using particulates

Compartment	Targets
Discrete compartments $(0.005–100)^{+}$	
Eye	Infection
Lung	Allergy
Joints	Arthritis
Gastrointestinal tract	Crone's disease, vaccination
Intralesional	(e.g. intratumour)
Bladder	Infection
Cerebral ventricles	Infection
Interstitial administration $(0.005–100)^{+}$	
Subcutaneous	Lymph node targeting (e.g. some cancers)
Intraperitoneal	Depot for anaesthetics, peptides
Intramuscular	
Intravascular targets Diseased macrophages $(0.1–1.0)^{+}$	Parasitic, fungal, viral, enzyme storage diseases; autoimmune diseases
Capillary filtration $(>10)^{+}$	Cancer, emphysema, thrombi
Circulating depot $(0.1–1.0)^{+}$	Anti-infectives, cytostatics, thrombolytics
Other blood cells $(0.1–1.0)^{+}$	Cancerous, platelets, gene therapy (bone marrow erythroblasts), immune cells (vaccination/adjuvant)
Extravascular targets Macrophage activation $(0.1–1.0)^{+}$	Abnormal cells (e.g. cancerous, virally infected)
Continuous endothelia $(<0.04)^{+}$	
Fluid-phase pinocytosis	
Receptor-mediated endo-/transcytosis	
Discontinuous endothelia $(<0.15)^{+}$	
Basement membranes	Spleen
Parenchymal cells	Liver
Diseased endothelia $(<0.5?)^{+}$	
Hyperpermeability	Inflammation (rheumatoid arthritis) Malignant hypertension
Proliferating endothelia	Invasive carcinoma
Denuded endothelia	Myocardial infarct, transluminal angioplasty
Basement membrane	Inflammation, wound healing
Ex vivo Cells	Cell separations (e.g. for neuroblastoma of bone marrow); cell targeting (e.g. for gene therapy)

$^{+}$Probable optimal diameter of particles, μm.

cases to parenchymal cells is within reach. The routes of administration will generally be parenteral, and it is likely that this will reduce their use, as will the need to perform costly safety pharmacology studies. Some opportunites do exist whereby particles can be considered for protecting the drug during gastrointestinal transit. Also such protection is useful for both low molecular weight and macromolecular drugs, avoiding both unwanted deposition and metabolism, as well as for helping to reduce immune responses to, for example, peptidergic mediators.

Although it is not easy to see how great uses will accrue from the use of particles, new ground is being broken all the time. Witness for example the use of liposomes to deliver genetic information [119, 120] or the incorporation of fusogenic viral sequences into liposomes to effect fussion with biological membranes [121] or the use of magnetic microspheres *in vitro* to sort diseased cells from normal ones [122]. Also this paper has only briefly discussed the role that particulate carriers can have as adjuvants in vaccination [123].

REFERENCES

[1] Tomlinson, E. (1986). (Patho)physiology and the temporal and spatial aspects of drug delivery. In: Tomlinson, E. & Davis, S. S. (eds) *Site-specific drug delivery. cell biology, medical and pharmaceutical aspects.* John Wiley, Chichester, pp. 1–26.

[2] Noble, J., Jones, A. G., Davis, M. S., Sledge, C. B., Kramer, R. I. & Livini, E. (1983). Leakage of radioactive particle systems from a synovial joint studied using a gamma camera: its application to radiation synovectomy. *J. Bone Joint Surg.* **65A** 381–389.

[3] Ratcliffe, J. H., Hunneyball, I. M., Wilson, C. G., Smith, A. & Davis, S. S. (1984). Microsphere systems for intrarticular drug administration. In: Davis, S. S., Illum, L., McVie, J. G. & Tomlinson, E. (eds) *Microspheres and drug therapy. pharmaceutical, immunological and medical aspects,* Elsevier, Amsterdam, pp. 345–346.

[4] Dingle, J. T., Gordon, J. C., Hazelman, B. L., Knight, C. G., Thomas, D. P. P., Phillips, N. C., Shaw, I. H., Fildes, F. J. T., Oliver, J. E., Jones, G., Turner, E. A. & Lowe, J. S. (1978). Novel treatment for joint inflammation. *Nature* **271** 327–373.

[5] Fehr, K., Velvart, M., Roos, K. & Weder, H. G. (1985). Intrarticular injection of corticosteroid-containing liposomes into normal and arthritic knee joints of rabbits. *Therapiewoche* **35** 2986–2998.

[6] Weinstein, J. N., Magin, R. L., Yatvin, M. B. & Zaharko, D. S. (1979). Liposomes and local hyperthermia: selective delivery of methotrexate to heated tumours. *Science* **204** 188–191.

[7] Carman-Meakin, B., Kellaway, I. W. & Farr, S. J. (1986). A liposomal sustained-release aerosol delivery system. *International Patent Application* Number WO 86/01714.

[8] Snipes, M. B., Chavez, G. T. & Muggenburg, B. A. (1984). Disposition of 3-, 7-, and 13-μm microspheres instilled into lungs of dogs. *Environ. Res.* **33** 333–342.

[9] Lehnert, B. E., Valdez, Y. E. & Stewart, C. C. (1986). Translocation of particles to the tracheobronchial lymph nodes after lung disposition: kinetics and particle-cell relationships. *Exp. Lung Res.* **10** 245–266.

[10] Juliano, R. L. & McCullough, H. N. (1980) Controlled delivery of an anti-

tumour drug: localized action of liposome encapsulated cytosine arabinoside administrated via the respiratory tract. *J. Pharmacol. Exp. Ther.* **214** 381–387.

[11] Farr, S. J., Kellaway, I. W., Parry-Jones, D. R. & Woolfrey, S. G. (1985). 99m-Technetium as a marker of liposomal deposition and clearance in the human lung. *Int. J. Pharmaceutics* **26** 303–316.

[12] Mufson, D. & Szoka, F. C. (1985). The application of liposome technology to targeted delivery systems. *Pharm. Technol.* 16–21.

[13] Gurny, R., Boye, T. & Ibrahim, H. (1985). Ocular therapy with nanoparticulate systems for controlled drug delivery used via the ocular route. *J. Controlled Release* **2** 353–361.

[14] Hara, S., Ishiguro, S. & Mizuno, K. (1985). Phagocytosis of polystyrene spheres in the rabbit corneal endothelium: contribution of lysosomal enzymes to the endothelial degeneration. *Ophthalmology and Visual Science* **26** 1631–1634.

[15] Algvere, P. & Martini, B. (1985). Sequelae of intravitreal phagocytic activity in response to microparticles. *Acta Ophthmalogica* **63** (Suppl. 173) 107–110.

[16] Klipstein, F. A., Engert, R. F. & Sherman, W. T. (1983). Peroral immunization of rats with *Escherichia coli* heat-labile enterotoxin delivered by microspheres. *Infection and Immunity* **39** 1000–1003.

[17] Matsuno, K., Schaffner, T., Gerber, H. A., Ruchti, C., Hess, M. W. & Cottier, H. (1983). Uptake by enterocytes and subsequent translocation to internal organs, e.g., the thymus, of percoll microspheres administered per os to suckling mice. *RES: J. Reticuloendothelial Soc.* **33** 263–273.

[18] Sanders, E. & Ashworth, C. T. (1961). A study of particulate intestinal absorption and hepatocellular uptake: use of polystyrene latex particles. *Exp. Cell Res.* **22** 137–144.

[19] Kimura, T. (1985). Intestinal absorption of liposomally-entrapped drugs. *Saishin Igaku* **40** 1818–1824.

[20] Patel, H. M., Tuzel, N. S. & Stevenson, R. W. (1985). Intracellular digestion of saturated and unsaturated phospholipid liposomes by mucosal cells. Possible mechanism of transport of liposomally entrapped marcomolecules across the isolated vascularly perfused rabbit ileum. *Biochim. Biophys. Acta* **839** 40–49.

[21] Nefzger, M., Kreuter, J., Voges, R., Liehl, E. & Czok, R. J. (1984). Distribution and elimination of polymethyl methacrylate nanoparticles after peroral administration to rats. *Pharm. Sci.* **73** 1309–1312.

[22] Owen, R. L., Pierce, N. F., Apple, R. T. & Cray, W. C., Jr. (1986). M cell transport of *Vibrio cholerae* from the intestinal lumen into Peyer's patches: a mechanism for antigen sampling and for microbial transepithelial migration. *J. Infect. Dis.* **153** 1108–1118.

[23] Bockman, D. E. & Cooper, M. D. (1973). Pinocytosis by epithelium associated with lymphoid follicles in the bursa of Fabricius, appendix and Peyer's patches. An electron microscopic study. *Am. J. Anat.* **136** 455–477.

[24] Wolf, J. L., Rubin, D. H., Finberg, R., Kauffman, R. S., Sharpe, A. H., Trier, J. S. & Fields, B. N. (1981). Intestinal M cells: a pathway for entry of reovirus into the host. *Science* **212** 471–472.

[25] Joel, D. D., Laissue, J. D. & LeFevre, M. E. (1978). Distribution and fate of ingested carbon particles in mice. *J. Reticuloendothelial Soc.* **72** 440–451.

[26] Weinstein, J. N. & Leserman, L. D. (1984). Liposomes as drug carriers in cancer chemotherapy. *Pharmac. Ther.* **24** 207–233.

[27] Leak, L. V. (1971). Studies on the permeability of lymphatic capillaries. *J. Cell. Biol.* **50** 300–323.

[28] Leak, L. V. (1986). Distribution of cell surface charges on mesothelium and lymphatic endothelium. *Microvasc. Res.* **31** 18–30.

[29] Bergqvist, L., Strand, S.-E. & Jonsson, P.-E. (1984). The characterisation of radiocolloids used for administration to the lymphatic system. In: Davis, S. S., Illum, L., McVie, J. G. & Tomlinson, E. (eds) *Microspheres and Drug Therapy. Pharmaceutical, Immunological and Medical Aspects,* Elsevier, Amsterdam, pp. 263–279.

[30] Taylor, A. E. & Granger, D. N. (1984). Exchange of macromolecules across the microcirculation. *Handbook Physiol.* **6** 467–520.

[31] Poste, G. (1983). Liposome targeting *in vivo:* problems and opportunities. *Biol. Cell* **47** 19–38.

[32] Casley-Smith, J. R. (1977). Lymph and lymphatics. In: Kaley, G. & Altura, B. M. (eds) *Microcirculation,* Vol. 1, University Park Press, Baltimore, pp. 423–502.

[33] Weinstein, J. N., Black, C. D. V., Barbet, J., Eger, R. R., Parker, R. J., Holton, O. D., Mulshine, J. L., Keenan, A. M., Larson, S. M., Carrasquillo, J. A., Sieber, S. M. & Covell, D. G. (1986). Selected issues in the pharmacology of monoclonal antibodies. In: Tomlinson, E. & Davis, S. S. (eds) *Site-specific Drug Delivery. Cell Biology, Medical and Pharmaceutical Aspects,* John Wiley, Chichester, pp. 81–91.

[34] Hirano, K., Hunt, C. A., Strubbe, A. & MacGregor, R. D. (1985). Lymphatic transport of liposome-encapsulated drugs following intraperitoneal administration — effect of lipid composition. *Pharm. Res.* 271–278.

[35] Mangat, S. & Patel, H. M. (1985). Lymph node localisation on non-specific antibody-coated liposomes. *Life Sci.* **36,** 1917–1925.

[36] Hashida, M. & Sezaki, H. (1984). Specific delivery of mitomycin C: combined use of prodrugs and spherical delivery systems. In: Davis, S. C., Illum, L., McVie, J. G. & Tomlinson, E. (eds) *Microspheres and Drug Therapy. Pharmaceutical, Immunological and Medical Aspects,* Elsevier, Amsterdam, pp. 281–293.

[37] Nakatsu, K. & Cameron, D. A. (1979). Uptake of liposome-entrapped mannitol by diaphragm. *Can. J. Physiol. Pharmacol.* **57,** 756–759.

[38] Ellens, H., Morselt, H. & Scherphof, G. (1981). *In vivo* fate of large multilamellar sphingomyelin-cholesterol liposomes after intraperitoneal and intraveneous injection into rats. *Biochim. Biophys. Acta* **674** 10–18.

[39] Davis, S. S., Illum, L., McVie, J. G. & Tomlinson, E. (eds) (1984). *Microspheres and Drug Therapy. Pharmaceutical, Immunological and Medical Aspects,* Elsevier, Amsterdam.

[40] McLaughlin, C. A. & Goldberg, E. P. (1983). Local chemo- and immunotherapy by intratumor drug injection: opportunities for polymer-drug compo-

sitions. In: Goldberg, E. P. (ed.) *Targeted Drugs,* John Wiley, New York, pp. 231–268.

[41] Martodam, R. R., Twumasi, D. Y., Liener, I. E., Powers, J. C., Nishino, N. & Krejcarek, G. (1979). Albumin microspheres as carrier of an inhibitor of leukocyte elastase: potential therapeutic agent for emphysema. *Proc. Natl. Acad. Sci. USA* **76** 2128–2132.

[42] Torchilin, V. P. (1983). Immobilized enzymes and the use of immobilization principles for drug targeting. In: Goldberg, E. P. (ed) *Targeted Drugs,* John Wiley, New York, pp. 127–152.

[43] Burger, J. J., Tomlinson, E., Mulder, E. M. A. & McVie, J. G. (1985). Albumin microspheres for intraarterial tumour targeting. I. Pharmaceutical aspects. *Int. J. Pharmaceutics* **23** 333–345.

[44] Lindberg, B., Lote, K. & Teder, H. (1984). Biodegradable starch microspheres. In: Davis, S. S., Illum, L., McVie, J. G. & Tomlinson, E. (eds) *Microspheres and Drug Therapy. Pharmaceutical, Immunological and Medical Aspects*, Elsevier, Amsterdam, pp. 153–189.

[45] Blanchard, R. J. W., Grotenhuis, I., LaFavre, J. W. & Perry, J. F. (1965). Blood supply to hepatic V2 carcinoma implants as measured by radioactive microspheres. *Proc. Soc. Exp. Biol. Med.* **118** 465–468.

[46] Lindell, B., Aronsen, K. F., Rothman, U. & Sjoegren, H. O. (1977). The circulation in liver tissue and experimental liver metastases before and after embolism of the liver artery. *Res. Exp. Med.* **171** 63–70.

[47] Gregoriadis, G., Senior, J., Wolff, B. & Kirby, C. (1985). Targeting of liposomes to accessible cells *in vivo. Ann. New York Acad. Sci.* **446**, 319–340.

[48] Hoefsmit, E. C. M., Duyvenstijn, A. M. & Kamperdijk, E. W. A. (1982). Relation between Langerhans cells, veiled cells and interdigitating cells. *Immunobiol.* **161**, 255–265.

[49] Brouwer, A. & Knook, D. L. (1983). The reticuloendothelial system and ageing: a review. *Mechanisms Ageing Develop.* **21** 205–228.

[50] Bradfield, J. W. (1984). The reticulo-endothelial system and blood clearance. In: Davis, S. S., Illum, L., McVie, J. G. & Tomlinson, E. (eds) *Microspheres and Drug Therapy. Pharmaceutical, Immunological and Medical Aspects*, Elsevier, Amsterdam, pp. 25–37.

[51] Lewis, J. C., Maldonado, J. E. & Mann, K. G. (1976). Phagocytosis in human platelets: localisation of acid-phosphatase-positive phagosomes following latex uptake. *Blood* **47** 833–840.

[52] Dobson, E. L. (1957). Factors controlling phagocytosis. In: Halpern, B. N., Benacerraf, B. & Delafresnaye, J. F. (eds) *Physiopathology of the reticulo-endothelial System,* Blackwell, Oxford, p. 97.

[53] Lehnert, B. E. & Tech, C. (1985). Quantitative evaluation of opsonin-independent phagocytosis by alveolar macrophages in monolayer using polystyrene microspheres. *J. Immunol. Methods* **78** 337–344.

[54] Chudwin, D. S., Artrip, S. G., Korenblit, A., Schiffman & Rao, S. (1985). Correlation of serum opsonins with *in vitro* phagocytosis of *Streptococcus pneumoniae. Infect. Immun.* **50**, 213–217.

[55] Czop, J. K., Fearon, D. T. & Austen, K. F. (1978). Opsonin-independent

phagocytosis of activators of the alternative complement pathway by human monocytes. *J. Immunol.* **120**, 1132–1138.

[56] Schwendener, R. A., Lagocki, P. A. & Rahman, Y. E. (1984). The effects of charge and size on the interaction of unilamellar liposomes with macrophages. *Biochim. Biophys. Acta* **772** 93–101.

[57] Abbracchio, M. P., Heck, J. D. & Costa, M. (1982). The phagocytosis and transforming activity of crystalline metal sulfide particles are related to their negative surface charge. *Carcinogenesis* **3** 175–180.

[58] Van Oss, C. J. (1978). Phagocytosis as surface phenomena. *Ann. Rev. Biochem.* **46** 669–722.

[59] Saad, A. H. & Williams, A. R. (1982). Effects of therapeutic ultrasound on clearance rate of blood borne colloidal particles *in vivo. Brit. J. Cancer* **45** Suppl. V, 202–205.

[60] Schroit, E. J., Hart, I. R., Madsen, J. & Fidler, I. J. (1983). Selective delivery of drugs encapsulated in lipsomes: natural targeting to macrophages involved in various disease states. *J. Biol. Response Modifiers* **2** 97–100.

[61] Territo, M. & Cline, M. J. (1976). Macrophages and their disorders in man. In: Nelson, D. S. (ed) *Immunobiology of the Macrophage,* Academic Press, New York, pp. 593–616.

[62] Lopez-Berenstein, G., Mehta, R., Hopfer, R. L., Mills, K., Kasi, L., Mehta, K., Fainstein, V., Luna, M., Hersh, E. M. & Juliano, R. L. (1983). Treatment or prophylaxis of disseminated infection due to *Candida albicans* in mice with liposome encapsulated amphotericin B. *J. Infect. Dis.* **5** 939–945.

[63] Juliano, R. L., Lopez-Berenstein, G., Hopfer, R., Mehta, R. & Mehta, K. & Mills, K. (1985). Selective toxicity and enhanced therapeutic index of liposomal polyene antibiotics in systemic fungal infections. *Ann. N. Y. Acad. Sci.* **446** 390–402.

[64] Poznansky, M. J. & Juliano, R. L. (1984). Biological approaches to the controlled delivery of drugs: A critical review. *Pharmacol. Revs.* **36** 277–336.

[65] Fidler, I. J. (1986). Immunomodulation of macrophages for cancer and antiviral therapy. In: Tomlinson, E. & Davis, S. S. (eds) *Site-specific Drug Delivery. Cell Biology. Medical and Pharmaceutical aspects,* John Wiley, Chichester, pp. 111–134.

[66] Umezawa, F., Eto, Y., Tokoro, F. & Maekawa, K. (1985). Enzyme replacement with liposomes containing beta-galactosidase fom charonia lumpas in murine globoid cell leukodystrophy (Twitcher). *Biochem. Biophys. Res. Comm.* **127** 663–667.

[67] Lynch, W. E., Sartiano, G. P., Rosenblum, S. L., Calkins, J. H. & Ramsey, C. B. (1985). The use of erythrocytes for delivery of chemotherapeutic agents to the reticuloendothelial system. *Biblthca Haemat. no. 51,* Karger, Basel, pp. 42–49.

[68] Adams, D. O. (1982). Macrophage activation and secretion. *Fed. Proc.* **41** 2193–2197.

[69] Poste, G. & Kirsch, R. (1982). Liposome-encapsulated macrophage activation agents and active non-specific immunotherapy of neoplastic disease. In:

Akoyounoglu, G., Evangelopoulos, A. E., Georgatsos, J., Palaiologos, G.,
Traketellis, A. & Tsiganos, C. P. (eds) *Cell Function and Differentiation, Part
A,* Alan R. Liss, New York, pp. 309–319.

[70] Gregoriadis, G., Neerunjub, D. E. & Hunt, R. (1977). Fate of liposome-
associated agents injected into normal and tumour-bearing rodents: attempts
to improve localization in tumour lines. *Life Sci.* **21** 357–370.

[71] Proffitt, R. T., Williams, L. E., Presant, C. A., Tin, G. W., Uliana, J. A.,
Gamble, R. C. & Baldeschweiler, J. D. (1983). Liposomal blockade of the
reticuloendothelial system; improved tumor imaging with small unilamellar
vesicles. *Science* **220** 502–505.

[72] Allen, T. M., Murray, L., MacKeigan, S. & Shah, M. (1984). Chronic
liposome administration in mice: effects on reticuloendothelial function and
tissue distribution. *J.Pharmacol. Exp. Therap.* **229** 267–275.

[73] Hopkins, C. R. (1986). Site-specific drug delivery — cellular opportunities and
challenges. In: Tomlinson, E. & Davis, S. S. (eds) *Site-specific Drug Delivery.
Cell Biology, Medical and Pharmaceutical Aspects,* John Wiley, Chichester,
pp. 27–48.

[74] Norde, W. (1984). Physicochemical aspects of the behaviour of biological
components at solid-liquid interfaces. In: Davis, S. S., Illum, L., McVie, J. G.
& Tomlinson, E. (eds) *Microspheres and Drug Therapy. Pharmaceutical,
Immunological and Medical Aspects,* Elsevier, Amsterdam, pp. 39–59.

[75] Wilkins, D. J. & Myers, P. A. (1966). Studies on the relationship between the
electrophoretic properties of colloids and their blood clearance and organ
distribution in rat. *Brit. J. Exp. Pathol.* **47** 569–576.

[76] Napper, D. H. & Netschey, A. (1971). Studies of the steric stabilisation of
colloidal particles. *J. Colloid Interface Sic.* **37** 528–535.

[77] Ottewill, R. H. (1977). Stability and instability in disperse systems. *J. Colloid
Interface Sci.* **58** 357–373.

[78] Abuchowski, A. & Davis, F. F. (1981). Soluble polymer-enzyme adducts. In:
Holcenberg, T. F. & Roberts, T. (eds) *Enzymes as Drugs,* John Wiley, New
York, pp. 367–384.

[79] Geyer, R. P. (1967). Studies on the metabolism of intravenous fat emulsion.
Fette Med. **6** 59–61.

[80] Jeppsson, R. & Rossner, S. (1975). The influence of emulsifying agents and
lipid soluble drugs on the fractional removal rate of lipid emulsion from the
blood stream of the rabbit. *Acta Pharmacol. Toxicol.* **37** 134–144.

[81] Davis, S. S. & Hansrasi, P. (1985). The influence of emulsifying agents on the
phagocytosis of lipid emulsions by macrophages. *Int. J. Pharm.* **23,** 69–77.

[82] Illum, L. & Davis, S. S. (1983). Effect of the nonionic surfactant poloxamer
338, on the fate and deposition of polystyrene microspheres following intravenous administration. *J. Pharm. Sci.* **72** 1086–1089.

[83] Illum, L. & Davis, S. S. (1984). The organ uptake of intravenously administered colloidal particles can be altered using a non-ionic surfactant (Poloxamer
338). *FEBS Letts.* **167** 79–82.

[84] Leu, D., Manthey, B., Kreuter, J., Speiser, P. & DeLuca, P. P. (1984).
Distribution and elimination of coated polymethyl[2–C^{14}]methacrylate nanoparticles after intravenous injections in rats. *J. Pharm. Sci.* **73** 1433–1437.

[85] Davis, S. S. & Illum, L. (1986). Colloidal delivery systems — opportunities and challenges. In: Tomlinson, E. & Davis, S. S. (eds) *Site-specific Drug Delivery. Cell Biology, Medical and Pharmaceutical Aspects,* John Wiley, Chichester, pp. 93–110.

[86] Utsumi, S., Shinomiya, H., Minami, J. & Sonoda, S. (1983). Inhibition of phagocytosis by erythrocyte membrane sialoglycoprotein on target liposomes. *Immunol.* **49** 113–120.

[87] Alpar, H. O. & Lewis, D. A. (1985). Therapeutic efficacy of asparaginase encapsulated in intact erythrocytes. *Biochem. Pharmacol.* **34** 257–261.

[88] Vidal, M., Sainte-Marie, J., Philippot, J. R. & Bienvenue, A. (1985). Low-density lipoprotein mediated targeting of liposomes to leukemic lymphocytes *in vitro. EMBO J.* **4** 2461–2468.

[89] Singhal, A. & Gupta, C. M. (1986). Antibody-mediated targeting of lipsomes to red cell *in vivo. FEBS Lett.* **201** 321–326.

[90] Laakso, T., Andersson, J., Artursson, P., Edman, P. & Sjoholm, I. (1986). Acrylic microspheres *in vivo.* X. Elimination of circulating cells by active targeting using specific monoclonal antibodies bound to microparticles. *Life Sci.* **38** 183–190.

[91] Machy, P., Barbet, J. & Leserman, L. D. (1982). Differential endocytosis of T and B lymphocyte surface molecules evaluated with antibody-bearing fluorescent liposomes containing methotrexate. *Proc. Natl. Acad. Sci. USA,* **79** 4148–4125.

[92] Stavridis, J. C., Deliconstantinos, G., Psallidopoulos, M. C., Armenakas, N. A., Hadjiminas, D. J. & Hadjiminas, J. (1986). Construction of transferrin-coated liposomes for *in vivo* transport of exogenous DNA to bone marrow erythrocytes in rabbits. *J. Exp. Cell. Res.* **164** 568–572.

[93] Auerbach, R., Alby, L., Morrissey, L. W., Tu, M. & Joseph, J. (1985). Expression of organ-specific antigens on capillary endothelial cells. *Microvasc. Res.* **29** 401–411.

[94] Rutgers, J. L., Wieczorek, R., Bonetti, F., Kaplan, K. L., Posnett, D. N., Friedman-Kein, A. E. & Knowles, D. M. (1986). The expression of endothelial cell surface antigens by AIDS-assocaited Kaposi's sarcoma. Evidence for a vascular endothelial cell origin. *Am. J. Pathol.* **122** 493–499.

[95] Smirnov, V. N., Domogatsky, S. P., Dolgov, V. V., Hvatov, V. B., Klibanov, A. L., Koteliansky, V. E., Muzykantov, V. R., Repin, V. S., Samokhin, B. V., Shekhonin, B. V., Smirnov, M. D., Sviridov, D. D., Tochilin, V. P. & Chazov, E. I. (1986). Carrier-directed targeting of liposomes and erythrocytes to denuded areas of vessel wall. *Proc. Natl. Acad. Sci. USA* **83** 6603–6607.

[96] Shoji, Y., Mizushima, Y., Yanagawa, A. & Yonaha, T. (1985). Electron microscopic studies on tissue distribution of lipid microspheres used as drug delivery carriers. *Drugs Exptl. Clin. Res.* **11** 601–609.

[97] Poste, G. (1985). Drug targeting in cancer therapy. In: Gregoriadis, G., Poste, G., Senior, J. & Trouet, A. (eds). *Receptor-mediated Targeting of Drugs,* Plenum, New York, pp. 427–474.

[98] Cleland, L. G., Roberts, B. V., Garrett, R. & Allen, T. M. (1982). Cortisol palmitate liposomes: enhanced antiinflammatory effect in rats compared with free cortisol. *Agents Actions* **12,** 348–352.

[99] Williams, B. D., O'Sullivan, M. M., Saggu, G. S., Williams, K. E., Williams, L. A. & Morgan, J. R. (1986). Imaging in rheumatoid arthritis using liposomes labelled with technetium. *Brit. Med. J.* **293** 1143–1144.

[100] Jellinek, H., Nagy, Z., Huttner, I., Balint, A., Kocze, A. & Kerenyi, T. (1969). Investigations of the permeability changes of the vascular wall in experimental malignant hypertension by means of a colloidal iron preparation. *Brit. J. Exp. Pathol.* **50** 13–18.

[101] Palmer, T. N., Caride, V. J., Fernandez, L. A. & Twickler, J. (1981). Liposome accumulation in ischaemic intestine following experimental mesenteric occlusion. *BioSci. Repts.* **1** 337–341.

[102] Mueller, T. M., Marcus, M. L., Mayer, H. E., Williams, J. K. & Hersmeyer, K. (1981). Liposome concentration in canine ischemic myocardium and depolarized myocardial cells. *Circ. Res.* **49** 405–410.

[103] Widder, K., Morris, R., Poore, G., Howard, D. & Senyei, A. E. (1981). Tumor remission in Yoshida sarcoma-bearing rats by selective targeting of magnetic albumin microsphere containing doxorubicin. *Proc. Natl. Acad. Sci. USA* **78** 579–581.

[104] Akimoto, M., Sugibayashi, K. & Morimoto, Y. (1985). Application of magnetic emulsions for sustained release and the targeting of drugs in cancer chemotherapy. *J. Controlled Release* **1** 205–215.

[105] Rettenmaier, M. A., Senyei, A. E. & Widder, K. J. (1985). *In vivo* alteration of RES phagocytosis by magnetic albumin microspheres. *J. Clin. Lab. Immunol.* **17** 99–103.

[106] Ghitescu, L., Fixman, A., Simionescu, M. & Simionescu, N. (1986). Specific binding sites for albumin restricted to plasmalemmal vesicles of continuous capillary endothelium: receptor-mediated transcytosis. *J. Cell. Biol.* **102** 1304–1311.

[107] Van Berkel, T. J. C., (1986). Kruijt, J. K., Harkes, L., Nagelkerke, J. F., Spanjer, H. & Kempen, H.-J. M. Receptor-dependent targeting of native and modified lipoproteins to liver cells. In: Tomlinson, E. & Davis, S. S. (eds) *Site-specific Drug Delivery. Cell Biology, Medical and Pharmaceutical Aspects*, John Wiley, Chichester, pp. 49–68.

[108] Kiwada, H., Nimura, H. & Kato, Y. (1985). Tissue distribution and pharmacokinetic evaluation of the targeting efficiency of synthetic alkyl glycoside vesicles. *Chem. Pharm. Bull.* **33** 2465–2482.

[109] Lees, R. S., Garabedian, H. D., Lees, A. M., Schumacher, D. J., Miller, A., Isaacsohn, J. L., Derksen, A. & Strauss, H. W. (1985). Technetium-99m low density lipoproteins: preparation and biodistribution. *J. Nucl. Med.* **26** 1057–1062.

[110] Halbert, G. W., Stuart, J. F. B. & Florence, A. T. (1985). A low density lipoprotein-methotrexate covalent complex and its activity against L1210 cells in vitro. *Cancer Chemother. Pharmacol.* **15** 223–227.

[111] Newman, S. A., Frenz, D. A., Tomasek, J. J. & Rabuzzi, D. D. (1985). Matrix-driven translocation of cells and non-living particles. *Science* **228** 885–889.

[112] Szymendera, J., Mioduszewska, O., Licinska, I., Czarnomska, A. & Lucka,

B. (1977). Pathologic changes in the lungs of mice following injection of human albumin microspheres. *J. Nucl. Med.* **18** 478–482.

[113] Nayar, R. & Schroit, A. J. (1985) Generation of pH-sensitive liposomes: use of large unilamellar vesicles containing *N*-succinyldioleoylphosphatidyletha-nolamine. *Biochemistry* **24** 5967–5971.

[114] Straubinger, R. M., Duzgunes, N. & Papahadjopoulos, D. (1985). pH-sensitive liposomes mediate cytoplasmic delivery of encapsulated macromole-cules. *FEBS Letts.* **179** 148–154.

[115] Bassett, J. B., Anderson, R. U. & Tucker, J. R. (1986). Use of temperature-sensitive liposomes in the selective delivery of methotrexate and cis-platinum analogues to murine bladder tumour. *J. Urol.* **135** 612–615.

[116] Magin, R. L. & Niesman, M. R. (1984). Temperature-dependent drug release from large unilamellar liposomes. *Cancer Drug Delivery* **1** 109–117.

[117] Liburdy, R. P. & Magin, R. L. (1985) Microwave-stimulated drug release from lipsomes. *Radiation Res.* **103** 266–275.

[118] Tomlinson, E. (1983). Microsphere delivery systems for drug targeting and controlled release. *Int. J. Pharm. Technol. Prod. Manuf.* **4** 49–57.

[119] Chernyavskii, V. A., Samarina, M. R. & Zerov, Yu, P. (1985). Liposomes as a carrier of genetic information. *Molek. Genetika, Mikrobiol. Virusol.* 3–12.

[120] Glushakova, S. E., Grodniskaya, N. A., Naroditskii, B. S., Kislina, O. S., Komarov, Yu. S., Tikhonenko, T. T., Mel'nikov, S. Ya. & Gendon, Yu. Z. (1985). Optimal transfer and incorporation of viral DNA into cells via liposomes containing influenza virus glycoproteins. *Molek. Genet., Mikro-biol. Virusol.* 32–36.

[121] Citovsky, V., Blumenthal, R. & Loyter, A. (1985). Fusion of Sendai virions with phosphatidylcholine-cholesterol liposomes reflects the viral activity required for fusion with biological membranes. *FEBS Lett.* **193,** 135–140.

[122] Treleaven, J. G., Gibson, F. M., Ugelstad, J., Rembaum, A., Philp, T., Caine, G. D. & Kemshead, J. T. (1984). Removal of neuroblastoma cells from bone marrow with monoclonal antibodies conjugated to magnetic micros-pheres. *Lancet* 70–73.

[123] Knudsen, R. C., Card, D. M. & Hoffman, W. W. (1986). Protection of guinea pigs against local and systemic foot-and-mouth disease after administration of synthetic lipid amine (Avridine) liposomes. *Antiviral Res.* **6** 123–133.

3

Therapeutic utility of liposomes

F. H. Roerdink, T. Daemen, I. A. J. M. Bakker-Woudenberg[†], G. Storm[‡], D. J. A. Crommelin[‡] and G. L. Scherphof, Laboratory of Physiological Chemistry, University of Groningen, Bloemsingel 10, 9712 KZ Groningen, [†]Department of Clinical Microbiology and Antimicrobial Therapy, Erasmus University, Rotterdam, 3000 DR Rotterdam and [†]Department of Pharmaceutics, State University of Utrecht, Catharijnesingel 60, 3511 GH Utrecht, The Netherlands

1. INTRODUCTION

In the past decade the application of liposomes as a potential controlled drug delivery system has gained wide interest [1,2]. Liposomes are microscopic structures consisting of one or more concentric lipid bilayers surrounding aqueous compartments within which water-soluble drugs can be entrapped. Lipophilic agents or lipophilic derivatives of water-soluble drugs can be incorporated into the lipid membranes.

Since 1972, when Gregoriadis and Ryman [3] proposed the use of liposomes as carriers of enzymes in the treatment of lysosomal storage diseases, the application of liposomes has been extended to a variety of drugs such as antineoplastic agents, antimicrobial compounds, immunomodulators, etc. [4]. The purpose of using liposomal carriers was to increase the uptake of drugs by specific cells or tissues, thereby enhancing the potency and/or reducing the toxicity of the encapsulated agents.

However, in the following years it soon became apparent that, in spite of some remarkable successes, liposomes are by no means a panacea for pharmacotherapy in general.

The purpose of this paper is to present a more balanced view on the potentialities and limitations of the use of liposomes as a drug delivery system. Emphasis will be given to the *in vivo* behavior of liposomes, targeting to specific tissues and some promising therapeutic applications in the field of immuno- and chemotherapy of metastatic cancer and infectious diseases.

2. BASIC ASPECTS OF LIPOSOME PREPARATIONS

Liposomes are formed spontaneously when amphipathic lipids are dispersed in excess water [5]. The lipid molecules arrange themselves by exposing their polar head groups towards the water phase, while the apolar hydrocarbon moieties stick together in the bilayer thus forming closed concentric bimolecular lipid leaflets separated by aqueous compartments.

Formation of stable liposomes from phospholipids is only possible at temperatures above the gel to liquid–crystalline phase transition temperature (T_c) which represents the melting point of the acyl chains. All phospholipids have a characteristic T_c, which depends on the nature of the polar head group and on length and degree of unsaturation of the acyl chains. Above T_c, phospholipids are in the liquid–crystalline phase, characterized by an increased mobility of the acyl chains. Decrease in temperature below T_c induces a transition to a more rigid state ('gel state') resulting in restrained mobility of tightly packed acyl chains. When the lipid molecules arrange themselves to form closed bilayer structures, water and solutes, e.g. drugs, are trapped between adjacent planes of polar head groups.

Liposomes can be formed from a variety of phospholipids. The lipid most widely used is phosphatidylcholine, either as such or in combination with cholesterol. Cholesterol is known to condense the packing of the phospholipids in bilayers above T_c, thereby reducing their permeability to encapsulate compounds. To confer surface charge to the liposomes, negatively charged lipids such as stearylamine are used.

Several types of liposomes are available now for application as a drug delivery system. Multilamellar vesicles (MLV) are formed spontaneously upon hydration of dry phospholipid in excess water. These vesicles are very heterogeneous in diameter (up to several microns) but can be 'sized' by extrusion through polycarbonate filters. The size of the liposomes can also be reduced by ultrasonication which ultimately results in a homogeneous suspension of small unilamellar vesicles (SUV) with diameters as small as 25 nm. Large unilamellar vesicles (LUV) of almost any lipid composition can be prepared by means of a reverse-phase evaporation method as described by Szoka et al. [6]. The relatively large entrapped aqueous volume of MLV and LUV (approximately 3 l/mol of lipid and 6 l/mol of lipid, respectively) vs SUV (approximately 0.3 l/mol of lipid) renders the former liposome types attractive candidates to serve as a delivery system for water-soluble drugs. Lipophilic drugs, on the other hand, can also be incorporated efficiently into SUV. See [7] for an extensive review.

3. LIPOSOMES *IN VIVO*

Among the various routes of administration of liposomes the intravenous injection is the most widely applied. The half-lives of liposomes in the blood stream can range from a few minutes to many hours depending on the size and lipid composition of the vesicles. Large-size vesicles like MLV or LUV are rapidly cleared from the blood and taken up by cells of the reticuloendothelial system (RES), especially macrophages in liver (Kupffer cells) and spleen [8–10]. Uptake occurs by way of endocytosis, thus causing the liposomes to end up in the lysosomal compartment of the cells. There the vesicles are degraded by lysosomal (phospho)lipases followed by release of lipo-some-encapsulated compounds [11–13]. In addition to liver and spleen macro-phages, circulating monocytes have been reported to take up significant amounts of liposomes. In the lung, the liposome-loaded monocytes can subsequently migrate to the alveoli to become alveolar macrophages [14].

Small-size vesicles like SUV are cleared much more slowly from the blood depending on the surface charge of the liposomes; neutral sphingomyelin/cholesterol vesicles, for example, have a half-life of approximately 24 h [15,16], whereas incorporation of a negatively charged lipid (phosphatidylserine) substantially increases the rate of blood elimination and concurrently stimulates the uptake of the vesicles by liver and spleen macrophages. Apparently, introduction of negative charge increases the affinity of the liposomes for the macrophages.

These data are compatible with results we obtained with isolated Kupffer cells cultured in monolayer. Neutral vesicles composed of cholesterol and equimolar amounts of phosphatidylcholine or sphingomyelin displayed a very low affinity for the cells. Incorporation of the positively charged stearylamine increased the uptake while negatively charged phosphatidylserine-containing vesicles were taken up even more efficiently [17].

Small unilamellar vesicles are not only taken up by phagocytic cells in liver and spleen upon IV injection but can also penetrate the 100 nm fenestrations in the endothelial cells lining the liver sinusoids, thus reaching the liver parenchymal cells. Accordingly, we found that after IV administration, substantial amounts of SUV are taken up by this cell type. Experiments with the lysosomotropic agent chloroquine, which effectively inhibits the activity of lysosomal phospholipases, indicate that uptake of the vesicles by the hepatocytes also occurs by way of an endocytic mechanism [10].

Incorporation of a glycolipid carrying a terminal non-reducing β-galactose, i.e. lactosylceramide in SUV, containing dimyristoylphosphatidylcholine as the bulk phospholipid, resulted in a two-fold increase in uptake of the vesicles by the hepatocytes. The increased uptake of these lactosylceramide vesicles could be inhibited by the administration of asialofetuin, a galactose-exposing glycoprotein, indicating that galactose receptors present on the hepatocyte membrane are involved in the uptake process [18].

However, penetration of IV injected liposomes to other tissues like the myocar-dium, skeletal muscles or the central nervous system is very poor because of the tight endothelium lining the capillaries in these organs preventing egress of the vesicles from the vascular compartment [14].

During their stay in the bloodstream, liposomes may be susceptible to destabiliz-ing effects of serum proteins, resulting in leakage of encapsulated water-soluble compounds. We and others found high density lipoproteins (HDL) to be mainly responsible for penetration into the liposomal bilayers, a process which was accom-panied by net loss of phosphatidylcholine from the liposomes to the HDL [19,20]. Very high susceptibility was found at the gel-to-liquid phase-transition temperature of the liposomal lipid, while both above and below that temperature the liposomes were relatively insensitive [21]. However, net loss of phospholipid could be pre-vented and, concomitantly, retention of encapsulated drugs was improved by incorporation of cholesterol in the liposomal membrane [21]. As discussed before, cholesterol is known to condense lipid membranes, thereby impeding penetration of serum (lipo)proteins, resulting in an increased stability of the liposomes.

4. THE LIPOSOME–DRUG CONCEPT

From the previous section it is obvious that successful targeting of liposomes to other cells than those belonging to the RES, with the exception of the hepatocytes and, possibly, circulating blood cells, is very unlikely. Although a high degree of specific liposome–cell association was obtained *in vitro* by coating the vesicles with cell-specific ligands like monoclonal antibodies or F(ab')$_2$ fragments, an efficient transfer of encapsulated drug was not always observed [22–24]. *In vivo,* the obstacles which have to be overcome are formidable. Firstly, the liposomes have to escape from non-specific clearance by the RES cells. Secondly, the vesicles have to cross the capillary endothelium and the basement membrane, and thirdly, many cell types, including most tumor cells, display only a very low endocytic capacity. Since endocytosis is the dominant mechanism of liposome–cell interaction, this circumstance means a serious limitation to the successful application of liposomes as a drug delivery system.

On the other hand, liposomes appear to be an ideal carrier system for the selective delivery of drugs to cells belonging to the RES. Small-size liposomes may also serve as carriers of drugs to be delivered to liver parenchymal cells by virtue of their capacity to penetrate the fenestrated liver endothelium. Once taken up by the cells the liposomes are degraded in the lysosomal compartment. Liposome-encapsulated drugs, when resistant to the intralysosomal environment, may slowly leak out of the lysosomes into the cytosol and could become available to exert their therapeutic action. The drug may also be released by the macrophages so as to maintain a therapeutic drug level in blood and/or tissues for a prolonged period of time. This 'sustained release' of drugs which may occur from circulating liposomes, liposomes adsorbed to cell membranes as well as from macrophages which have engulfed drug-loaded liposomes, may be an important application of liposome delivery systems [2]. Particularly during administration of cell-cycle-specific antitumor drugs like cytosine arabinoside, sustained exposure of the tumor cells to the drug will enhance the therapeutic effect by continuously killing the cells entering the S-phase.

Another interesting aspect of the liposome–drug concept is the reduction of the toxicity of liposome-encapsulated agents. This might be particularly true for anti-neoplastic agents like Adriamycin or antimicrobial drugs like amphotericin B. The decrease in toxicity is thought to be accomplised by altered pharmacokinetics and tissue distribution of the drugs applied, as will be discussed in the following sections.

5. LIPOSOMES AS CARRIERS OF ANTIMICROBIAL AGENTS

Although very effective antimicrobial drugs have been available for more than 50 years now, therapeutic failures still occur, especially in immunocompromised individuals such as patients with underlying malignant disease or patients receiving immunosuppressive drugs. Besides inadequate host defense, toxicity of the administered drug or poor penetration into affected cells in cases of intracellular infections can contribute considerably to failure of antimicrobial treatment. Application of liposomes as a drug delivery system might offer an excellent approach to overcome these problems by increasing the selective delivery of applied drugs to the affected cells and/or by decreasing drug toxicity.

The first reports on this approach were published independently by three different groups using liposomes as carriers of antimonial drugs like meglumine antimoniate in experimental Leishmaniasis infection [25–27]. The Leishmania parasites are lodged inside the lysosomes of phagocytic cells, precisely the intracellular site where liposomes end up after IV injection. Encapsulation of the antimonial drug within MLV resulted in a nearly 1000-fold increase in therapeutic efficacy of this highly toxic drug. We obtained similar results with the use of liposome-encapsulated ampicillin in the treatment of experimental *Listeria monocytogenes* infection in mice [28]. Entrapment of the antibiotic within MLV resulted in a 90-fold increase in therapeutic activity of the drug (Fig. 1). The increase in therapeutic index appeared

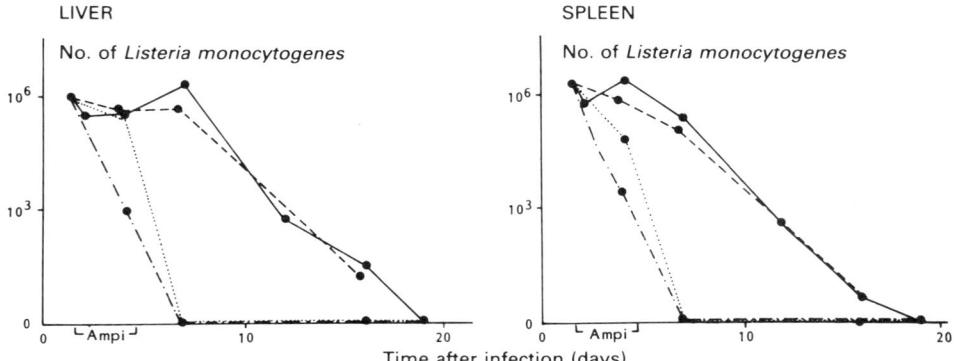

Fig. 1 — Effect of liposome-entrapped and non-entrapped ampicillin on the numbers of *Listeria monocytogenes* in the liver and spleen at different intervals after intravenous inoculation of 5×10^3 bacteria. Antibiotic was administered intravenously, starting 40 h after bacterial inoculation: two doses of 0.27 mg ampicillin encapsulated in 2 μmol lipid each at 72-h intervals (·····); two doses of 0.27 mg amplicillin plus 2 μmol lipid each at 72-h intervals (– – –); eight doses of 6 mg free ampicillin each at 12-h intervals (–·–·); untreated controls (———). Data are median values (*n*=5).

to be accomplished, at least partly, by an increased delivery of the ampicillin to the sites of infection, i.e. the liver and spleen. In addition, we found with murine peritoneal macrophages infected with *Listeria monocytogenes* that encapsulation of the ampicillin within MLV resulted in an increased availablility of the antibiotic to the intracellular bacteria; liposomal ampicillin killed 99% of the bacteria whereas a similar concentration of free ampicillin plus empty liposomes only inhibited intracellular bacterial growth [29].

Besides application of liposomes as drug carriers in the treatment of intracellular infections, the vesicles have also been used as carriers of amphotericin B in the treatment of mycotic infections such as histoplasmosis [30], cryptococcosis [31] and candidiasis, both in mice with an intact host-defense system and in leukopenic mice [32,33]. In a preliminary clinical study Lopez-Berestein and colleagues found that liposomal amphotericin B was effective in the treatment of *Candida* and *Aspergillus* infections in leukemia patients, who had previously failed to respond to treatment with the non-encapsulated drug [34]. The increase in therapeutic efficacy of amphotericin by encapsulation in liposomes apparently results from a reduction of toxicity of the drug. In a recent study Juliano and coworkers [35] found that, while free amphotericin is extremely toxic to both fungal cells and mammalian cells *in vitro*, the liposomal drug remains toxic to fungal cells but has little effect on mammalian cells. It is well known that amphotericin interacts with ergosterol in fungal cell membranes forming transmembrane channels resulting in extracellular release of ions and metabolites. On the other hand the drug also interacts with cholesterol in mammalian cell membranes, which is probably the basis of its toxicity. Incorporation of the lipophilic amphotericin within liposomes might result in a facilitated transfer of the drug to fungal cells, while transfer to mammalian cells is hampered. This selective transfer of amphotericin from liposomes to fungal cells may form the molecular basis of the reduced toxicity in addition to other factors such as altered kinetics or tissue distribution [36].

Another interesting example of enhancement of antibacterial activity by liposome encapsulation was published by Sunamoto and coworkers [37]. They showed that uptake of IV injected liposomes by circulating monocytes and alveolar macrophages can be increased by coating the vesicles with a palmitoyl derivative of amylopectin. After IV injection the amylopectin-modified liposomes were found to distribute with high preference to the lungs. This observation was elegantly applied in the treatment of experimental lung infection caused by *Legionella pneumophila* in guinea pigs by the systemic administration of a mixture of free and liposome-encapsulated sisomycin. When the infection was treated with free sisomycin alone all animals died within 6 days, while a 100% survival was attained when treated with the mixture of free and liposome-encapsulated antibiotic.

6. LIPOSOMES AS CARRIERS OF IMMUNOMODULATORS

The natural avidity of macrophages for liposomes can also be exploited in the application of the vesicles as carriers of immunomodulators to render these cells cytotoxic to metastatic tumor cells. Macrophages appear to be an important barrier against the proliferation and metastatic spread of tumor cells [38]. Activation of macrophages to tumor cytotoxicity occurs as a result of exposure to a variety of immunomodulating substances such a lymphokines, γ-interferon and muramyl dipeptide (MDP). By a hitherto unknown mechanism, activated macrophages are capable of selectively killing tumor cells, thereby leaving normal cells unharmed. This approach may open new perspectives in the treatment of patients with metastatic cancer which is often seriously hampered by the biological heterogeneity of the tumor cells with respect to growth rate, sensitivity to various cytotoxic drugs, etc.

After *in vivo* administration of free MDP no enhancement of macrophage-mediated cytotoxicity can be achieved since the drug is rapidly excreted via the kidneys [39,40]. Encapsulation of the MDP within liposomes (MLV), however, greatly potentiated the ability of the drug to render mouse peritoneal and alveolar macrophages tumoricidal *in vivo* [41]. Studies by Fidler and coworkers [42], for example, have shown that administration of MDP, encapsulated in liposomes, results in a significant reduction of experimental lung metastases in mice bearing syngeneic B16-melanoma cells. Similar results were published by Thombre and Deodhar [43] on the inhibition of liver metastases from murine colon adenocarcinoma by IV administration of liposome-encapsulated C-reactive protein or lymphokines. This therapeutic effect was thought to be mediated by the activation of hepatic macrophages (Kupffer cells). Since the liver is a major site for metastatic cells originating from, for example, colorectal tumors, activation of Kupffer cells to tumorcytotoxicity would present an interesting approach to the effective treatment of early stages of liver metastases. At that time the tumor burden is relatively low and — taken together with the dominant uptake of IV injected liposomes by the Kupffer cells — this would provide optimal conditions for efficient eradication of liver (micro)metastases.

We have studied the tumoricidal properties of Kupffer cells *in vitro* following incubation of the cells with free or liposome-encapsulated MDP (Table 1). The

Table 1 — Potentiation of tumoricidal activity of rat liver macrophages by muramyl dipeptide (MDP) in liposomes

Macrophage treatment[a]	Liposomal lipid (mM)	MDP (μg/ml)	% of cytotoxicity[b]
Free MDP	—	50	31
	—	25	31
	—	12.5	30
MDP-liposomes	0.375	0.375	54
(1 μg MDP/μmol	0.250	0.250	57
lipid)	0.050	0.050	38

[a] Rat liver macrophages were isolated by pronase perfusion of the liver and purified by centrifugal elutriation. Cells (25×10^4) were incubated with medium (RPMI) containing 10% heat-inactivated fetal calf serum (FCS), free MDP or MDP encapsulated in liposomes (MLV, lipid composition: PC/PS/CHOL, molar ratio 4:1:5). After 4 h [^{3}H]thymidine-labeled B16 melanoma cells were added to each well. After a 48-h co-culture period cytotoxicity was assayed by measuring the release of [^{3}H]label from the melanoma cells into the medium.
[b] Per cent cytotoxicity was calculated according to the formula: $100 \times (A-B)/(C-B)$, in which A = radioactivity in supernatant of tumor cells co-cultured with treated macrophages, B = radioactivity in supernatant of tumor cells co-cultured with control macrophages and C = radioactivity in the total amount of tumor cells added per well.
PC = phosphatidylcholine; PS = phosphatidylserine, CHOL = cholestrol.

results show that Kupffer cells can indeed be activated to a tumorcytotoxic state against B16-melanoma cells after exposure to free, non-encapsulated MDP. The percentage of cytotoxicity induced by relatively high concentrations (up to $50\,\mu g$ MDP/ml) reached a maximum of about 30%. However, as little as $0.05\ \mu g$ MDP/ml, encapsulated within MLV, was required to obtain a comparable extent of cytotoxicity. From these data it can be concluded that a 250- to 1000-fold potentiation of the MDP-induced cytotoxicity is achieved by encapsulating the drug within liposomes. The data shown in Table 1 also demonstrate that exposure of the cells to liposome-encapsulated MDP resulted in a higher maximal degree of cytotoxicity (50–60%) than exposure to free MDP, which resulted in a maximal cytotoxicity of 30%.

Although these preliminary results (see also ref. [44]) are encouraging, successful application of liposome-encapsulated immunomodulators in the treatment of patients with liver metastases may be hampered by unfavourable macrophage:tumor cell ratios in many metastatic tumors. Therefore, therapeutic regimens designed to stimulate macrophage-mediated tumor cytotoxicity almost certainly will have to be used in combination with other treatment modalities such as chemotherapy to reduce the tumor load, while activated macrophages could eradicate surviving tumor cells.

7. LIPOSOMES AS CARRIERS OF ANTINEOPLASTIC DRUGS

As discussed in sections 3 and 4, successful targeting of liposomes, at least to solid tumors located outside the bloodstream, is very unlikely to be achieved. Therefore, selective introduction of antineoplastic drugs into tumor cells *in vivo* by means of liposomes would seem to be an impossible task at the present time. On the other hand, application of liposomes as a drug delivery system for antitumor drugs may be of great benefit in diminishing toxicity of encapsulated compounds by altering the pharmacokinetics and/or tissue distribution. In addition, as pointed out before, liposomes can serve as a sustained- or controlled-release system for cytostatic drugs such as cytosine-arabinoside. The therapeutic effect of this cell-cycle-specific drug is enhanced by liposomal encapsulation probably by maintaining therapeutically favourable drug levels for a prolonged period of time following leakage from the liposomes or, alternatively, from macrophages which have phagocytosed drug-loaded liposomes (see section 4).

A promising example of a liposomal delivery system for antitumor drugs is the use of doxorubicin (DXR) in liposome-encapsulated form. Doxorubicin, an anthracycline antibiotic, has a well-established position in the treatment of a variety of solid neoplasms, lymphomas and leukaemias, Its clinical use, however, is limited by its cardiotoxicity, which sharply rises after a cumulative dose of 550 mg/m^2. Several groups have shown that entrapment of DXR within liposomes markedly reduces its cardiotoxicity without loss of antitumor activity [45–48]. However, the mechanism responsible for the increased therapeutic index is not fully understood. Low uptake of the liposomal DXR by the myocardium in addition to depot formation in macrophages leading to sustained release of the drug into the circulation or directly to target tumor cells might be held responsible for the reduction in (cardio)toxicity and preservation of antitumor activity.

We studied the therapeutic effect of liposome-encapsulated DXR in rats bearing an experimental solid tumor, i.e. an IgM immunocytoma. We used two different liposome preparations: 'fluid' liposomes, containing egg–phosphatidylcholine (PC, $T_c < 0°C$) as the bulk phospholipid and relatively low amounts of cholesterol (CHOL) vs 'solid' liposomes containing distearoyl phosphatidylcholine (DSPC, T_c: +58°C) and relatively high amounts of cholesterol. Both liposome preparations were of the MLV-type and negatively charged by incorporating phosphatidylserine (PS) and dipalmitoyl phosphatidylglycerol (DPPG), respectively. (See for molar ratios legend to Table 2.) For comparison a saline-treated and a 'free' DXR-treated animal group

Table 2 — Antitumor activity of free DXR and DXR-liposomes in solid IgM immunocytoma-bearing LOU/M Wsl rats. Values are tumour size (mm±S.D.)

Treatment group	0	3	Day 7	10	14
Saline	24.1±2.7	34.4±2.5	—[a]	—[a]	—[a]
Free DXR	24.6±2.6	21.7±2.2	14.8±1.4	13.5±2.0	—[a]
PC/PS/CHOL (10/1/4)	25.8±2.8	22.3±2.3	14.6±2.5	13.7±2.3	8.8±4.2
DSPC/DPPG/ CHOL (10/1/10)	24.1±2.7	26.9±3.7[b]	13.7±2.3	8.9±3.7	5.0±0.0

Groups of ten tumor-bearing animals were formed at random. Treatment was started approximately 17 days after tumor cell inoculation when the tumor had reached a diameter of 2 cm or more (= day 0). The dose per injection was 2 mg DXR/kg body weight. Injections were performed IV (tail vein) on 5 consecutive days (day 0–4) followed by one or more injections on day 11. Tumor size was measured with vernier callipers and expressed as mean value of three perpendicular measurements.
[a] Day of death of treated animals.
[b] $p < 0.001$ versus each of the other treatment groups (students' t-test, two-sided).
See text for abbreviations.

were included. From the data shown in Table 2 it is clear that, with the dosage schedule used, both free DXR and DXR entrapped in the two liposome preparations, induced a strong regression of the tumor. However, a marked difference in the expression of the antitumor activity of the two liposome types could be observed. While during the first 3 days after starting therapy the solid DSPC/DPPG/CHOL liposomes did not induce a significant tumor regression, treatment with the fluid PC/PS/CHOL liposomes was already as effective as the free DXR. Apparently, treatment with the solid liposome type causes a delay in antitumor activity as compared to treatment with the fluid liposome type. Different kinetics of drug release from circulating liposomes induced by serum proteins could be excluded as a major contribution to the observed differences in therapeutic activity (not shown).

Therefore, the delayed antitumor effect taken together with the absence of any significant uptake of either liposome type by the tumor tissue itself (results not shown) led us to believe that the mechanism underlying the different therapeutic activities of the two liposome preparations involves different rates of sustained release of DXR from liposome-loaded macrophages. We reasoned that upon uptake of IV injected DXR-liposomes by macrophages, especially in liver and spleen, the kinetics of the intracellular degradation of the vesicles and, consequently, the rate of extracellular release of the drug is dictated by the physical state of the liposomal membranes; 'solid' liposomes, by virtue of the tightly packed acyl chains in the lipid membranes, might be less susceptible to lysosomal enzyme activities than 'fluid' membranes, causing a delay in the release of liposomal DXR.

To provide evidence in favour of this hypothesis we injected either of the two liposome preparations, labeled in the aqueous phase with [^{3}H]inulin and in the lipid phase with cholesteryl-[^{14}C]oleate, intravenously into rats. [^{3}H]inulin was used as a parameter of liposome up-take, since it is metabolically inert and, if administered in free form, it is not taken up by liver and spleen but rapidly excreted via the kidneys. Cholesteryl-[^{14}C]oleate, on the other hand, is susceptible to intracellular esterase activity resulting in the liberation of the labeled oleate from the cholesterol moiety. Consequently, degradation of the liposomes in liver and spleen cells will result in an increase in the ^{3}H/^{14}C ratio, if release of oleate from the cells occurs.

Table 3 shows that both markers were cleared at similar rates from the circulation

Table 3 — *In vivo* retention of integrity of DXR-containing liposomes

Liposome type	Tissue	Ratio ^{3}H/^{14}C		Initial ratio ^{3}H/^{14}C of the liposome preparation
		1 h	4 h	
PC/PS/CHOL	Blood	5.0±0.1	—[a]	5.1±0.1 (*n*=3)
(10/1/4)	Liver	ND	7.9±0.6	
	Spleen	ND	53.3±14.2	
DSPC/DPPG/CHOL	Blood	5.4±0.1	5.7±0.1	5.3±0.1 (*n*=3)
(10/1/10)	Liver	ND	4.8±0.4	
	Spleen	ND	6.9±0.4	

DXR-containing liposomes, labeled with [^{3}H]inulin as a marker of the aqueous phase and cholesteryl-[^{14}C]oleate as a marker of the lipid phase were administered IV to rats (2 mg DXR/kg body weight). The results are expresed as the mean±S.D. of four animals.
[a] Amounts of radioactivity too low for accurate determination.
ND = not determined.
See text for abbreviations.

as the observed ^{3}H/^{14}C ratios equal those of the liposome preparations before injection up to at least an hour, indicating that the vesicles remained intact during their stay in the bloodstream. However, whereas in the case of the 'fluid' liposomes the ^{3}H/^{14}C ratio in liver and spleen increased substantially at 4 h after injection, the ratio did not increase at all in the case of the 'solid' liposomes. These observations were taken to indicate that the 'fluid' PC/PS/CHOL vesicles are much more susceptible to intracellular degradation than the 'solid' DSPC/DPPG/CHOL vesicles. The relatively slow degradation of the solid liposomes correlates well with the delayed antitumor activity displayed by these vesicles. Liposome degradation within macrophages seems to be the rate-limiting step in the expression of antitumor activity. Following intralysosomal degradation of DXR-liposomes the drug is released into the blood, thereby preventing high-peak concentrations which appeared to be very toxic towards cardiac tissue.

The difference in susceptibility to intracellular degradation of the two liposome preparations could also be demonstrated by incubating the vesicles, labeled with cholesteryl-[^{14}C]oleate, with cultured Kupffer cells: the 'fluid' vesicles were degraded considerably faster than the 'solid' liposomes. Similar results were found by incubating the two preparations at pH 4.8 with lysosomal fractions isolated from rat liver homogenates. PC/PS/CHOL liposomes were much more sensitive to lysosomal esterase activity than DSPC/DPPG/CHOL vesicles (results not shown).

In summary, uptake and processing of DXR-liposomes by mononuclear phagocytes of the RES seem to be important determinants of the *in vivo* therapeutic action of the drug. The beneficial effect of liposomal encapsulation (reduction in cardiotoxicity along with preservation of antitumor activity) is thought to be the result of prolonged DXR levels maintained by 'infusion' of DXR (or active metabolites) into the blood from these depot cells. By manipulating the lipid composition of the liposomes rates of intracellular degradation can be influenced, which, in turn, will determine the rate of release of the drug and thereby, conceivably, its therapeutic effect [17,49]. Crucial for such a drug delivery system is of course that DXR is released in a cytotoxic form from the macrophages. Recent observations with peritoneal macrophages revealed that this is a real possibility [50].

8.   CONCLUDING REMARKS

Although liposomes possess a number of favourable properties which would enable them to function as a drug delivery system, it is obvious that there are also severe limitations. As discussed in section 4, the major one is the inability of the vesicles to cross the capillary endothelial cells in most organs except the liver. Another obstacle is the limited potency of many cell types to phagocytose particles like liposomes while, by the same token, fusion with the plasma membrane has proven to be of little if any significance thus far for any cell type.

On the other hand, liposomes seem to be attractive carriers of drugs to macrophages, which is demonstrated by the application of liposomes in the treatment of certain infectious diseases or in the immunotherapy of cancer. Besides that, the use of liposomes appears to be of great benefit in the reduction of the toxicity of certain drugs such as amphotericin or adriamycin. In addition, interesting results have been published on the application of liposomes for the local delivery of drugs, e.g. the intra-articular injection of liposome-associated cortisol palmitate in the treatment of arthritis [51], the intrapulmonary application in the therapy of the respiratory distress syndrome [52] or the intralymphatic administration for the diagnosis or treatment of lymph node metastases [53].

Finally, problems concerning large-scale production of liposomes as a pharmaceutical product, acute and chronic toxicity and immunogenicity of liposome preparations require rigorous attention before clinical application of the vesicles as a drug delivery system can be considered.

ACKNOWLEDGEMENTS

The authors wish to thank Dr P. A. Steerenberg, RIVM, for his cooperation, Joke Regts, Aletta Veninga, Bert Dontje, Jan Wijbenga, August Lokerse and Joke Vink-Van den Berg for skilful technical assistance and Rinske Kuperus for typing the manuscript.

REFERENCES

[1] Gregoriadis, G. (1980). The liposome drug-carrier concept: its development and future. In: Gregoriadis, G. & Allison, A. C. (eds) *Liposomes in Biological Systems*, John Wiley & Sons Ltd, New York.

[2] Juliano, R. L. (1981). Liposomes as a drug delivery system. *Trends in Pharmacol. Sci.* **2** 39–41.

[3] Gregoriadis, G. and Ryman, B. E. (1972). Fate of protein-containing liposomes injected into rats. An approach to the treatment of storage diseases. *Eur. J. Biochem.* **24** 485–491.

[4] Gregoriadis, G., Senior, J. & Trouet, A. (eds) (1983). *Targeting of Drugs*, NATO-ASI series A, vol. 47, Plenum Press, New York/London.

[5] Leserman, L. D. & Barbet, J. (eds) (1982). *Liposome Methodology*, vol. 107, editions INSERM, Paris.

[6] Szoka, F., Olson, F., Heath, T., Vail, W., Mayhew, E. & Papahadjopoulos, D. (1980). Preparation of unilamellar liposomes of intermediate size (0.1–0.2 μm) by a combination of reverse phase evaporation and extrusion through polycarbonate membranes. *Biochim. Biophys. Acta* **601** 559–571

[7] Juliano, R. L. & Layton, D. (1980). Liposomes as a drug delivery system. In: Juliano, R. L. (ed.) *Drug Delivery Systems*, Oxford University Press, pp. 189–236.

[8] Roerdink, F. H., Dijkstra, J., Hartman, G., Bolscher, B. & Schlerphof, G. (1981). The involvement of parenchymal, Kupffer and endothelial liver cells in the hepatic uptake of intravenously injected liposomes. Effects of lanthanum and gadolinium salts. *Biochim. Biophys. Acta* **677** 79–89.

[9] Roerdink, F. H., Dijkstra, J., Spanjer, H. H. & Scherphof, G. L. (1984). *In vivo* and in vitro interaction of liposomes with hepatocytes and Kupffer cells. *Biochem. Soc. Trans.* **12** 335–336.

[10] Roerdink, F. H., Regts, J. Van Leeuwen, B. & Scherphof, G. (1984). Intrahepatic uptake and processing of intravenously injected small unilamellar phospholipid vesicles in rats, *Biochim. Biophys. Acta* **770** 195–202.

[11] Dijkstra, J., Van Galen, W. J. M., Hulstaert, C. E., Kalicharan, D., Roerdink, F. H. & Scherphof, G. L. (1984). Interaction of liposomes with Kupffer cells *in vitro*. *Exp. Cell Res.* **150** 161–176.

[12] Dijkstra, J., Van Galen, M. & Cherphof. G. (1984). Effects of ammoniumch-

loride and chloroquine on endocytic uptake of liposomes by Kupffer cells *in vitro. Biochim. Biophys. Acta* **804** 58–67.

[13] Dijkstra, J., Van Galen, M., Regts, J. & Sherphof, G. (1985). Uptake and processing of liposomal phospholipids by Kupffer cells *in vitro. Eur. J. Biochem.* **148** 391–397.

[14] Poste, G., Bucana, C., Raz, A., Bugelski, P., Kirsh, R. & Fidler, I. J. (1982). Analysis of the fate of systemically administered liposomes and implications for their use in drug delivery. *Cancer Res.* **42** 1412–1422.

[15] Gregoriadis, G. & Senior, J. (1980). The phospholipid component of small unilamellar liposomes controls the rate of clearance of entrapped solutes from the circulation. *FEBS Lett.* **119** 43–46.

[16] Spanjer, H. H. (1985). Targeting of liposomes to liver cells *in vivo*. PhD Thesis, State University Groningen.

[17] Roerdink, F., Regts, J. & Scherphof, G. (1986). Effect of lipid composition on the uptake and intracellular degradation of liposomes by Kupffer cells. In: Kirn, A., Knook, D. L. & Wisse, E. (eds) *Cells of the Hepatic Sinusoid*, vol. 1, Kupffer Cell Foundation, pp. 131–136.

[18] Spanjer, H. H. & Scherphof, G. (1983). Targeting of lactosylceramide-containing liposomes to hepatocytes *in vivo. Biochim. Biophys. Acta* **734** 40–47.

[19] Krupp, L., Chobanian, A. V. & Brecher, P. I. (1976). The *in vivo* transformation of phospholipid vesicles to a particle resembling HDL in the rat. *Biochim. Biophys. Res. Commun.* **72** 1251–1258.

[20] Scherphof, G., Roerdink, F., Waite, M. & Parks, J. (1978). Distintegration of phosphatidylcholine liposomes in plasma as a result of interaction with high-density lipoproteins. *Biochim. Biophys. Acta* **542** 296–307.

[21] Scherphof, G., Morselt, H., Regts, J. & Wilschut, J. (1979). The involvement of the lipid phase transition in the plasma-induced dissolution of multilammelar phosphatidylcholine vesicles. *Biochim. Biophys. Acta* **556** 196–207.

[22] Weinstein, J. N., Leserman, L. D., Henkart, P. A. & Blumenthal, R. (1982). Antibody-mediated targeting of liposomes. In: Gregoriadis, G., Senior, J. & Trouet, A. (eds) *Targeting of Drugs*, Plenum Press, New York, pp. 185–202.

[23] Toonen, P. A. H. M. & Crommelin, D. J. A. (1983). Immunoglobulins as targeting agents for liposome-encapsulated drugs. *Pharmac. Weekblad, Scientific Edition,* 269–280.

[24] Connor, J., Sullivan, S. & Huang, L. (1985). Monoclonal antibody and liposomes. *Pharmac. Ther.* **28** 341–365.

[25] Alving, C. R., Steck, E. A., Chapman Jr., W. L., Waits, V. B., Hendricks, L. D., Swartz Jr., G. M. & Hanson, W. L. (1978). Therapy of Leishmaniasis: superior efficacies of liposome-encapsulated drugs. *Proc. Natl. Acad. Sci. USA* **75** 2959–2963.

[26] Black, C. D. V., Watson, G. J. & Ward, R. J. (1977). The use of pentostam liposomes in the chemotherapy of experimental Leishmaniasis. *Trans. Roy. Soc. Trop. Med. Hyg.* **71** 550–552.

[27] New, R. R. C., Chance, M. L., Thomas, S. C. & Peters, W. (1978). Antileishmanial activity of antimonials entrapped in liposomes. *Nature* **272** 55–56.

[28] Bakker-Woudenberg, I. A. J. M., Lokerse, A. F., Roerdink, F. H., Regts, D.

& Michel, M. F. (1985). Free versus liposome-entrapped ampicillin in treatment of infection due to *Listeria monocytogenes* in normal and athymic (nude) mice. *J. Infect. Dis.* **151** 917–924.

[29] Bakker-Woudenberg, I. A. J. M., Lokerse, A. F., Vink-Van den Berg, J. C., Roerdink, F. H. & Michel, M. F. (1986). Effect of liposome-entrapped ampicillin on the survival of *Listeria monocytogenes* in murine peritoneal macrophages. *Antimicrob. Agents Chemother.* (in press).

[30] Taylor, R. L., Williams, D. M., Craven, P. C., Graybill, J. R., Drutz, D. J. & Magee, W. E. (1982). Amphotericin B in liposomes: a novel therapy for histoplasmosis. *Am. Rev. Respir, Dis.* **125** 610–611.

[31] Graybill, J. R., Craven, P. C., Taylor, R. L., Williams, D. M. & Magee, W. E. (1982). Treatment of murine cryptococcosis with liposome-associated amphotericin B. *J. Infect. Dis.* **145** 748–752.

[32] Lopez-Berestein, G., Mehta, R., Hopfer, R. L., Mills, K., Kasi, L., Mehta, K., Fainstein, V., Luna, M., Hersh, E. M. & Juliano, R. (1983). Treatment and prophylaxis of disseminated infection due to *Candida albicans* in mice with liposome-encapsulated amphotericin B. *J. Infect. Dis.* **147** 939–945.

[33] Lopez-Berestein, G., Hopfer, R. L., Mehta, R., Mehta, K., Hersh, E. M. & Juliano, R. L. (1984). Liposome-encapsulated amphotericin B for treatment of disseminated Candidiasis in neutropenic mice. *J. Infect. Dis.* **150** 278–283.

[34] Lopez-Berestein, G., Fainstein, V., Hopfer, R. L., Mehta, K., Sullivan, M. P., Keating, M., Rosenblum,. M. G., Mehta, R., Luna, M., Hersh, E. M., Reuben, J., Juliano, R. L. & Bodey, G. P. (1985). Liposomal amphotericin B for the treatment of systemic fungal infections in patients with cancer: a preliminary study. *J. Infect. Dis.* **151** 704–710.

[35] Mehta, R., Lopez-Berestein, G., Hopfer, R. L., Mills, K. & Juliano, R. L. (1984). Liposomal amphotericin B is toxic to fungal cells but not to mammalian cells. *Biochim. Biophys. Acta* **770** 230–234.

[36] Juliano, R. L. & Lopez-Berestein, G. (1985). New lives for old drugs: liposomal drug delivery systems reduce the toxicity but not the potency of certain chemotherapeutic agents. *Pharmac. Internat.* **6** 164–167.

[37] Sunamoto, J., Goto, M., Iida, T., Hara, K., Saito, A. & Tomonaga, A. (1984). Unexpected tissue distribution of liposomes coated with amylopectin derivatives and successful use in the treatment of experimental Legionnaires' disease. In: Gregoriadis, G., Poste, G., Senior, J. & Trouet, A. (eds) *Receptor-mediated Targeting of Drugs*, Plenum Press, New York, pp. 359–371.

[38] Fidler, I. J. (1985). Macrophages and metastases. A biological approach to cancer therapy: presidential address. *Cancer Res.* **45** 4714–4726.

[39] Parant, M., Parant, F., Chedid, L., Yapo, A., Petit, J. F. & Lederer, E. (1979). Fate of synthetic immunoadjuvant, muramyl dipeptide (^{14}C-labeled) in the mouse, *Int. J. Immunopharmacol.* **1** 35–47.

[40] Fogler, W. E., Wade, R., Brundish, D. E. & Fidler, I. J. (1985). Distribution and fate of free and liposome-encapsulated ^{3}H nor-muramyl dipeptide and ^{3}H muramyl tripeptide phosphatidyl ethanolamine in mice. *J. Immunol.* **135** 1372–1377.

[41] Poste, G., Bucana, C. & Fidler, I. J. (1982). Stimulation of host response

against metastatic tumours by liposome-encapsulated immunomodulators. In: Gregoriadis, G., Senior, J. & Trouet, A. (eds) *Targeting of Drugs*, Plenum Press, New York, pp. 261–284.

[42] Fidler, I. J., Sone, S., Fogler, W. E. & Barnes, Z. L. (1984). Eradication of spontaneous metastases and activation of alveolar macrophages by intravenous injection of liposomes containing muramyl dipeptide. *Proc. Natl. Acad. Sci. USA* **78** 1680–1684.

[43] Thombre, P. S. & Deodhar, S. D. (1984). Inhibition of liver metastases in murine colon adenocarcinoma by liposomes containing human C-reactive protein or crude lymphokines. *Cancer Immunol. Immonother.* **16** 145–150.

[44] Daemen, T., Veninga, A., Roerdink, F. H. & Scherphof, G. L. (1986). *In vitro* activation of rat liver macrophages to tumoricidal activity by free or liposome-encapsulated muramyl dipeptide. *Cancer Res.* (in press).

[45] Forssen, E. A. & Tokes, Z. A. (1983). Improved therapeutic benefits of doxorubicin by entrapment in anionic liposomes. *Cancer Res.* **43** 546–550.

[46] Gabizon, A., Dagan, A., Goren, D., Barenholz, Y. & Fuks, Z. (1982). Liposomes as *in vivo* carriers of adriamycin: reduced cardiac uptake and preserved antitumor activity in mice. *Cancer Res.* **42** 4734–4739.

[47] Rahman, A., White, G., More, N. & Schein, P. S. (1985). Pharmacological, toxicological, and therapeutic evaluation in mice of doxorubicin entrapped in cardiolipin liposome. *Cancer Res.* **45** 796–803.

[48] Van Hoesel, Q. G. C. M., Steerenberg, P. A., Crommelin, D. J. A., Van Dijk, A., Van Oort, W., Klein, S., Douze, J. M. C., De Wildt, D. J. & Hillen, F. C. (1984). Reduced cardiotoxicity and nephrotoxicity with preservation of antitumor activity of doxorubicin entrapped in stable liposomes in the LOU/M Wsl rat. *Cancer Res.* **44** 3698–3705.

[49] Roerdink, F. H., Daemen, T., Regts, D., Veninga, A., De Boer, O. & Scherphof, G. L. (1986). Delivery of macrophage activating factors by means of liposomes. In: Illum, L., Davis, S. S. & Tomlinson, E. (eds) *Advanced Drug Delivery System for Peptides and Proteins*, Plenum Press, London/New York (in press).

[50] Storm, G., Steerenberg, P. A., Emmen, F., Van Borssum-Waalkes, M. & Crommelin, D. J. A. Release of doxorubicin from peritoneal macrophages exposed *in vivo* to doxorubicin-containing liposomes. Submitted for publication.

[51] De Silva, M., Hazleman, B. L., Page Thomas, D. P. & Wraight, P. (1979). Liposomes in arthritis: a new approach. *Lancet* **1** 1320–1322.

[52] Fujiwara, T., Maeta, H., Chida, S., Morita, T., Watabe, Y. & Abe, T. (1980). Artificial surfactant therapy in hyaline-membrane disease. *Lancet* **1** 55–59.

[53] Kaledin, V. I., Matienko, N. A., Nikolin, V. P., Gruntenko, Y. V. & Budker, V. G. (1981). Intralymphatic administration of liposome-encapsulated drugs to mice: possibility for suppression of the growth of tumor metastases in the lymph nodes. *J. Natl. Cancer Inst.* **66** 881–887.

4

Monoclonal antibodies as carriers for drug delivery

G. F. Rowland, Biotechnology Division, S.A. Druggists Ltd, Department of Biochemistry, University of Stellenbosch, Stellenbosch, Republic of South Africa

1. INTRODUCTION

In any discussion of the benefits that may be derived from methods for drug delivery, the principle of directing a drug to a specific target site is of considerable importance. Drug side-effects and toxicity are generally associated with drug action at non-target sites and this limits the amount of a drug that can be administered, thereby reducing its potential effectiveness. For this reason, any substance with inherent target-site specificity offers attractive possibilities as a drug delivery agent. Antibodies are excellent example of substances with inherent specificity and are paramount in the wide range of specificities exhibited. It is thus not surprising that they have been considered as candidates for drug delivery since their discovery at the beginning of the century [1].

2. ANTIBODIES AS CARRIERS

A major difficulty in the use of antibodies for drug delivery has been their heterogeneity. An antiserum derived from a rabbit immunized with a well-defined simple chemical antigen will nevertheless contain a complex mixture of immunoglobulin molecules recognizing the antigen. These antibodies will vary in their amino acid sequence and as a result will be heterogeneous with respect to their size, charge antigen specificity and affinity. They will also vary in their ability to bind drug molecules that one may wish to couple for delivery. Heterogeneity will also be displayed if such antibodies are administered *in vivo,* either alone or with agents coupled to them. Some of the antibody molecules will be rapidly degraded and excreted whereas others will have a longer biological half-life. Without doubt, many of the difficulties associated with the early attempts to use polyclonal antibodies for drug targeting were the result of this heterogeneity, a difficulty further compounded by the lack of reproducibility of one polyclonal antiserum by another (see for example [2, 3]).

Despite these problems the exquisite specificity that can be achieved by antibodies led research workers to investigate their use for drug targeting even before the modern techniques became available for making virtually unlimited amounts of homogeneous monoclonal antibodies of defined specificity. Moreover, certain features of polyclonal antibodies may still offer advantages for drug delivery. Thus, the polyclonality can result in recognition of more than one specific location at a given target site thereby providing a greater drug delivery capacity, although this could also be achieved by mixtures of monoclonal of predefined specificity.

Another possible advantage for polyclonal antibodies is the wide range of species that can be used to produce them. Production of monoclonal antibodies is at present confined to mice, rats and to a very limited extent humans as the species. The *in vivo* performance of antibodies as target site delivery agents varies according to the species of origin and this may be an overriding feature in determining whether or not the system functions successfully [4].

3.   ANTICANCER DRUG DELIVERY

Most research workers in the field of antibody drug targeting have focussed their attention on the delivery of anticancer drugs. It is in this field of chemotherapy that the greatest need arises for target site specificity. Anticancer drugs tend to be highly toxic and their effectiveness limited by a very small therapeutic ratio. A major aim of work in anticancer drug delivery with antibodies should therefore be to increase the therapeutic ratio with known drugs in clinical use. This simple but strict criterion for efficacy of a drug delivery system has rarely been adopted. One problem is that in order to demonstrate it, one should be dealing with real clinical situations and not with experimental animal models. The dilemma then arises that clinical trials may not be justified until there is sufficient evidence that the materials being tested are safe and effective in animals. Since antibodies used in drug targeting recognize targets that are generally species specific, preclinical efficiency data must be obtained with model preparations and not with the actual materials that will be used in man, unlike preclinical tests with conventional drugs.

Early work using experimental animal systems and polyclonal antibodies involved the use of those few anticancer drugs in clinical use which appeared to lend themselves to covalent chemical coupling to antibodies by simple means. It is interesting to note that nearly 30 years after Mathé [5] described the conjugation of methotrexate to anti-mouse leukaemic antibodies for drug targeting, the first human clinical trials of monoclonal antibody drug conjugates are taking place using methotrexate as the drug [6]. It would be tempting to think that these trials have arisen by direct development of those early experiments but this is far from the reality. Following the experiments of Mathé, almost no work was carried out in this field for 14 years and when it began again it involved entirely different drugs and antibodies [7]. The alkylating agent chlorambucil, now rarely used in chemotherapeutic regimens, was coupled to polyclonal goat or rabbit antitumour antibodies. These were produced by immunization with tumour cells and absorbing the resultant antiserum with normal cells until only residual antitumour activity remained. This technique was the only one available in days before monoclonal antibodies were 'invented' and was the method used in many studies by the research group at the Research Laboratories of G. D. Searle & Co. in High Wycombe. Using a model system involving rabbit antibodies against a mouse lymphoma, drug targeting was investigated using chlorambucil, methotrexate, melphalan, daunomycin and Adria-mycin [8]. Various methods of coupling were employed and in order to try and increase the amount of drug delivered by each antibody molecule, the idea of using a polymeric carrier of the drugs was devised [9, 10]. A drug–carrier complex was first prepared and subsequently coupled to the antibody by analogy with railway carriages being loaded with goods and coupled to a locomotive for transport.

Similar studies were in progress during the same period in the laboratories of the Weizmann Institute in Israel, both groups independently inventing the polymeric carrier or bridge principle [11]. In the Weizmann studies, initial work was focussed on daunomycin and Adriamycin [12]. Subsequently, this group has coupled metho-trexate, cytosine arabinoside and platinum to both polyclonal and monoclonal antibodies against both animal and human tumour targets [13].

4.   MONOCLONAL ANTIBODIES FOR ANTICANCER DRUG TARGETING

With the development of hybridoma technology to obtain monoclonal antibodies [14], the entire field of immunoconjugate targeting has expanded considerably. Many research groups in academic hospital and industrial laboratories have entered the field of making monoclonals aimed at detecting or treating human cancer. Antigens associated with haematological malignancies and others found in solid tumours have been identified by monoclonals generated using cells or crude tumour suspensions and screened subsequently for tumour specificity by examining the reactivity of the antibodies with tumour and non-tumour cells [15]. The choice of normal cells and the method of screening are important if the ultimate aim is to use the antibodies for therapeutic immunotargeting. It is not sufficient to examine a restricted range of normal cells by a single method such as immunofluorescence binding. Minor components of normal cells may express the antigen seen by the monoclonal but these may be important cells whose destruction can have grave consequences. It is also important that *in vitro* screening methods can indicate the quantity of antigen per tumour cell and relate this to the normal cells. By this technique it was shown that the melanoma antigen p97 as detected by monoclonal antibody was present on melanoma cells at levels orders of magnitude higher than on a very extensive range of normal cells [16]. This gave the confidence needed to use the antibodies *in vivo* in melanoma patients coupled to radioactive iodine, first at low doses for imaging [17] and subsequently at doses that could be therapeutic [18].

The production of useful monoclonals for anticancer targeting has been subject to different approaches. The method most widely adopted is that used by Brown *et al.* [19] in which the appropriate type of malignant cell is used as the immunogen. After screening and selection for tumour cell selectivity, the work leads to the isolation and characterization of the antigen recognized. The method of screening will dictate the type of antigen and hence antibody that is found. Thus reactivity with intact cells as determined by immunofluorescence or immunocytochemistry at the cell membrane will help to ensure that the antigen is expressed on cell surfaces and so be available as a target to circulating immunoconjugates. Test systems often rely heavily on isolated cells from tissue culture but this may be a poor indication of the expression of antigen in solid tumours, especially where there is antigenic heterogeneity [20]. It is therefore very important to screen with sections (frozen to preserve antigenic structure) of tumour and normal tissue [21].

Occasionally monoclonals produce surprising reactivities that can be beneficial. Thus the antibody designated 791T/36 was produced after immunizing with human osteogenic sarcoma cells but on screening it was found to react also with carcinoma of the colon and some other carcinoma cells [22]. The reactivity in colorectal carcinoma is however not at the cell surface but associated with a 72 000 dalton glycoprotein expressed in tumour stroma [23]. Such a pattern of antigen expression may not be ideal for all types of targeting but if it allows quantities of immunoconjugate to be trapped within a solid tumour mass then possibilities exist for the drug to be released locally albeit outside the target cell.

This target situation may also apply to an antigen such as carcino-embryonic antigen (CEA). The production of anti-CEA monoclonals exemplifies an alternative approach to that using crude cellular immunogens. Carcino-embryonic antigen belongs to a family of glycoproteins identified as being associated mainly with gastrointestinal malignancies [24]. Techniques for isolation and purification of CEA have been available for some time and this has enabled monoclonals to be produced using purified immunogen. Screening is now simpler, being based on reactivity with the purified antigen as the main criterion. However, this has proved to be a trap for the unwary. Reactivity with a 'pure' antigen such as CEA does itself not eliminate unwanted cross-reactivities *in vivo*. Preparations of CEA contain CEA-like normal glycoproteins and monoclonals may react with shared epitopes. Failure to screen a promising monoclonal with an extensive range of normal tissues can result in a dangerous cross-reactivity with normal human granulocytes which will be damaged if an immunoconjugate is administered. The systemic clinical toxicity described by Dillman *et al.* [25] using a radio-labelled monoclonal anti-CEA for imaging is most probably due to this unwanted reactivity.

Anti-CEA monoclonals that do not bind granulocytes have however been obtained. One of the most promising in terms of specific tumor reactivity is the antibody designated 11.285.14, produced by collaboration between the research groups originally located at the Surgical Immunology Unit, Birmingham and the Lilly Research Centre, Windlesham. This antibody has been extensively tested by a number of laboratores using ELISA techniques [26], immunocytochemistry [20, 21, 27] and *in vivo* radioimmunolocaliztion in patients with gastrointestinal malignancies [28]. It is this antibody that has been used as a carrier for the vinca alkaloid vindesine in the experimental treatment of human tumour cell lines and xenografts as described below.

5.   THE COUPLING OF DRUGS TO MONOCLONAL ANTIBODIES

In order to achieve delivery of a drug to its target site by means of antibody, the coupling procedure should fulfil certain generally agreed criteria. These include the need for both the drug and the antibody to retain their respective activities and for the conjugate or complex to remain stable in transit to the target site. Thus although a wide range of chemical coupling methods exists for attaching small molecules to macromolecules, many of these will be unsuitable for drug–antibody targeting by being too harsh or by producing linkages that are unstable *in vivo*.

The earliest coupling method used for drug–antibody conjugation was diazotization [5], a technique which favours coupling to tyrosine residues of proteins. The general belief that tyrosines are commonly involved in the antigen-combining site of antibodies and are therefore unsuitable as sites for extensive drug coupling has produced a tendency to avoid this type of reaction in subsequent studies. It should be noted, however, that radioactive iodine labelling of antibodies is performed by hundreds of laboratories without significant loss of antigen-binding capacity, despite the fact that it is usually the tyrosine residues that are derivatized.

Lysine residues are generally present in abundance in immunoglobulins and the epsilon amino side chain is commonly the preferred site for drug conjugation. This has largely dictated the type of drug that is attached. The formation of a carboxyamide link between drug and antibody can be achieved by a variety of methods in which a carboxylic group on the drug is activated to allow attack of the lysine amino group. If the drug contains a carboxylic group which is not important for its drug action then conjugation can be achieved. Chlorambucil, used by Ghose *et al.* [7], fulfils this criterion but it appears likely that in this early study an ionic complex not a covalent link was obtained [2].

The amino sugars of Adriamycin and daunomycin are also suitable groups for coupling to lysine amino groups. The early studies by the Weizmann Institute team showed that periodate oxidation was the most successful of a variety of coupling methods. More recently several other methods of coupling daunomycin have been investigated and it was again found that coupling through the amino sugar, this time using a *cis*-aconityl linkage, gave the most effective conjugate [29].

A difficulty in drawing general conclusions about drug-to-antibody coupling methods when using monoconals is that one monoclonal may behave quite differently from another. Studies using an active azide derivative of a vinca alkaloid to produce vindesine–monoclonal antibody conjugates illustrate this point [30]. Four monoclonals recognizing different human tumour-associated antigens were conjugated. The highest molar drug-to-antibody conjugation ratio obtained varied from 3:1 to 10:1 depending on the antibody used. In addition, the percentage of antibody activity retained was as high as 98% for one antibody coupled at 6:1, whereas another retained only 2% activity at a conjugation ratio of 4:1. These results were reproducible and probably reflect differences in the ternary structure of the immunoglobulin. The antibody which retained only 2% activity probably contains exposed lysine residues at or near the antigen-combining site, making it unsuitable for this type of conjugation procedure.

One of the antibodies in the study described above was the anti-CEA monoclonal 11.285.14. Using the azide method, no more than 3:1 was obtained without loss of material but at this ratio 96% of the activity was retained. It was interesting to discover that by using an alternative method of coupling in which an active ester of the alkaloid was formed, preparations with a conjugation ratio of 10:1 and 80% activity were regularly achieved [31]. It is likely that the same lysine residues are coupled by the two methods but in this case the difference in reaction product is due to the active site on the drug and activation method.

It has become clear that in using highly homogeneous monoclonal preparations, each antibody must be individually evaluated for any particular type of drug coupling procedure requiring chemical manipulation. Similar conclusions have been reached by other workers, for example in attempting to couple cytosine arabinoside to a monoclonal recognizing a human T cell [13].

6. BIOLOGICAL EFFECTS OF DRUG–ANTIBODY CONJUGATES

Most research workers in the field of immunoconjugate targeting have used *in vitro* test systems to evaluate the potential of their preparations. The advantages are obvious; many variables can be tested using small quantities of conjugate over wide ranges. Results can be obtained in a few days and many different target cells can be tested. Unfortunately, the *in vitro* data do not always give a true picture of what may happen *in vivo*. Thus two similar immunoconjugates based on the same drug coupled to two different monoclonals with identical specificity and affinity may well produce identical *in vitro* cytotoxicity results. They could however behave very differently *in vivo* with one conjugate being more rapidly cleared. Rapid clearance of antibody is one factor that can reduce drug accumulation at the target site [4].

Calculations regarding potential effectiveness when based on *in vitro* cytotoxicity may also be misleading when comparing free drug and conjugate. Many drug–antibody conjugates, although highly specific, are less potent than free drug when tested on cells *in vitro*. When tested *in vivo,* this loss of potency can be fully compensated for by a much longer target site residence time. Clear examples of this have come from the studies using the vinca alkaloids coupled to monoclonals recognizing human tumour-associated antigens. The vincas were originally chosen for coupling because of their very high molar activity. It appeared likely that if drug potency could be fully retained in immunoconjugates, then effective doses could be delivered even though the site density on the target cell was not high. When a vindesine–monoclonal conjugate was compared with free vindesine over 24 h of culture with the osteogenic sarcoma target cell 791T, it appeared that the free drug was 2000 times more potent than conjugate [32]. However, if exposure of the cells to the preparations was limited to 15 min, followed by longer culture in drug media, sensitivity of cells to free or conjugated drug was similar. More recently an extensive study of vindesine conjugated to monoclonal anti-CEA was carried out in which nine different human cell lines were examined for target cytotoxicity *in vitro* [33]. In these studies, 24-h exposure was used and free vindesine was again found to be considerably more potent than conjugate. Specificity was however obtained. Conjugates did not affect cells lacking the target antigen, CEA, whereas free vindesine did not discriminate between them.

Since a major objective of drug delivery using antibodies is *in vivo* therapy, it is important to test preparations *in vivo* even if the *in vitro* potency of conjugates appears poor in comparison with free drug. An extensive series of studies using vindesine conjugated to the anti-CEA-monoclonal 11.285.14 has been carried out. In an early experiment using a human CEA-expressing tumour xenograft (MAWI) in athymic mice, marked suppression of tumour growth could be obtained with repeated injections of VDS-11.285.14 at 5 mg/kg in terms of vindesine content [34,35]. Subsequently a number of experiments were carried out over a range of dose levels and comparisons made between free and conjugated drug [36]. The results are revealing from several aspects. Firstly it is clear that the potency *in vivo* of the free and conjugated drug is not very different. An inhibition of tumour growth of 50% was obtained by free vindesine at 1.5 mg/kg and by vindesine–monoclonal at 2.5 mg/kg. Secondly, the toxicity of the conjugate was considerably less than that of free drug. Thus at dose levels of 3 mg/kg free vindesine, toxicity resulted in death of 30% of recipient mice whereas repeated dose of conjugate containing vindesine at 15 mg/kg caused no appreciable toxicity. Thirdly, despite being able to administer higher doses of drug in a conjugated form, tumour suppression reached a maximum of about 85% which was maintained over a range of dose levels. In other words, improving the therapeutic index does not guarantee a cure.

Experiments in the use of vindesine conjugated to 11.285.14 have recently been extended to a wider range of human tumour xenografts [37]. These experiments have been aimed at questions of target antigen density. Are the tumour-suppressive effects observed related to target site antigens? The results show that growth of a human tumour lacking CEA (Colo 320 DM) is not suppressed with vindesine–anti-CEA, whereas tumour LS174T, expressing high levels of antigen, is suppressed.

7.   EVIDENCE FOR SITE-SPECIFIC DRUG DELIVERY BY DRUG–ANTIBODY CONJUGATES

The selectivity of *in vivo* action of vindesine anti-CEA on cells expressing the target antigen is thus demonstrated in two ways. Firstly by a reduced systemic toxicity giving rise to an improved therapeutic index, and secondly by a lack of effect on a tumour not expressing CEA. These results clearly support the view that target site-specific drug delivery has been achieved. However, direct evidence for this was until recently not available. To overcome this, a series of experiments was carried out in which the *in vitro* distribution of radioactively labelled drug was determined in tumour-bearing mice using either free vindesine, vindesine conjugated to monoclonal anti-CEA or to an irrelevant monoclonal [36]. The results confirmed that drug delivery was target site selective, if not completely specific, when using the anti-CEA antibody. When tumour or tissue to plasma ratios of labelled drug were examined, it was found that up to ten times as much drug accumulated in the tumour as in most normal tissues when delivered in the form of specific antibody conjugate. By contrast no selective tumour uptake was observed with either free drug or conjugate to an irrelevant antibody.

Several aspects of the results obtained using labelled drug are of considerable importance. Firstly, the concentration of drug accumulated at the target site was found to remain high for several days. This is probably a reflection of the long biological half-life of the antibody. Thus free drug was rapidly cleared, only 0.01% of the injected dose remaining per ml of plasma by 3 days. Vindesine–anti-CEA showed levels above 10% at this time and 4% after day 9. Secondly, the high tumour selectivity for conjugated drug was observed over a wide range of injected dose levels. Whereas most previous studies, aimed at demonstrating tumour site selectivity, utilized microgram amounts of labelled antibody per injection into a mouse, in the vindesine–anti-CEA study, selective uptake could be demonstrated at dose levels of 2.0 mg/kg in terms of drug, which is 55 mg/kg in terms of antibody or 1.375

mg per 25 g mouse. From such experiments it was possible to calculate the amount of drug delivered to the tumour in a conjugated form compared with that in a free form. Six days after injection of conjugate at a dose of 2 mg/kg in terms of vindesine, approximately 9 μg of drug was present per gram of tumour. By contrast free vindesine was present at a concentration of only 0.009 μg/g by day 3, a factor of 1000 less. It appears likely that the greatly increased amount of drug delivered to tumour as an antibody conjugate will compensate for apparent loss of potency due to conjugation. Perhaps this is why the *in vivo* effective dose levels of free and conjugated drug are much closer than those obtained *in vitro*.

8.   TOXICITY STUDIES WITH DRUG–ANTIBODY CONJUGATES

Although the dose of conjugated vindesine that can be administered is considerably higher than that of free drug in the various studies using human tumour xenografts, it is important to determine the acute toxicity from which an LD_{50} dose can be calculated. Single injections of free or conjugated vindesine into Balb/c strain mice showed that the LD_{50} value for conjugated drug was more than 15 times higher than for free drug [35]. Moreover the type of toxicity normally associated with many anticancer drugs, namely bone marrow depression, damage to cells of the gastrointestinal mucosa or neutrotoxicity was completely absent from mice treated with very high doses of conjugated vindesine. Mice receiving a single dose of 90 mg/kg vindesine conjugated to antibody all survived, although a transient weight loss was observed [35].

It is likely that the limiting toxicity of most drug–antibody conjugates would be in tissues of the reticuloendothelial system. The experiments performed using radiolabelled vindesine–antibody conjugates show that at higher dose levels the relative accumulation of drug increases in the liver and spleen [36].

9.   CLINICAL STUDIES

Although polyclonal and monoclonal antibodies have been used for radioimmunoimaging in increasing numbers in recent years, clinical studies with drug–antibody conjugates have been considered with much greater caution. One possible reason is that radiolabelling an antibody is a relatively commonplace procedure that can be carried out by a hospital laboratory. Drug conjugation is by no means a routine procedure and in the case of drugs under patent will involve collaboration with or approval by a pharmaceutical company partner. Responsibility for safety is thus shared by both clinician and industry, the latter being under particular pressure to ensure that no untoward side-effects can be ascribed to the drug. Despite such pressures, clinical studies have been performed and others are in the planning phase. An early study with conjugated vindesine was carried out by Ford *et al.* [38] using a polyclonal sheep anti-CEA preparation that had been shown previously to localize in the tumours of patients with gastrointestinal malignancies [39]. This study demonstrated several valuable points. Firstly it showed that radiolocalization of the antibody was still possible despite the presence of conjugated drug. If this result is taken together with the labelled drug localization studies in nude mice described above, it appears likely that antibody (polyclonal or monoclonal) capable of imaging a patient's tumour will also deliver a drug such as vindesine to the target site. It is also important to note that in one patient with very high circulating levels of CEA, biopsy of tumour 3 days after injection of iodine-labelled antibody conjugate showed nearly five times the radioactivity in the tumour than in surrounding normal tissue. Thus presence of circulating CEA does not prevent localization of conjugate.

The second important feature of this study is that by careful use of escalating dose levels in different patients it was possible to show that a vindesine–antibody conjugate produced no obvious toxicity or hypersensitivity when given as a single dose of up to 40 mg antibody containing 1.8 mg drug. Although this dose was somewhat less than that given clinically as free drug, it shows that at least the antibody conjugate approach is not more hazardous to man than free drug therapy. Results of this nature taken together with animal toxicity studies of drug–monoclonal conjugates have paved the way for the phase I and phase II clinical studies being planned.

Studies with the monoclonal antibody designated 791T/36 have advanced to the stage that phase I clinical trials have recently been carried out on ten colorectal cancer patients using a methotrexate conjugate [6]. As with the polyclonal antibody vindesine study of Ford *et al*. [38], the object was to check that drug conjugation of an antibody did not destroy its ability to localize at a tumour site. The results were very similar. The biodistribution of labelled conjugate as determined by scintigraphy was the same as for free antibody and there was an increase of almost four-fold in the uptake of conjugate by tumour compared with normal colon.

In this study it was also possible to measure the biological half-life of the conjugate. Clearance was biphasic with a half-life of 22 h. This is similar to the clearance rate described by Armitage *et al*. [40] for the same unconjugated monoclonal antibody. An initial rapid clearance was followed by a slower second phase during which the percentage of labelled antibody in the blood fell from 28% on day 1 to 9% on day 5. This second phase probably corresponds to clearance and excretion of the antibody with a half-life of about 2 days.

In the study using a methotrexate–monoclonal conjugate [6], dose levels were very low, only trace amounts being administered in order to determine localization and clearance. Escalation of dose to ensure safety may be necessary before tests of efficiency can be carried out.

10. CONCLUSIONS AND FUTURE DIRECTIONS

It is clear that work on the use of monoclonal antibodies for drug targeting is progressing steadily towards clinical utility. The applications at present envisaged are mostly in cancer chemotherapy where the greatest need arises for site-specific drug delivery. It may indeed be premature to speculate on other applications until cancer therapy with drug antibody conjugates is clearly shown to work in the clinic. The elimination of specific populations of immunoreactive cells in patients undergoing rejection of tissue transplants or in certain severe autoimmune disease states may be the next category of applications. Beyond that, applications in the fields of infectious disease and nervous system disease become much more speculative and of less obvious benefit when compared with conventional therapy.

Future work is less likely to be in the direction of new applications than in improvments of the present situation. Monoclonal antibodies with greater selectivity could help, but although in the cancer field this may be achieved through identification of oncogene products, it should be remembered that target antigen density and location may be less favourable for drug targeting as specificity increases. Thus an oncogene product present inside a cancer cell at low levels may be a highly specific marker of cancer in that organism but quite useless as a target for delivery of drug–antibody conjugates.

Improvements in the method of coupling of drugs to antibody could be of great value. If in the case of vindesine, a method was achieved which gave a stable conjugate with no loss of potency as determined *in vitro* and yet allowed accumulation of drug to proceed at the levels observed with the existing preparations, it is possible that a very effective product could be obtained.

Modifications that can increase the tumour residence time of a drug–antibody conjugate would probably make a major impact on its effectiveness. Evidence for this comes from studies in which antibodies have been used to deliver radioactive isotopes for cancer therapy [4]. It was found that the tumour residence time of labelled antibodies is directly related to the biological half-life and that this varies according to the species in which the antibody is raised. Thus rabbit, pig and monkey antibodies labelled with ^{131}I had tumour-effective half-lives of 3–4 days and were associated with remissions in the treatment of human cancers able to bind antiferritin antibodies. Other species, including mouse, from which monoclonals are derived, had shorter half-lives and did not induce remissions. It is possible that mouse monoclonal antibodies conjugated to drugs may also fail to produce the desired biological effect in man unless they can be induced to remain longer at the target site.

One avenue of approach to overcome this possible limitation is the use of human monoclonal antibodies. To date, the production of human monoclonals of predefined human target site specificity by hybridoma technology has met with very limited success. As may be anticipated the immunogenicity of human target structures is very different in man than in other species and although *in vitro* immunization techniques can work, they have so far failed to produce useful antitumour human monoclonals.

It is more likely that modern techniques of molecular gene cloning will be used to produce the required structures. Experiments have been described which demonstrate the feasibility of using recombinant DNA technology to produce chimaeric antibody molecules in which the antigen-combining site is derived from a mouse myeloma and the constant region of the molecule from human immunoglobulin. Morrison *et al.* [41] prepared IgG chimaeras in this way and Boulianne *et al.* [42] described the preparation of chimaeric IgM. The *in vivo* biological properties of such chimaeras are not easy to predict but since the *in vivo* fate of immunoglobulin molecules is largely regulated by that part of the molecule encoded for by constant-region genes, it is quite possible that they would behave more like human than mouse antibodies.

As such techniques become routine it is also likely that they will include steps that encompass the drug moiety that one wishes to deliver. This may be in the form of specific receptor sites on the molecule for drug coupling, or the drug itself if it can be biologically synthesized by such techniques. An example being actively pursued by some biotechnology companies is the total synthesis of immunotoxin for cancer therapy. The immunotoxin consisting of antibody and the active polypeptide chains of plant toxins such as ricin can be defined in terms of total amino acid sequences and hence prepared by recombinant DNA technology. This provides a chimaeric protein molecule with dual biological functions. An example of such chimaeric molecules was described by Neuberger *et al.* [43] in which the constant-region portion of a mouse myeloma was replaced by a polypeptide sequence with enzyme activity.

In conclusion it is clear that the specificity conferred by antibody molecules is now being actively exploited for novel methods of therapy. Without doubt, advances in cellular and molecular biology will also be applied to this area in order to produce useful site-specific drug delivery systems.

REFERENCES

[1] Ehrlich, P. (1900). A general review of the recent work in immunity. In: *Collected Papers of Paul Ehrlich Vol. 2: Immunology and Cancer Research* (1956), Pergamon Press, London, p. 442.

[2] O'Neill, G. J. (1979). The use of antibodies as drug carriers. In: Gregoriadis, G. (ed.) *Drug Carriers in Biology and Medicine,* Academic Press, London, pp. 23–41.

[3] Rowland, G. F. (1983). The use of antibodies and polymer conjugates in drug targeting and synergy, In: Golberg, E. (ed.) *Targeted Drugs,* John Wiley, New York, pp. 57–72.

[4] Order, S. E. (1985). Analysis, results and future prospective of the therapeutic use of radiolabelled antibody in cancer therapy. In: Baldwin, R. W. & Byers, V. S. (eds) *Monoclonal Antibodies for Cancer Detection and Therapy,* Academic Press, London, pp. 304–306.

[5] Mathé, G., Loc, T. B. & Bernard, J. (1958). Effet sur la leucemie L1201 de la souris d'une combinaison par diazotation d'A-methopterine et de gamma-globulines de hamsters porteur de cette leucemie par heterogreffe. *Comptes Rendues* **246** 1626–1628.

[6] Ballantyne, K. C., Perkins, A. C., Pimm, M. V., Garnett, M. C., Armitage, N. C., Baldwin, R. W. & Hardcastle, J. D. (1986). Localisation of monoclonal antibody-drug conjugate 791T/36-methotrexate in colorectal cancer. *J. Clin. Oncol.* (in press).

[7] Ghose, T., Norwell, S., Guclu, A., Cameron, D., Bodurtha, A. & Macdonald, A. S. (1972). Immunochemotherapy of cancer with chlorambucil-carrying antibody. *B. Med. J.* **iii** 495.

[8] Rowland, G. F., Davies, D. A. L., O'Neill, G. J., Newman, C. E. & Ford, C. H. J. (1977). Specific cancer therapy by drugs synergising with or attached to tumour-specific antibodies: experimental background and clinical results. In: Rainer, H. (ed.) *Immunotherapy of Malignant Diseases,* Schattauer-Verlag, Stuttgart, pp. 316–322.

[9] Rowland, G. F., O'Neill, G. J. & Davies, D. A. L. (1975). Suppression of tumour growth in mice by a drug–antibody conjugate using a novel approach to linkage. *Nature* **255** 487–488.

[10] Rowland, G. F. (1977). Effective antitumour conjugates of alkylating drug and

antibody using dextran as the intermediate carrier. *Europ. J. Cancer* **13** 593–596.

[11] Hurwitz, E., Maron, R., Bernstein, A., Wilcheck, M., Sela, M. & Arnon, R. (1978). The effect *in vivo* of chemotherapeutic drug–antibody conjugates in two murine experimental tumour systems. *Int. J. Cancer* **21** 747–755.

[12] Hurwitz, E., Maron, R., Wilchek, M., Arnon, R. & Sela, M. (1975). The covalent binding of daunomycin and adriamycin to antibodies with retention of both drug and antibody activities. *Cancer Res.* **35** 1175–1181.

[13] Arnon, R. & Hurwitz, E. (1985). Monoclonal antibodies as carriers for immunotargeting of drugs. In: Baldwin, R. W. & Byers, V. S. (eds) *Monoclonal Antibodies for Cancer Detection and Therapy*, Academic Press, London, pp. 367–383.

[14] Köhler, G. & Milstein, C. (1975). Continuous cultures of fused cells secreting antibody of predefined specificity. *Nature* **256** 495.

[15] Rowland, G. F. (1983). Use of antibodies to target drugs to tumour cells. *Clinics in Allergy and Immunology,* vol. 3, no. 2, pp. 235–257.

[16] Brown, J. P., Woodbury, R. G., Hart, C. E., Hellström, I. & Hellström, K. E. (1981). Quantitative analysis of melanoma associated antigen p97 in normal and neoplastic tissues. *Proc. Nat. Acad. Sci. USA* **78** 539–543.

[17] Larson, S. M., Brown, J. P., Wright, P. W., Carrasquillo, J. A., Hellström, I. & Hellström, K. E. (1983). Imaging of melanoma with ^{131}I-labelled monoclonal antibodies. *J. Nuclear Med.* **24** 123–129.

[18] Hellström, K. E. & Hellström, I. (1985). Monoclonal anti-melanoma antibodies and their possible clinical use. In: Baldwin, R. W. & Byers, V. S. (eds) *Monoclonal Antibodies for Cancer Detection and Therapy*, Academic Press, London, pp. 17–51.

[19] Brown, J. P., Nishiyama, K., Hellström, I. & Hellstroℑm, K. E. (1981). Structural characterisation of human melanoma-associated antigen p97 with monoclonal antibodies. *J. Immunol.* **127** 539–546.

[20] Hockey, M. S., Stokes, H. J., Thompson, H., Woodhouse, C. S., Macdonald, F., Fielding, J. W. L. & Ford, C. H. J. (1984). Carcinoembryonic antigen (CEA) expression and heterogeneity in primary and autologous metastatic gastric tumours demonstrated by a monoclonal antibody. *B. J. Cancer* **49** 192–233.

[21] Gatter, K. C., Abdulaziz, Z., Beverley, P., Corvalan, J. R. F., Ford, C., Lane, E. B., Mota, M., Nash, J. R. G., Pulford, K., Stein, H., Taylor-Papadimitriou, J., Woodhouse, C. & Mason, D. Y. (1982). Use of monoclonal antibodies for the histopathological diagnosis of human malignancy. *J. Clin. Path.* **35** 1253–1267.

[22] Embleton, M. J., Gunn, B., Byers, V. S. & Baldwin, R. W. (1981). Antitumour reactions of monoclonal antibody against a human osteogenic-sarcoma cell line. *B. J. Cancer* **43** 582–587.

[23] Pimm, M. V. & Baldwin, R. W. (1985). Localization of an anti-tumour monoclonal antibody in human tumour xenografts: kinetic and quantitative studies with the 791T/36 antibody. In: Baldwin, R. W. & Byers, V. S. (eds) *Monoclonal Antibodies for Cancer Detection and Therapy*, Academic Press, London, pp. 98–129.

[24] Rogers, G. T. (1983). Carcinoembryonic antigen and related glycoproteins. Molecular aspects and specificity. *Biochim. Biophys. Acta* **695** 227–232.

[25] Dillman, R. O., Beauregard, J. C., Sobol, R. E., Royston, I., Bartholomew, R. M., Hagen, P. S. & Halper, S. P. (1983). Complications associated with *in vivo* administration of anti-CEA murine monoclonal antibodies in patients with advanced colorectal carcinoma. *Proc. Am. Ass. Cancer Res.* 217.

[26] Woodhouse, C. S. (1982). An investigation of human lung tumour antigens. *PhD Thesis,* University of Birmingham.

[27] Corvalan, J. R. F., Axton, C. A., Brandon, D. R., Smith, W. & Woodhouse, C. (1984). Classification of anti-CEA monoclonal antibodies. *Protides of the Biol. Fluids* **31** 921–924.

[28] Hockey, M. S., Ford, C., Newman, C., Corvalan, J. R. F., Rowland, G., Stokes, H., Thompson, H., Woodhouse, C. S. & Fielding, J. W. L. (1983). The immunohistochemical localization of carcinoembryonic antigen (CEA) with monoclonal antibody in gastric adenocarcinomas. *B. J. Surgery* **70** 300.

[29] Gallego, J., Price, M. R. & Baldwin, R. W. (1984). Preparation of four daunomycin–monoclonal antibody 791T/36 conjugates with anti-tumour activity. *Int. J. Cancer* **33** 737–744.

[30] Rowland, G. F., Simmonds, R. G., Corvalan, J. R. F., Baldwin, R. W., Brown, J. P., Embleton, M. J., Ford, C. H. J., Hellström, K. E., Hellström, I., Kemshead, J. T., Newman, C. E. & Woodhouse, C. S. (1983). Monoclonal antibodies for targeted therapy with vindesine. *Protides of the Biol. Fluids* **30** 375–379.

[31] Rowland, G. F. & Simmonds, R. G. (1985). Effects of monoclonal antibody–drug conjugates on human tumour cell cultures and xenografts. In: Baldwin, R. W. & Byers, V. S. (eds) *Monoclonal Antibodies for Cancer Detection and Therapy,* Academic Press, London, pp. 345–364.

[32] Embleton, M. J., Rowland, G. F., Simmonds, R. G., Jacobs, E., Marsden, C. H. & Baldwin, R. W. (1983). Selective cytotoxicity against human tumour cells by a vindesine–monoclonal antibody conjugate. *B. J. Cancer* **47** 43–49.

[33] Ford, C. H. J., Bartlett, S. E., Casson, A. G., Marsden, C. H. & Gallant, M. E. (1986). Vindesine monoclonal anti-CEA conjugate efficacy and specificity with 9 human cancer cell lines. *NCI Monographs* (in press).

[34] Rowland, G. F., Corvalan, J. R. F., Axton, C. A., Gore, V. A., Marsden, C. H., Smith, W. & Simmonds, R. G. (1984). Suppression of growth of a human colorectal tumour in nude mice by vindesine–monoclonal anti-CEA conjugates. *Protides of the Biol. Fluids* **31** 783–786.

[35] Rowland, G. F., Axton, C. A., Baldwin, R. W., Brown, J. P., Corvalan, J. R. F., Embleton, M. J., Gore, V. A., Hellström, I., Hellström, K. E., Jacobs, E., Marsden, C. H., Pimm, M. V., Simmonds, R. G. & Smith, W. (1985). Antitumour properties of vindesine–monoclonal antibody conjugates. *Cancer Immunol. Immunother.* **19** 1–7.

[36] Rowland, G. F., Simmonds, R. G., Gore, V. A., Marsden, C. H. & Smith, W. (1986). Drug localisation and growth inhibition studies of vindesine–monoclonal anti-CEA conjugates in a human tumour xenograft. *Cancer Immunol. Immunother.* **21** 183–187.

[37] Casson, A. G., Ford, C. H. J., Marsden, C. H., Gallant, M. E. & Bartlett, S. E.

(1986). Efficacy and selectivity of vindesine monoclonal anti-CEA antibody conjugates on human tumour cell lines grown as xenografts in nude mice. *NCI Monographs* (in press).

[38] Ford, C. H. J., Newman, C. E., Johnson, J. R., Woodhouse, C. S., Reeder, T. A., Rowland, G. F. & Simmonds, R. G. (1983). Localisation and toxicity study of a vindesine–anti-CEA conjugate in patients with advanced cancer. *B. J. Cancer* **47** 35–42.

[39] Dykes, P. W., Hine, K. G., Bradwell, A. R., Blackburn, J. C., Reeder, T. A., Drolc, Z. & Booth, S. N. (1980). Localisation of tumour deposits by external scanning after injection of radiolabelled anti-carcinoembryonic antigen. *Br. Med. J.* **280** 220–222.

[40] Armitage, N. C., Perkins, A. C., Hardcastle, J. D., Pimm, M. V. & Baldwin, R. W. (1985). Monoclonal antibody imaging in malignant and benign gastrointestinal diseases. In: Baldwin, R. W. & Byers, V. S. (eds) *Monoclonal Antibodies for Cancer Detection and Therapy*, Academic Press, London, pp. 130–158.

[41] Morrison, S. L., Johnson, M. J., Herzenberg, L. A. & Oi, V. T. (1984). Chimaeric human antibody molecules: mouse antigen-binding domains with human constant region domains. *Proc. Natl. Acad. Sci. USA* **81** 6851–6855.

[42] Boulianne, G. L., Hozumi, N. & Shulman, M. J. (1984). Production of functional chimaeric mouse/human antibody. *Nature* **312** 643–646.

[43] Neuberger, M. S., Williams, G. T. & Fox, R. O. (1984). Rcombinant antibodies possessing novel effector functions. *Nature* **312** 604–608

5

Soluble polymers as targetable drug carriers

John B. Lloyd, Biochemistry Research Laboratory, Department of Biological Sciences, University of Keele, Staffordshire ST5 5BG, UK

1. INTRODUCTION

Soluble synthetic polymers are emerging as drug delivery vehicles of great promise. They are undoubtedly more versatile than microparticulate carriers, owing to the much greater number of potential target sites in the body. Also, and perhaps surprisingly at first sight, they have many advantages over natural macromolecules.

My work in this area stemmed from a meeting in October 1972 with Professor Helmut Ringsdorf of the University of Mainz. Ringsdorf was visiting Keele University under the auspices of the British Council, at the invitation of (now Emeritus Professor) Peter Plesch, a distinguished polymer chemist in our Chemistry Department. Ringsdorf had, and has, interests in many aspects of polymer science, but was particularly developing the concept of pharmacologically active polymers. My own interests are in pinocsytosis and lysosome function, and it was quickly clear to Ringsdorf and I that there was scope for fruitful collaboration between our laboratories. My first idea was that synthetic polymers, with their scope for systematic variation in parameters such as molecular size, charge and hydrophobicity, could be invaluable in unravelling the substrate-specifying of pinocytosis. Drs Alan Moore and Ken Williams were at that time obtaining some fascinating data at Keele on the rate of pinocytosis of variously modified bovine serum albumin by rat yolk-sac cells [1,2]. Ringsdorf and I were able to develop our plans further in May 1974, when I was invited to lecture at his Institute in Mainz. I was later pleased to see endocytosis and lysosomes accorded a prominent place in the published version of a lecture given by him in May 1975 [3].

Another encounter of great significance for my work was a brief meeting in July 1978 with Dr Jindřich Kopeček of the Institute of Macromolecular Chemistry, Czechoslovak Academy of Sciences. Ringsdorf had drawn my attention to experiments Kopeček had published on the effects of proteolytic enzymes on short oligopeptide sequences covalently attached to the soluble polymer polyhydroxypropylmethacrylamide (polyHPMA). Kopeček and I met at the Dresden meeting of the Federation of European Biochemical Societies, where I suggested to him that his conjugates should be tested against lysosomal enzymes, since these would be the enzymes they would encounter in pinocytic uptake by cells. That meeting in Dresden was followed, in February 1980, by the first of many visits by myself and my colleagues to Prague and by visits by Dr Kopeček and members of his team to Keele.

This historical introduction has been included for two reasons. First, it allows me to make clear at the start that almost all of the work I shall describe has been a collaborative effort between the Keele team and either Ringsdorf's laboratories or Kopeček's. The references to published papers will amply demonstrate the extent of these collaborations. Secondly, I can acknowledge gratefully my indebtedness to the British Council and the Royal Society for their support of these collaborative studies. The British Council, through its Academic Links scheme, has funded numerous visits to Mainz and Prague by myself and members of the Keele team, while the Royal Society, by formalizing our link with Prague under its agreement with the Czechoslovak Academy of Sciences, and by numerous travel grants, has facilitated many visits in both directions. These meetings, for assessment and planning of the research programme, as well as sometimes for a specific piece of experimental work, have been of the utmost importance.

In proceeding now to describe the results of our research programme, I shall begin with the general concept and its foundation in cell biology. I shall then describe the progress we have made in developing a particular carrier system, one based on polyHPMA. I shall place more stress on the general than on the particular, both because it is probably more important in looking to the future and also because we have already published several recent summaries of our work [4–6]. References [7] and [8] are brief general accounts of the concept of drug delivery using soluble macromolecules.

2.　ENDOCYTOSIS AND LYSOSOMES

Biological membranes are effective barriers to macromolecules. The cell's plasma membrane prevents the loss from the cytoplasm of enzymes and other biopolymers, while the intracellular membranes delineate functionally distinct subcellular compartments, each with its own metabolic pattern, determined in turn by its enzyme complement. Mechanisms for translocation of macromolecules across membranes do exist, but these are specific and sophisticated, such as the use of signal peptides to direct secretory proteins into the cisternae of the endoplasmic reticulum and the routes by which the genetic material of viruses and bacteria can enter cells.

Although macromolecules cannot in general cross the plasma membrane, they can be captured by cells and taken to an intracellular site. Endocytosis, a term that subsumes two related phenomena, pinocytosis and phagocytosis, involves the formation and inward migration of vesicles comprising invaginated plasma membrane and containing engulfed substrates. The contents of these vesicles are channelled to the lysosomes, resident cellular organelles containing hydrolytic enzymes, without traversing any membranes. A cell's lysosomes may be thought of as its digestive tract, and indeed the analogy is apt, for the lysosomes are the site of digestion of exogenous macromolecules and thus the source of many nutritionally valuable metabolites for the cytoplasm. The lysosome membrane allows the passage of these digestion products but prevents the escape of undigested macromolecules or of the lysosomal enzymes.

I have elsewhere [9,10] recently reviewed the current understanding of endocytosis and lysosomes, and will not repeat most of that material here. Two aspects deserve an explicit mention, however. The first is a major difference between pinocytosis and phagocytosis. Pinocytosis, the capture of extracellular liquid, is seemingly a constitutive activity of all nucleated animal cells, whereas phagocytosis, the capture of small particles, is the preserve of a few specialized cell types such as the mononuclear phagocytes (macrophages) and neutrophils. Secondly, pinocytosis, although apparently the non-specific uptake of ambient fluid, can be highly substrate-specific. The external face of the plasma membrane bears many binding sites or receptors for specific solutes which can be avidly captured by the membrane internalization involved in pinocytosis. In some cases the type or density of a receptor will be characteristic of some particular cell type.

3.   THE IDEAL MACROMOLECULAR DRUG CARRIER

It is possible to introduce the concept of the targetable drug–polymer conjugate (see Fig. 1). It will be a soluble macromolecule to which a drug is covalently attached by a

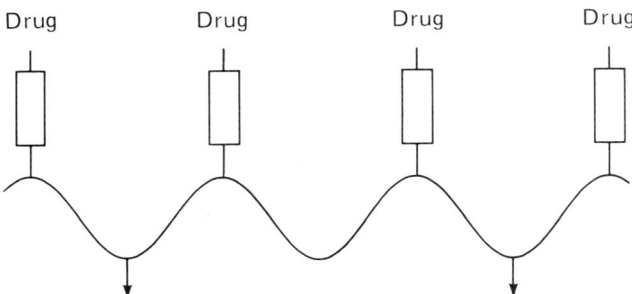

Fig. 1 — Diagrammatic representation of a macromolecular drug carrier. Drug molecules are attached to the polymer by linkages (□) susceptible to degradation in the lysosomes. The macromolecule also incorporates features (↓) that recognize and bind to target cells. Reproduced from ref. [7] with permission of Elsevier Science Publishers B.V., Amsterdam.

'spacer' moiety susceptible to degradation by lysosomal enzymes. The polymer will also bear 'targeting' moieties which, by mimicking some physiological substrate, will bind to a receptor present on the target cell. There are few restrictions on the nature of the drug to be conjugated, other than the chemical feasibility of suitably attaching it to the polymer and the requirement that, after release from the carrier in the lysosome, it should be able to penetrate the lysosome membrane and enter the cytoplasm. In theory at least, there are also many potential target cells: accessibility via the bloodstream following parenteral injection is clearly a requirement but, as explained above, most cell types of the body are active in pinocytosis.

So what kind of macromolecule can serve? In Table 1 I list some of the properties

Table 1 — Properties of the ideal macromolecular drug carrier

(1) Adequate drug-loading capacity.
(2) Retention of water-solubility when drug-loaded
(3) Molecular weight too large to permit glomerular filtration, but small enough to reach all cell types.
(4) Unmodified carrier not captured by adsorptive pinocytosis
(5) Carrier–drug linkage stable in body fluids but degradable in the lysosomes
(6) Carrier slowly biodegradable in extracellular compartment or degraded in the lysosomes
(7) Non-toxic, non-immunogenic and generally 'biocompatible'.

I consider important. Most of these are self-explanatory, but one (the fourth) perhaps deserves some amplification. It is important that the carrier itself is not captured by absorptive or receptor-mediated pinocytosis., If it were, the effectiveness of any specific targeting moiety would be much reduced. This, parenthetically, is a besetting problem for targeting with particulate carriers: they are so effectively captured by the mononuclear phagocyte (reticuloendothelial) system that a targeting moiety has rather little influence on the body distribution.

At this point we can consider the relative advantages of natural and synthetic macromolecules. I can again refer to a more extended treatment of this theme [11], but the essentials are summarized in Table 2. Except in the matter of biodegradabi-

Table 2 — Drug targeting with soluble macromolecules: synthetic polymers vs natural macromolecules

Advantages of synthetic polymers

(1) Can be tailor-made to predetermined specifications: molecular size, charge, hydrophobicity and capacity for drug attachment can all be optimised.
(2) More robust and consequently more stable during manipulation and storage.
(3) Chemistry of drug and targeting-moiety attachment less laborious.
(4) Easier and cheaper to produce in quantity and high purity.
(5) Less immunogenic.

Advantages of natural macromolecules

(1) Monodisperse (proteins)
(2) Generally more biodegradable

lity, synthetic polymers emerge well ahead of their natural counterparts. Perhaps the most exciting feature of synthetic polymers is the wide choice available, limited only by the imaginative powers and synthetic ingenuity of the polymer chemists. In addition to the homopolymers, which consist of chains of identical repeating units, there are many types of copolymer. Two (or even three) different monomers may be copolymerized in a defined ratio: the resultant copolymer may have its component monomers arranged randomly or as regularly repeating dimers (or trimers). Block copolymers consist of pieces of two homopolymers (A and B) joined end-to-end: these may have many possible structures, A–B and A–B–A for example. There is also the possibility of attaching several polymer chains together by cross-links (see also below), although this process frequently leads to loss of water solubility.

As explained above, a useful polymer will be one that does not adhere non-specifically to cells. We have found that this means in practice avoiding excessive charge or hydrophobicity. Many authors have reported that polymers with a high density of positive charges, such as polylysine and polyornithine, bind tightly to cell membranes. Even a much lower charge-density has profound effects: a copolymer comprising 93% vinylpyrrolidone units and 7% (cationic) vinylamine adhered to mammalian cell surfaces, whereas the homopolymer polyvinylpyrrolidone did not [12]. Conversely, a synthetic polyanion, pyran copolymer (DIVEMA), was found to adsorb to rat peritoneal macrophages and to enter these cells by pinocytosis 100 times as rapidly as polyvinylpyrrolidone [13]. We have studied the effect of hydrophobic residues in some detail. Polyhydroxypropylmethacrylamide does not absorb to cell membranes, but its rate of pinocytosis increases dramatically if 10–20% of the monomer residues are substituted with a phenolic residue [14]. Similarly the incorporation of 10–20% phenolic side-chains greatly increases the cell-binding of another polymer, polyhydroxyethylaspartamide [15,16]. Polymers that bind to cell surfaces are also likely to bind to plasma proteins: this will inevitably alter the interactions with cells and, *in vivo*, may lead to intravascular aggregate formation.

We have reported one study on a block copolymer [17]. It comprised a hydrophilic portion, polyethyleneoxide, and a hydrophobic, polylysine whose ε-amino group were substituted to 50% with palmitoyl residues. The rate of pinocytosis by rat peritoneal macrophages was similar to that of the homopolymer polyethyleneoxide, showing that here the major hydrophobic domain is without much effect. This result is probably explained by observations indicating that in an aqueous environment the copolymer forms a unimolecular micelle, and that only its hydrophilic portion is seen by the cell.

Thus far the best molecules available are polyvinylpyrrolidone (polyVP) and polyHPMA, with the latter preferred because of the ease of adding substituent groups. Derivatization of polyHPMA with low percentages of oligopeptides [18] or phenolic residues [14] is possible without causing adherence to cells. These two polymers are water-soluble even to high degrees of polymerization, but non-specific cell adherence is seen with both at high molecular weight [19,20]. Another advantage of these two polymers is their biocompatibility. The two homopolymers polyVP and polyHPMA have, in the past, both undergone extensive testing *in vivo* as potential plasma expanders, and both were found satisfactory. The amount administered in these tests was of course greatly in excess of that needed for drug delivery. A recent investigation [21] showed that polyHPMA is barely immunogenic in mice.

4.   TARGETED DRUG DELIVERY WITH polyHPMA

As explained earlier, a targetable drug–polymer conjugate must bear both targeting and drug moieties. Using polyHPMA we have been able to demonstrate both targeting and intracellular drug delivery.

Targeting has been accomplished by derivatizing polyHPMA with glycylglycylgalactosamine (Gly-Gly-CalNH$_2$) [22,23]. This moiety appears, perhaps surprisingly, to be recognized by the asialoglycoprotein receptor on hepatocytes. The polymer, when injected into the rat bloodstream, is very efficiently removed by the liver parenchymal cells and taken into their lysosomes. Only 5–10% of the hydroxypropyl residues on the polymer need to be replaced by Gly-Gly-CalNH$_2$ to achieve maximal targeting. In these experiments ^{125}I-labelled tyrosine residues, attached to the polymer by a lysosomally degradable spacer (see below), were also present in low amount. Monitoring the tissue localization of the radiolabel at different times after administration provided convincing evidence that the labelled moiety, which can be considered a drug analogue, was released from its carrier by the action of the lysosomal enzymes. Some evidence of targeting to L1210 cells using their fructose receptor has recently been obtained (see below).

Although the natural substrates for the lysosomal enzymes are themselves macromolecules, it is far from self-evident that these enzymes would attack linkages in non-natural polymers. We are therefore gratified to find that an enzyme mix from rat liver lysosomes can in appropriate circumstances cleave *p*-nitroaniline from conjugates with polyHPMA [24–26]. The crucial factor is the size and nature of the spacer moiety linking the leaving group to the polymer. *p*-Nitroaniline conjugated directly by amide-link to methacryloyl moieties was not released, but interposition of a suitable oligopeptide renders the distal amide linkage susceptible. The nature of the oligopeptide greatly influences the rate of enzymic attack: in order of susceptibility, tetrapeptide > tripeptide > dipeptide linkages, and inclusion of hydrophobic amino acids enhances digestibility. The identity of the enzyme(s) responsible has not been firmly established, but in most cases release of *p*-nitroaniline is largely or entirely thiol-dependent. The lysosomal enzymes not only release a terminal chromophore such as *p*-nitroaniline; they can also partially digest the oligopeptide itself. This was evident from the kinetics of *p*-nitroaniline release from certain oligopeptide side-chains [26], and also from some parallel experiments using a tissue cultured *in vitro*, in which digestion took place in the cells following pinocytic uptake of the conjugate [18]. In these experiments the terminal amino acid was tyrosine, permitting the conjugate to be labelled with ^{125}I and digestion to be monitored by the generation of free [^{125}I]iodotyrosine. With susceptible side-chains, such as -Gly-Gly-Tyr-nitroanilide, free [^{125}I]iodotyrosine was released by the tissue into the culture medium; with resistent side-chains, such as -Gly-βAla-nitroanilide, radioactivity accumulated in the tissue without production of radiolabelled breakdown product.

Oligopeptides can also be used as lysosomally digestible components of cross-links between polymer chains. Short lengths of polyHPMA can be linked by di(oligopeptidyl) diamines, as shown in Fig. 2, to yield a larger macromolecule. If such cross-linked molecules were used for targeted delivery of a cytotoxic drug, intralysosomal processing would not only release the drug but also degrade the cross-links. The polymer fragments released from the target cell on its demise would be

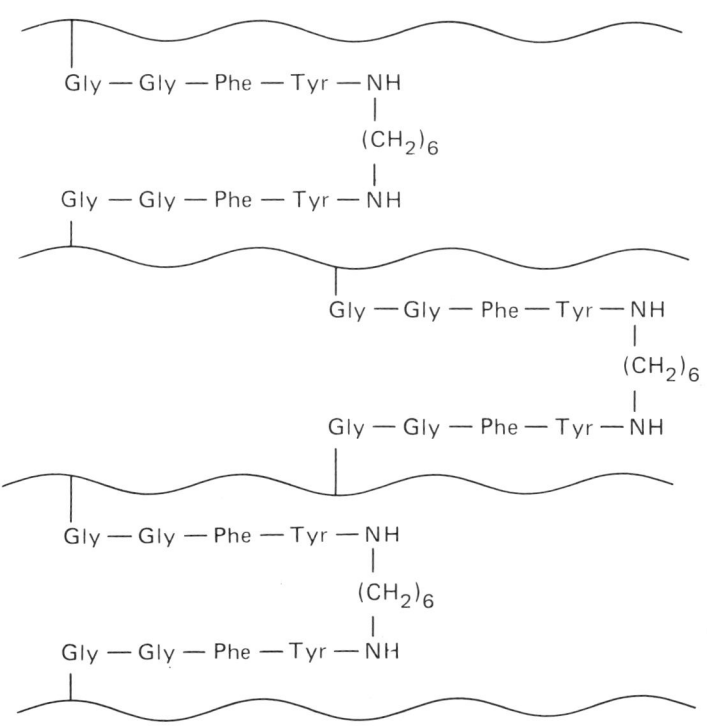

Fig. 2 — Semi-schematic representation of the structure of a cross-linked polyHPMA. The short polymer chains (wavy lines) are cross-linked by di(oligopeptidyl)hexamethylenediamine to produce a larger molecule. Diamines other than hexamethylenediamine can and have been used.

small enough to enter the glomerular filtrate, thus obviating the accumulation of undegradable polymer within the body. The degradation of oligopeptide-containing cross-links, such as those in the polymer shown in Fig. 2, by lysosomal enzymes has been demonstrated [20,27].

As indicated in Table 1, a drug carrier must not release its drug prematurely. This means that the drug–spacer linkage must not be susceptible to degradation in the body fluids. Although there are amidases active in the bloodstream, it is possible to design oligopeptide spacers that retain drug during transit through the bloodstream but release it under the influence of the lysosomal enzymes [28].

Having demonstrated that polyHPMA can in model systems satisfy all the requirements for a targetable drug carrier, we have recently proceeded to test its capacity to deliver bioactive compounds to relevant cell types [29,30]. The system is in principle applicable to the delivery of many types of drug, but we have concentrated initially on the delivery of cytotoxic anticancer drugs, not least because the need for targeted delivery is most pressing here. Conjugates of daunorubicin with polyHPMA were synthesized, again using oligopeptides as spacers. It was tiresome, if not surprising, to discover that the nature of the attached drug altered the structural requirements in the spacer. Whereas tyrosinamide was cleaved effectively from a glycylglycine spacer [9], daunorubicin was not, requiring a tetrapeptide spacer such as Gly-Phe-Leu-Gly or Gly-Phe-Phe-Leu for acceptable rates of enzymic attack. The conjugates were also cytotoxic to a murine leukaemia cell line L1210, both *in vitro* and *in vivo*. Although it is plausible that the observed cytotoxic effects result from pinocytosis of the conjugate and intracellular release of daunorubicin, other possible explanations such as an effect of the conjugate at the cell surface have not been conclusively eliminated. A significant observation in this context is the low cytotoxicity of the polymer bearing glycylglycyl-daunorubicin side-chains which, as noted above, are resistant to the action of lysosomal enzymes. The possibility of targeting the cytotoxic conjugates has been demonstrated by incorporating fucosyla-mine-terminating side-chains: L1210 cells have a fucose-recognizing receptor and are somewhat more susceptible to conjugates bearing the targeting moiety.

5. SUMMARY AND CONCLUSION

The work reported above has demonstrated the following:

(1) Lysosomal amidases can release bioactive substances from oligopeptide side-chains of polyHPMA.
(2) Different rates of release can be achieved by designating appropriate oligopeptide spacers.
(3) Targeting to a chosen cell type can be achieved by incorporation of moieties that are recognized by receptors specific to these cells.
(4) After uptake by pinocytosis, the polymer releases its charge of drug in the lysosome. The drug then passes into the cytoplasm and thence into the extracellular fluid.
(5) Polymers with lysosomally digestible cross-links can be used to overcome the problem of residue accumulation in the body.

There is thus every indication that the system described has the potential to become a clinically valuable drug delivery system. It has recently been patented [31]. The major obstacle is a fundamental one that applies to all approaches to targeting. We do not yet know whether the various cell types of the body have surface features sufficiently specific to those cells. If not, positive targeting is an unrealizable dream. On this question I am hopeful: new receptors are constantly being reported, and it seems realistic to believe that at least some of these will be exploitable for targeted drug delivery.

ACKNOWLEDGEMENTS

Grants from the Cancer Research Campaign and the Science and Engineering Research Cuncil are gratefully acknowledged. The international collaborations were sponsored and supported by the British Council and the Royal Society.

REFERENCES

[1] Moore, A. T., Williams, K. E. & Lloyd, J. B. (1974). The Effect of chemical treatment of [^{125}I]iodinated bovine serum albumin on its rate of pinocytosis by 17.5-day rat yolk-sac cultured *in vitro*. *Biochem. Soc. Trans.* **2** 648–650.

[2] Moore, A. T., Williams, K. E. & Lloyd, J. B. (1977). The effect of chemical treatments of albumin and orosomucoid on rate of clearance from the rat bloodstream and rate of pinocytic capture by rat yolk sac cultured *in vitro*. *Biochem. J.* **164** 607–616.

[3] Ringsdorf, H. (1975). Structure and properties of pharmacologically active polymers. *J. Polymer Sci. Polymer Symp.* **51** 135–153.

[4] Lloyd, J. B., Duncan, R., Kopeček, J. & Rejmanová, P. (1984). Targeting and lysosomal handling of polymethacrylamide–oligopeptide conjugates. In: Gregoriadis, G., Poste, G., Senior, J. & Trouet, A. (eds) *Receptor-mediated Targeting of Drugs* Plenum Press, New York & London, pp. 417–425.

[5] Lloyd, J. B., Duncan, R. & Kopeček, J. (1984). Synthetic polymers as targetable carriers for drugs. *Pure & Appl. Chem.* **56** 1301–1304.

[6] Kopeček, J., Rejmanová, P., Duncan, R. & Lloyd, J. B. (1985). Controlled release of drug model from N(-2-hydroxypropyl)-methacrylamide copolymers. *Ann. N.Y. Acad. Sci.* **446** 93–103.

[7] Lloyd, J. B. (1985). Macromolecules as vehicles for intracellular drug delivery. *Pharmacy International* **6** 252–255.

[8] Lloyd, J. B., Duncan, R. & Kopeček, J. (1986). Synthetic polymers as carriers for chemotherapeutic agents. *Biochem. Soc. Trans.* **14** 391–392.

[9] Lloyd, J. B. (1986). Endocytosis and lysosomes: recent progress in intracellular traffic. In: Gregoriadis, G. & Senior, J. (eds) *Targetting of Drugs with Synthetic Systems*, Plenum Press, New York, pp. 000–000.

[10] Lloyd, J. B. & Forster, S. (1986). The lysosome membrane. *Trends Biochem. Sci.* **11** 365–368.

[11] Lloyd, J. B. (1986). Targeting with synthetic polymers: a realistic goal. In: *Gregoriadis G. & Senior, J. (eds) Targeting of Drugs with Synthetic Systems*, Plenum Press, New York, pp. 000–000.

[12] Prattern, M. K., Cable, H. C., Ringsdorf, H. & Lloyd, J. B. (1982). Adsorptive pinocytosis of polycationic copolymers of vinylpyrrolidone with vinylamine by rat yolk sac and rat peritoneal macrophage. *Biochem. Biopphys. Acta* **719** 424–430.

[13] Prattern, M. K., Duncan, R., Cable, H. C., Schnee, R., Ringsdorf, H. & Lloyd, J. B. (1981). Pinocytic uptake of divinyl ether-maleic anhydride (pyran copolymer) and its failure to stimulate pinocytosis. *Chem.-Biol. Interactions* **35** 319–330.

[14] Duncan, R., Cable, H. C., Rejmanová, P., Kopeček, J. & lloyd, J. B. (1984).

Tyrosinamide residues enhance pinocytic capture of N-(2-hydroxypropyl) methacrylamide copolymers. *Biochem. Biophys. Acta* **799** 1–8.

[15] Duncan, R., Starling, D., Rypaček, F., Drobník, J. & Lloyd, J. B. (1982). Pinocytosis of poly(α,β-(N-2-hydroxyethyl))-DL-aspartamide and a tyramine derivative by rat visceral yolk sacs cultured *in vitro*. Ability of phenolic residues to enhance the rate of pinocytic capture of a macromolecule. *Biochem. Biophs. Acta* **717** 248–254.

[16] Duncan, R., Cable, H. C., Rypaček, F., Drobník, J. & Lloyd, J. B. (1985). Characterization of the adsorptive pinocytic capture of a polyaspartamide modified by the incorporation of tyramine residues. *Biochim. Biophys. Acta* **840** 291–293.

[17] Pratten, M. K., Lloyd, J. B. Hörpel, G. & Ringsdorf, H. (1985). Micelle-forming block copolymers: pinocytosis by macrophages and interaction with model membranes. *Macromol. Chem.* **186** 725–733.

[18] Duncan, R. D., Rejmanová, P. Kopeček, J. & Lloyd, J. B. (1981). Pinocytic uptake and intracellular degradation of N-(2-hydroxypropyl)methacrylamide copolymers. *Biochim. Biophys. Acta.* **678** 143–150.

[19] Duncan, R., Prattern, M. K., Cable, H. C., Ringsdorf, H. & Lloyd, J. B. Effect of molecular size of ^{125}I-labelled poly(vinylpyrrolidone) on its pinocytosis by rat visceral yolk sacs and rat peritoneal macrophages. *Biochem. J.* **196** 49–55.

[20] Cartlidge, S. A., Duncan, R., Lloyd, J. B., Rejmanová, P. & Kopeček, J. (1986). Soluble, crosslinked N-(2)-hydroxypropyl)methacrylamide copolymers as potential drug carriers. 1. Pinocytosis by rat visceral yolk sacs and rat intestine cultured *in vitro*. Effect of molecular weight on uptake and intracellular degradation. *J. Controlled Release* 3 55–66.

[21] Ríhová, B., Ulbrich, K., Kopeček, J. & Mančal, P. (1983). Immunogenicity of N-(2-hydroxypropyl)methacrylamide copolymers — potential hapten or drug carriers. *Folia Microbiol.* **28** 217–227.

[22] Duncan, R., Kopeček, J., Rejmanová, P. & Lloyd, J. B. (1983). Targeting of N-(2-hydroxypropyl)methacrylamide copolymers to liver by incorporation of galactose residues. *Biochem. Biophys. Acta* **755** 518–521.

[23] Duncan, R., Seymour, L. C. W., Scarlett, L., Lloyd, J. B., Rejmanová, P. & Kopeček, J. (1986). Fate of N-(2-hydroxypropyl)methacrylamide copolymers with pendent galactosamine residues after intravenous administration to rats. *Biochim. Biophys. Acta* **880** 62–71.

[24] Duncan, R., Lloyd, J. B. & Kopeček, J. (1980). Degradation of side chains of N-(2-hydroxypropyl)methacrylamide copolymers by lysosomal enzymes. *Biochem. Biophys. Res. Comm.* **94** 284–290.

[25] Duncan, R., Cable, H. C., Lloyd, J. B., Rejmanová, P. & Kopeček, J. (1982). Degradation of side-chains of N-(2-hydroxypropyl)methacrylamide copolymers by lysosomal thiol-proteinases. *Bioscience Reports* **2** 1041–1046.

[26] Duncan, R., Cable, H. C., Lloyd, J. B., Rejmanová, P. & Kopeček, J. (1983). Polymers containing enzymatically degradable bonds, 7. Design of oligopeptide side-chains in poly[N-(2-hydroxypropyl)methacrylamide] copolymers to promote efficient degradation by lysosomal enzymes. *Makromol. Chem.* **184** 1997–2008.

[27] Rejmanová, P., Kopeček, J., Pohl, J., Baudyš, M. & Kostka, V. (1983).

Polymers containing enzymatically degradable bonds, 8. Degradation of oligo-peptide sequences in N-(2-hydroxypropyl)methacrylamide copolymers by bovine spleen cathepsin B. *Makromol. Chem.* **184** 2009–2020.

[28] Rejmanová, P., Kopeček, J., Duncan, R. & Lloyd, J. B. (1985). Stability in rat plasma and serum of lysosomally degradable oligopeptide sequences in N-(2-hydroxypropyl)methacrylamide copolymers. *Biomaterials* **6** 45–48.

[29] Duncan, R., Kopečkova-Rejmanová, P., Strohalm, J., Hume, I., Cable, H. C., Pohl, J., Lloyd, J. B. & Kopeček, J. (1987). Increased therapeutic potential of anticancer agents coupled to N-(2-hydroxypropyl)methacrylamide copo-lymers. 1. Evaluation of daunomycin and puromycin conjugates *in vitro. Brit. J. Cancer* (in press).

[30] Duncan, R., Koečkova,-Rejmanova, P., Strohalm, J., Hume, I. C., Lloyd, J. B. & Kopeček, J. (1987). Increased therapeutic potential of anticancer agents coupled to N-(2-hydroxypropyl)methacrylamide copolymers. 2. Evaluation of daunomycin conjugates *in vivo* against L1210 leukaemia. *Brit. J. Cancer* (submitted).

[31] Kopeček, J., Rejmanová, P., Stohalm, J., Ublrich, K., Říhová, B., Chytry, V., Lloyd, J. B. & Duncan, R. (1985). Synthetic polymeric drugs. *European Patent Appl.* 85309560.2 (31.12.85).

6

Design of biodegradable polymers for controlled release

F. G. Hutchinson and **B. J. A. Furr**, Imperial Chemical Industries plc, Pharmaceuticals Division, Mereside, Alderley Park, Macclesfield, Cheshire SK10 4TG, UK

1. INTRODUCTION

In recent years there have been major advances in genetic engineering and consequently the production of many interesting and pharmacologically active polypeptides. There have also been concurrent improvements in procedures for total chemical synthesis of lower molecular weight peptides such as 'Zoladex'† (ICI 118630; D-Ser (Bu^t)^6-Azgly^{10}-LHRH; Fig. 1), which is a highly potent, synthetic

$$\overline{|}Glu\text{-}His\text{-}Trp\text{-}Ser\text{-}Tyr\text{-}Gly\text{-}Leu\text{-}Arg\text{-}Pro\text{-}Gly\text{-}NH_2$$

LHRH

$$\overline{|}Glu\text{-}His\text{-}Trp\text{-}Ser\text{-}Tyr\text{-}D\text{-}Ser(Bu^t)\text{-}Leu\text{-}Arg\text{-}Pro\text{-}Azgly\text{-}NH_2$$

Zoladex ICI 118630

Fig. 1 — Structures of LHRH and 'Zoladex'.

analogue of luteinizing hormone-releasing hormone (LHRH). However, the therapeutic and commercial potential of this and other polypeptide drugs will only be fully realized if these advances are accompanied by improvement in the design of dosage forms, leading to practical and effective formulations.

The use of polypeptides in human and animal diseases is frought with problems.

---

† 'Zoladex' is a trademark, the property of Imperial Chemical Industries plc.

These macromolecular drugs are usually ineffective by the oral route as they are rapidly degraded and deactivated by proteolytic enzymes in the alimentary tract. Even if stable to enzymatic digestion, their molecular weights are too high for absorption through the intestinal wall to occur. Other routes of administration including intranasal [1,2], buccal [3], intravaginal [4–7] and rectal have been used, but these are all associated with a low and variable bioavailability and none of these offers a general solution applicable to all polypeptides. Consequently, polypeptides and proteins are normally administered parenterally (subcutaneous, intramuscular and intravenous injection) but since these drugs have very short elimination half-lives frequent injections are required to produce an effective therapy. For polypeptide hormones, where the pharmacology of the agent is compatible with sustained release, the most appropriate dosage form is one that is capable of releasing drug continuously at a controlled rate over a period of weeks or even months. If the carrier providing for such release is polymeric then it is preferred that it should be biodegradable and so would ultimately disappear from the site of administration. Currently, a number of biodegradable polymers are being evaluated as carriers for the sustained release of low molecular weight drugs (Fig. 2).

*⎧ Polylactic acid (polylactide)

⎨ Polyglycolic acid (polyglycolide)

⎪ Poly (lactic acid—co—glycolic acid)

⎩ Poly (lactide—co—glycolide)

Poly (ε—caprolactone)

Poly (hydroxybutyric acid)

Poly ortho—esters

Poly acetals

Poly dihydropyrans

Synthetic polypeptides

Cross—linked proteins

Poly cyanoacrylates

Hydrogels (i) cross—linked

*   (ii) amphipathic block copolymers

Fig. 2 — Biodegradable polymers used in drug delivery.

Long experience with homo- and copolymers of lactic and glycolic acids has shown that these materials are inert and biocompatible in the physiological environment and degrade to toxicologically acceptable products [8]. Consequently, these polymers are invariably the materials of choice in the initial design of parenteral sustained-delivery systems using a biodegradable carrier, particularly when release over many weeks is required. We have adopted this approach and were the first group to identify and characterize the mechanisms of transport which allow movement of these polypeptide drugs from biodegradable formulations based on these polyesters [9]. This work has been extended latterly to include release of polypeptides and proteins from biodegradable hydrogels derived from amphipathic block copolymers and based in part on these (co-)polyesters [10].

2. RATIONALE

The succesful development of sustained-release biodegradable delivery systems for peptide drugs such as 'Zoladex' requires recongition and resolution of a number of major problems posed by these macromolecular drugs. Firstly, the mechanism most commonly used to achieve sustained release, namely controlled diffusion through a matrix or membrane, may not be appropriate for a high molecular weight polypeptide. Design of a sustained-release dosage form must take into account both the properties of the rate-controlling polymer and the drug. For diffusion of the drug to occur it must have some limited solubility in the polymer; this is often the case with low molecular weight drugs. In contrast, it is well established that, in the absence of specific chemical interactions, polypeptides will either be insoluble in, or incompatible with, any polymer such as polyester, which has a totally dissimilar structure, because of entropic and enthalpic factors [11]. Consequently, low or negligible solubility of the macromolecular drug in a polymer, such as a polyester, will prevent diffusional transport of the agent through the polymer phase. With regard to the properties of the drug the most important of these are its size, shape and solubility [12]. There is an approximate log–log correlation between molecular weight (M) and diffusion coefficient (D) where: $\log D = a - b \log M$ (where a and b are arbitrary constants) such that D decreases as molecular weight increases. For polypeptides M is large and the diffusion coefficient becomes vanishingly small because the diffusant cannot be accommodated by the free volume of polymer arising from rotational or translational segmental mobility. Consequently, polymers such as polyesters are not likely to allow partition-dependent diffusion of polypeptides through the polyester to occur.

Secondly, polypeptides are biologically labile and can be readily degraded by tissue enzymes. They must, therefore, be effectively protected at the depot site if active drug is to be released continuously. The difficulty of achieving this is emphasized by the fact that synthetic polypeptides have actually been used as biodegradable carriers for drugs such as steroids and narcotic antagonists [13, 14].

Thirdly, excipients used to achieve sustained relese of macromolecular drugs might provoke an adjuvant-induced immunological response, which may be related to the nature of the excipient, the delivery rate, or profile of release. There is some evidence that sustained release of large proteins may be an effective means of raising antibodies to them [15]. Finally, long-lasting depots might become encapsulated by fibrous tissue, thus inhibiting further release of drug. This is certainly the case for non-degradable silicone elastomer implants [16].

These imposing problems opposing sustained polypeptide delivery have been resolved by the design of biodegradable delivery systems based on polyesters such as poly (d,l-lactide) and poly (d,l-lactide-co-glycolide) to give formulations which allow release of polypeptides over an extended period of time. This work has been extended to include amphipathic polymers consisting in part of biodegradable polyesters and which in a physiological environment behave as hydrogels. Although emphasis is focussed on the LHRH analogue, 'Zoladex', it has been shown that these technologies can also be applied to high molecular weight polypeptides.

3. LACTIC/GLYCOLIC ACID POLYMERS

These simple biodegradable homo- and copolymers were prepared at elevated temperature by the ring-opening polymerization of dry, freshly prepared acid dimers. d,l-lactide and glycolide, by using organo-tin compounds as catalysts. Control of molecular weight was achieved by using a chain transfer agent such as d,l-lactic acid. In this way polymers (Fig. 3) of variable composition, having intrinsic

Polyesters

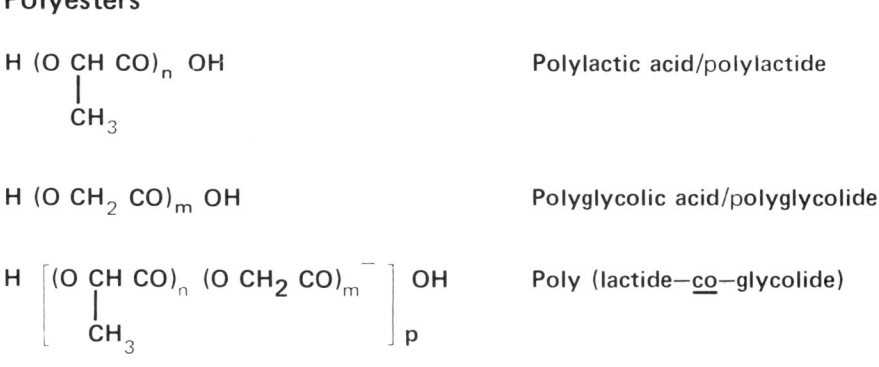

Fig. 3 — Polymers and copolymers of lactic and glycolic acids.

viscosities from 0.1 to >1, can be prepared. The polymers can be further characterized by size exclusion chromatography relative to polystyrene standards to define number average molecular weight (M_n), weight average molecular weight (M_w) and polydispersity ($P=M_w/M_n$). Additionally, the polymers can be characterized by ^{13}C-NMR to define the distribution of comonomers and polymer structure (that is, the average value for n and m of copolymers shown in Fig. 3).

3.1   Degradation studies on poly (d,l-lactide-co-glycolide)

Because polypeptides have high molecular weight and are water soluble, their release from these polyesters by classical partition-dependent diffusion is unlikely to occur. Consequently, degradation of the poly (d,l-lactide) or poly (d,l-lactide-co-glycolide) will be a critical factor in determining transport of the high molecular weight polypeptide from the dosage form. The degradation of these polymers in the absence of drug has been characterized in terms of molecular weight and its distribution, weight loss, water uptake and morphology of the hydrated and degraded polymer.

Degradation of the polymer *in vitro* in buffer at pH 7.4 results in progressive changes in molecular weight and molecular weight distribution. Under these conditions degradation is not enzyme mediated and must occur by simple hydrolytic cleavage of ester groups; the profile of weight loss and change in molecular weight are consistent with this. High molecular weight polymers degrade to lower molecuar weights, as measured by viscosity, yet retain their water insolubility. Only after an extended time of degradation does any weight loss occur. In contrast, very low molecular weight polymers can degrade with weight loss immediately. Similar results are obtained with high lactide-containing polymers except that the time scale of events is more extended for these more hydrolytically stable polymers. These results are consistent with bulk hydrolysis in the *in vitro* condition and this correlates broadly with degradation of these polymers *in vivo* suggesting that even in subcutaneous tissue, enzyme-mediated degradation is significantly less important than simple hydrolysis. In this event, polylactides could effectively protect polypeptides at the depot site from the influence of degradative enzymes.

For these degradation experiments, if the logarithm of the number average molecular weight is plotted as a function of time, then for high molecular weight polymers an essentially linear relationship is seen to hold except at extended times of degradation where a discontinuity arises (Fig. 4).

Pitt and Schindler [17], studying poly (d,l-lactide), have seen a similar behaviour but have ignored the nature of, and reasons for, the discontinuity. In fact, this arises because of water uptake by the degrading polymer. For an amorphous polyester, water uptake will be governed, empirically, by the intrinsic hydrophilicity of the repeat units and by end-group effects. For these polyesters the end groups are alkoxylic and carboxylic and these increase as molecular weight falls, that is, as degradation proceeds the essentially hydrophobic polymer becomes more hydrophilic. The profile of water uptake at 37°C in buffer at pH 7.4, for polymers which have been dried rigorously, has been studied as a function of time. For these, water uptake is determined by two events. The first is simple diffusional ingress into the dried material and in the absence of degradation this would occur to a level that would be characteristic of the equilibrium swelling of this kind of material. However, these polymers are hydrolytically unstable and following, or even during this initial diffusional phase, the polymer can degrade and so take up more water. For high molecular weight polymers, having a normal distribution ($P\sim2$), these two phases of water uptake are separated by an interval during which water uptake increases hardly at all. In contrast, low molecular weight polymers have an essentially continuous water uptake.

It can be shown empirically that the water uptake for a thin polymer film having a molecular weight M_n and a polydispersity P, in the absence of significant hydrolytic degradation, is described approximately by the hyperbolic function:

$$[H_2O] = a + \frac{b}{P\,M_n}$$

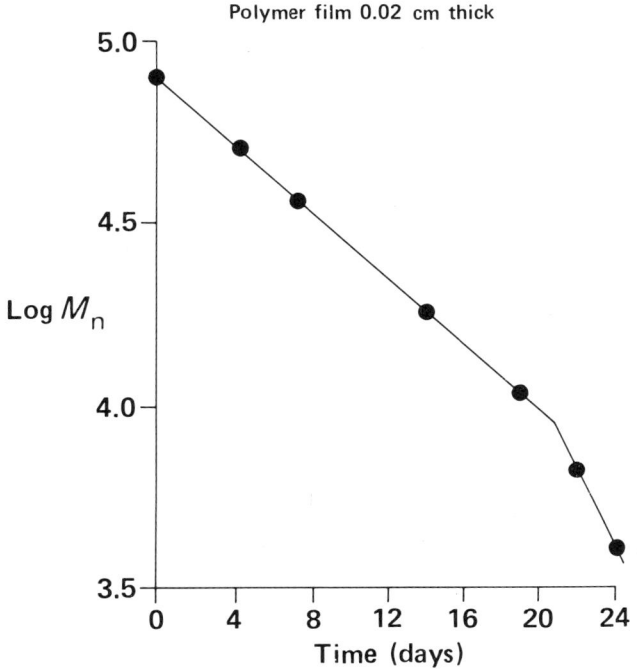

Fig. 4 — *In vitro* degradation of poly (*d*,*l*-lactide-co-glycolide) at 37°C in buffer at pH 7.4. Number average molecular weight of degrading polymer as function of time.

where a and b are constants related to polymer composition.

If the initial diffusional ingress into thin films is assumed to be instantaneous then approximate expressions can be derived for degradation-induced change of molecular weight and water uptake with time using a similar but modified model proposed by Pitt and Schindler [17].

Degradation of poly (lactide-co-glycolide) proceeds by hydrolytic scission of ester groups generating polymers containing one terminal carboxyl group/chain. Defining degradation as appearance of -CO_2H and applying the normal kinetic equation governing ester hydrolysis:

$$d\frac{[CO_2H]}{dt} = K[H_2O][ester][CO_2H] \qquad (1)$$

and $[CO_2H] \alpha \dfrac{1}{M_n^t}$

where M_n^t is the number average molecular weight at time t.

For all practical purposes [ester] can be considered a constant and as

$$[H_2O] = a + \frac{b}{P\,M_n}$$

equation (1) reduces to

$$d\,[1/M_n^t] = k.\,a + \frac{b}{P\,M_n^t}\cdot\frac{1}{M_n^t} \tag{2}$$

where $k = K$ [ester].

At $t = 0$, $M_n^t = M_n^0$ where M_n^0 is initial number average molecular weight and the solution to equation (2) is:

$$M_n^t = M_n^0\,e^{-akt} + b\frac{(e^{-akt} - 1)}{aP} \tag{3}$$

and

$$[H_2O]_t = a\left[1 + \frac{b}{a\,P\,M_n^0\,e^{-akt} + b\,(e^{-akt} - 1)}\right] \tag{4}$$

It should be noted that these derived expressions relate to the condition where the polymers have initially a normal distribution (i.e. $P \sim 2$) and hydrolysis of the polymer chains is essentially a random process.

It can be seen from Fig. 5 that the derived equation for water uptake correlates broadly with experimentally determined events. Thus, hydrolytic degradation is characterized by reduction in molecular weight, enhanced water uptake and ultimately weight loss of polymer, All these events occur at a temperature which is below or near the glass transition temperature of the polyester. This in turn implies that morphological changes are likely to occur within the polymer whilst hydrolysis is occurring. This is confirmed by scanning electron-microscopy of the degraded products which shows the development of porosity within the degrading polyester.

These studies have shown that degradation of poly (d,l-lactide) and poly (d,l-lactide-co-glycolide) is dependent on molecular weight, polydispersity geometry, polymer composition and polymer structure and ultimately leads to enhanced water uptake and the generation of porosity.

Thus, water-soluble polypeptides may be released from these biodegradable polyesters since enhanced water uptake and the generation of porosity should facilitate transport of polypeptide from the dosage form. This is likely to involve diffusion through aqueous pores generated in the drug polymer matrix. In this event, the release of polypeptide will differ mechanistically from the processes thought to occur during release of steroids, narcotic antagonists and antimalarials from poly (d,l-lactide) and poly (d,l-lactide-co-glycolide) [8]. Whereas these low molecular weight drugs will diffuse, by a simple partition-dependent process, through intact polymer membranes in diffusion cell experiments, these same polymer membranes are totally impermeable to polypeptides.

Polymer film 0.02 cm thick

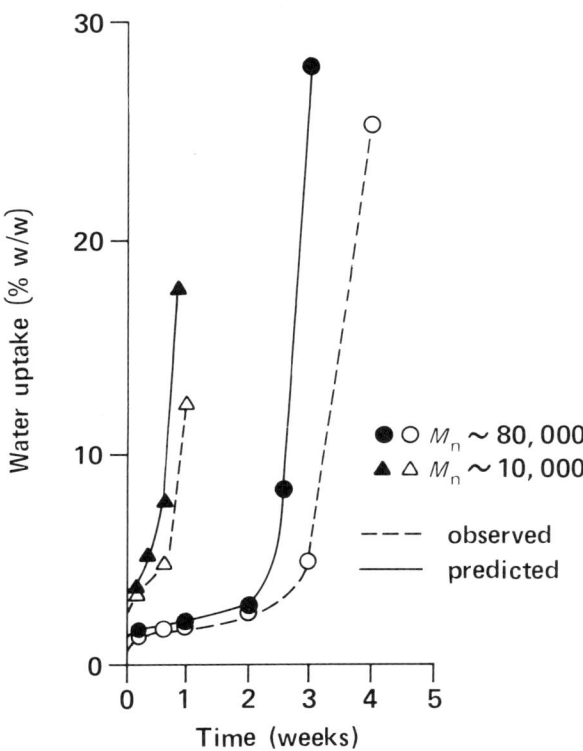

Fig. 5 — *In vitro* degradation of poly (*d,l*-lactide-co-glycolide) at 37°C in buffer ap pH 7.4.
Water uptake of degrading polymer as function of time.

3.2   Release studies with 'Zoladex'

Chronic administration of LHRH analogues such as 'Zoladex' has been shown to cause a reversible chemical castration which leads to regression of hormone-responsive animal and human mammary and prostate tumors [18].

Because of low oral potency, the drugs have usually been administered once or more times daily. A biodegradable formulation, based on poly (lactide-co-glycolide), either as a subdermal depot or as an injectable suspension, which will deliver the drug over a period of 28 days or even longer, would be more clinically acceptable. Research was focussed on 'Zoladex' (molecular weight 1269) from solid depots because this was thought more likely to afford a clearer understanding of the physicochemical parameters which allow transport of drug from the dosage form. In this respect 'Zoladex' is a particularly useful drug as studies both *in vitro* and *in vivo* can be undertaken. In the *in vitro* situation absorption of the drug into an external aqueous medium can be measured by high performance liquid chromatographic analysis of the aqueous phase to give a quantitative measure of the amount released.

Continuous release of the polypeptide *in vivo* can be measured qualitatively by the biological effect elicited in regularly cycling adult female rats. Normally, these rats have an oestrus cycle of 4 days and the occurrence of oestrus is indicated by the presence of cornified cells in vaginal smears. In rats given subdermal depots of 'Zoladex', release of drug at an effective rate will cause a fall in circulating oestrogens, which in turn leads to a suppression of oestrus and absence of cornified smears. Rats therefore show an extended period of dioestrus.

On the basis of degradation studies, transport of drug from these depots is likely to be governed by various properties of the rate-controlling polyester. These properties include polymer composition, molecular weight and distribution, level of drug incorporation, morphology of the drug/polymer mixture, degradation characteristics of the polymer and geometry. It can be shown that release of polypeptide from these biodegradable polyesters occurs by diffusion through aqueous pores generated in the dosage form. These aqueous channels, which facilitate drug release, are generated by two distinct and separate mechanisms. The first involves leaching of drug from polypeptide domains at or near the surface of the delivery system and essentially is a dissolution/diffusion-controlled event. However, drug within the body of the depot, existing in isolated domains not continuous or contiguous to the surface, cannot be released until the second mechanism becomes operative. This second mechanism involves degradation of the polyester and is associated with the generation of microporosity in, and enhanced water uptake by, the degrading polymer.

Typical parameters controlling the initial phase of release are, for example, drug loading and geometry, whereas the second phase is intrinsically related to the degradation properties of the polyester. When these two phases of release do not overlap, discontinuous release is observed (Fig. 6(a)).

However, by controlling the properties of the polymer the initial phase of release can be made to overlap with the second phase and depots can be defined which give continuous release over 28 days both *in vitro* and *in vivo* (Fig. 6(b)). These depots have been used to induce a castration-like effect in rats and thereby to inhibit growth of mammary and prostate tumours [18].

The effect of a single subcutaneous depot containing 500 μg 'Zoladex' on the growth of rat dimethylbenzanthracene-induced mammary tumours is shown in Fig. 7. This experiment is a model for advanced mammary cancer and in control animals given placebo depots tumours have doubled in size in 4 weeks. In contrast, tumours regress markedly in rats given the single depot.

If rats are given depots at the start of the experiment and then at weeks 4 and 8 a far more profound regression occurs (Fig. 8). By week 11 none of the tumours present at the start of the experiment is palpable. As the effect of the final depot becomes exhausted, around week 16, recovery in growth of the tumours occurs.

These depots are equally effective in animal models for prostate ciarcinoma. Single depots containing 1 mg 'Zoladex' given every 28 days to male rats bearing hormone-responsive Dunning R3327, transplantable prostate tumours cause a marked inhibition of tumour growth. Chemical castration using 'Zoladex' depots is

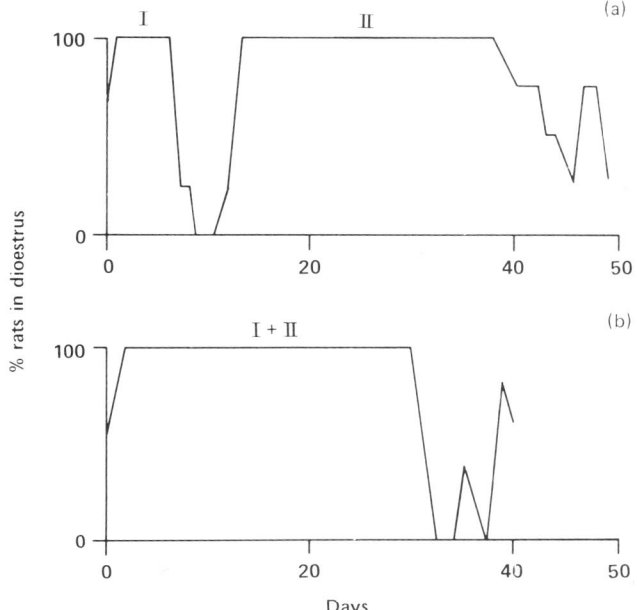

Fig. 6 — Effect of subdermal depots containing 300 μg of 'Zoladex' administered to regularly
cycling adult female rats.
(a) Depots containing 3% (w/w) 'Zoladex' in high molecular weight polymer. (b) Depots
containing 20% (w/w) 'Zoladex' in low molecular weight polymer. I = Initial release due to
leaching from surface. II = degradation-induced release.

shown in this animal model to cause an inhibition of tumour growth to values
indistinguishable from those in surgically castrated animals (Fig. 9).

These promising results achieved in animal studies have now been substantiated
in clinical trials in patients suffering form prostatic carcinoma [19,20] and in
premenopausal women with advanced breast cancer [21].

4.   CONCLUSION

Using acceptable biodegradable polymers such as lactide/glycolide materials it is
possible to design a diversity of polymer types which allow continuous release of
polypeptides, an objective that some 5–6 years ago was thought to be virtually
impossible. However, from our work this design must accommodate, at a fundamental level, and understanding and an appreciation of polymer and materials science of
the polymer alone and in association with the polypeptide, as well as the biology and
pharmacology of the drug. Inevitably this means research teams that are broadly
based and comprised of many different types of specialist. Without such interaction
and cooperation advanced delivery systems for drugs, whatever their nature, are
unlikely to be optimized.

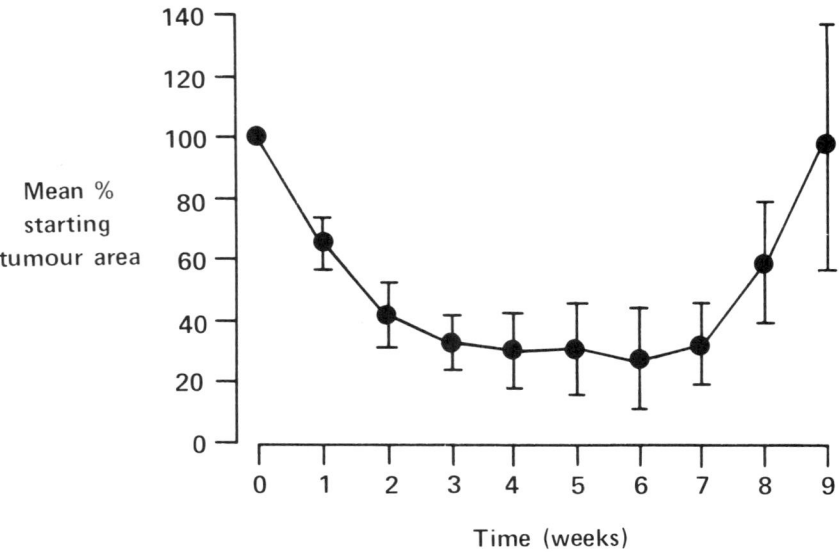

Fig. 7 — Effect of a single subcutaneous depot containing 500 μg of 'Zoladex' on the growth of dimethylbenzanthracene-induced mammary tumors.

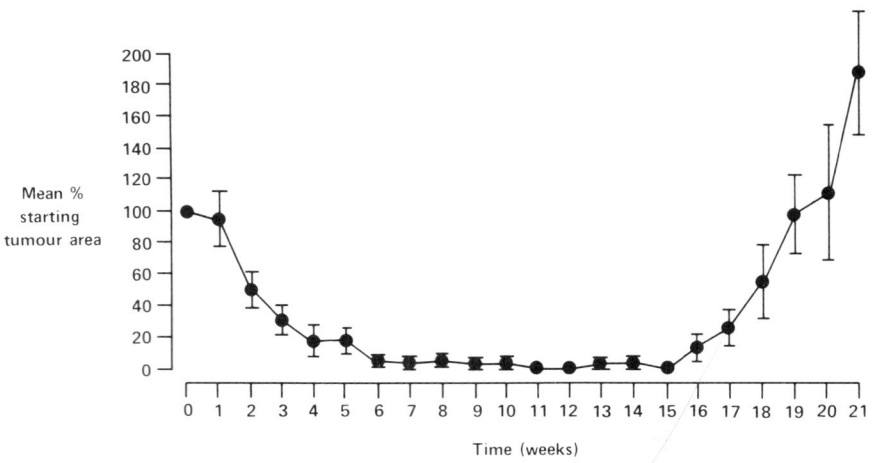

Fig. 8 — Effect of a single subcutaneous depot containing 500 μg 'Zoladex' given at weeks 0, 4 and 8 on the growth of rat dimethylbenzanthracene-induced mammary tumors.

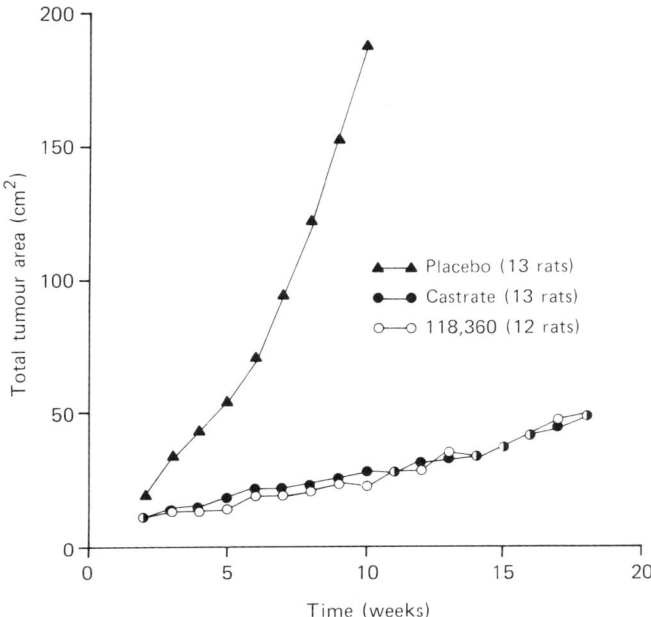

Fig. 9 — Effect of a single subcutaneous depot containing 1 mg of 'Zoladex' given every 4 weeks on the growth of hormonal-responsive, transplantable, Dunning R3327, prostate tumours. Treatment groups are placebo controls (▲; 13 rats), 'Zoladex' (○; 12 rats) and surgically castrated animals (●; 13 rats).

REFERENCES

[1] Anik, S. T., Sanders, L. M., Chaplin, M. D., Kushinsky, S. & Nerenberg, C. (1984). Delivery systems of LHRH and analogs. In: Vickery, B. H., Nestor Jr., J. J. & Hafez, E. S. E. (eds) *LHRH and its Analogs: Contraceptive and Therapeutic Applications*, MTP Press Limited, Boston, USA, pp. 421–435.

[2] Petri, W., Seidel, R. & Sandow, J. (1984). Pharmaceutical approach to long-term therapy with peptides. *Int. Cong. Series — Excerpta Medica* **656** 63–76.

[3] Anders, R., Merkle, H. P., Schurr, W. & Ziegler, R. (1983). Buccal absorption of protirelin: an effective way to stimulate thyrotropin and prolactin. *J. Pharm. Sci.* **72**, 1481–1483.

[4] Okado, H., Zamazaki, I., Ogava, Y., Hirai, S., Yashiki, T. & Mima, H. (1982). Vaginal absorption of a potent luteinizing hormone-releasing hormone analog (Leuprolide) in rats I: absorption by various routes and absorption enhancement. *J. Pharm. Sci.* **71** 1367–1371.

[5] Okado, H., Zamazaki, I., Yashiki, T. & Mima, H. (1983). Vaginal absorption of a potent luteinizing hormone-releasing hormone analog (Leuprolide) in rats II: mechanism of absorption enhancement with organic acids. *J. Pharm. Sci.* **72** 75–78.

[6] Okado, H., Yashiki, T. & Mima, H. (1983). Vaginal absorption of a potent luteinizing hormone-releasing hormone analog (Leuprolide) in rats III: effect of estrous cycle on vaginal absorption of hydrophilic model compounds. *J. Pharm. Sci.* **72** 173–176.

[7] Okado, H., Zamazaki, I., Yashiki, T., Shimamoto, T. & Mima, H. (1982). Vaginal absorption of a potent luteinizing hormone-releasing hormone analog (Leuprolide) in rats IV: evaluation of the vaginal absorption and gonadotrophin responses by radioimmunoassay. *J. Pharm. Sci.* **73** 298–302.

[8] Wise, D. L., Fellman, T. D., Sanderson, J. E. & Wentworth, R. L. (1979). Lactic/glycolic acid polymers. In: Gregoriadis, G. (ed.) *Drug Carriers in Biology and Medicine*, Academic Press, London, England, pp. 237–270.

[9] Hutchinson, F. G. (1982). Continuous release pharmaceutical compositions. European Patent Application 58481.

[10] Churchill, J. R. & Hutchinson, F. G. (1985). Continuous release formulations. United States Patent 4526938.

[11] Bohn, L. (1975). Compatible polymers. In: Brandtup, J. & Immrgut, E. H. (eds) *Polymer Handbook,* 2nd edn, John Wiley and Sons, New York, III, p. 211.

[12] Baker, R. W. & Lonsdale, H. R. (1974). Controlled release; mechanisms and rates. In: Tanquary, A. C. & Lacey, R. E. (eds) *Controlled Release of Biologically Active Agents*, vol. 47, *Advances in Experimental Medicine and Biology*, Plenum Press, New York, pp. 15–71.

[13] Mitra, S., Van Fress, M., Anderson, J. M., Peterson, R. V., Gregonis, D. & Feijen, J. (1979). Pro-drug controlled release from polygutamic acid. Polymer Preparation, American Chemical Society, Division Polymer Chemistry **20**(2) 32–35.

[14] Sidman, K. R., Schwope, A. D., Steber, W. D. & Rudolph, S. E. (1981). Use of synthetic polypeptides in the preparation of biodegradable delivery systems for narcotic antagonists. *NIDA Research Monographs* **28** 214–231.

[15] Langer, R. (1981). Polymer for the sustained release of macromolecules: their use in a single-step method of immunisation. *Methods in Enzymol.* **73**, 57–75.

[16] Anderson, J. M., Niven, H., Pelagalli, J., Olanoff, L. S. & Jones, R. D. (1981). The role of the fibrous capsule in the function of implanted drug–polymer sustained release systems. *J. Biomed. Mat. Res.* **15** 889–902.

[17] Pitt, C. G. & Schindler, A. (1980). The design of controlled drug delivery systems based on biodegradable polymers. In: Hafez, E. S. E. & van Os, W. A. A. (eds) *Progress in Contraceptive Delivery Systems*, vol. 1, MTP Press, Lancaster, England, pp. 17–46.

[18] Furr, B. J. A. & Hutchinson, F. G. (1985). Biodegradable sustained relase formulations of the LH-RH analogue 'Zoladex' for the treatment of hormone responsive tumours. EORTC Genitourinary Group Monograph 2, Part A: *Therapeutic Principles in Metastatic Prostate Cancer*, Alan R. Liss, Inc., pp. 143–153.

[19] Walker, K. J., Turkes, A. O., Zwink, R., Beacock, C., Buck, A. C., Peeling, W. B. & Griffiths, K. (1984). Treatment of patients with advanced cancer of the prostate using a slow-release (depot) formulation of the LH-RH agonist ICI 118630. *J. Endocrinol.* **103** R1–R4.

[20] Robinson, M. R. G., Denis, L., Mahler, C., Walker, K., Stitch, R. & Lunglmayr, G. (1985). An LH-RH analogue ('Zoladex') in the management of carcinoma of the prostate; a preliminary report comparing daily subcutaneous injections with monthly injections. *Eur. J. Surg. Oncol.* **11** 159–165.

[21] Williams, M. R., Walker, K. J., Turkes, A., Blamey, R. W. & Nicholson, R. I. (1986). The use of an LH-RH agonist (ICI 118630; 'Zoladex') in advanced premenopausal breast cancer. *Brit. J. Cancer* **53** 629–636.

[22] Hutchinson, F. G. & Furr, B. J. A. (1985). Biodegradable polymers for the sustained release of peptides. *Biochem. Soc. Trans.* **13** 520–523.

7

Implantable osmotically powered drug delivery systems

Nigel Ray and **Felix Theeuwes**, Alza Corporation, 950 Page Mill Road, PO Box 10950, Palo Alto, California 94303–0802, USA

Designed as research tools, a series of miniature osmotic pumps deliver a variety of test solutions or suspensions at zero-order rates for periods of hours, days, weeks, or months. The osmotic pumps consist of a cylindrical reservoir for the test solution, surrounded by a layer of the osmotic driving agent, which in turn is encased in a semipermeable membrane.

The pumping rates of such devices are determined by the hydraulic permeability of the membrane, its dimensions, and the osmotic properties of the driving agent. As such, the delivery profiles are independent of the drug formulations dispensed. Drugs of various molecular configurations, including ionized drugs and macromolecules, can be dispensed in a variety of vehicles.

Devices of this type have been used with a diversity of biologically active substances in several animal species. Besides serving as subcutaneous and intraperitoneal implants for systemic treatment, the pumps can be used for site-specific delivery of agents by directing the effluent via a catheter attachment. Examples of systemic and local delivery will be reviewed. In addition to constant (zero-order) delivery, patterned administration has also been accomplished by the use of a programmed catheter attachment. Miniature osmotic pumps have made contributions to numerous areas of biomedical research. Examples will be reviewed dealing with the process of drug scheduling, toxicology, targeted delivery, and patterned administration.

1. INTRODUCTION

A series of miniature, self-powered, osmotic pumps are designed to deliver test solutions continuously at controlled rates into laboratory animals. When implanted subcutaneously or intraperitoneally, these pumps serve as a constant source for prolonged drug delivery. In addition to systemic applications, site-specific administration can be achieved by directing via a catheter the drug solutions which are released by these pumps.

Depending on the model selected, delivery rates of test solutions from 0.5 to 10 μl per hour can be maintained for as long as 4 weeks following a simple implantation procedure. For more prolonged administration, pumps may be serially implanted. Multiple pumps may be implanted simultaneously to achieve higher rates of delivery than are attainable with a single pump. During delivery, no external connections are required and animals remain untethered and unrestrained. Use of these devices can reduce the stress placed on laboratory animals by the repeated animal handling that is necessary for serial injections or gavages. This paper reviews the current systems available and several types of research applications represented by selected examples.

2.   DESIGN AND OPERATION OF THE MINIATURE OSMOTIC PUMP [1]

Miniature osmotic pumps are capsular in shape and are manufactured in several sizes (Fig. 1):

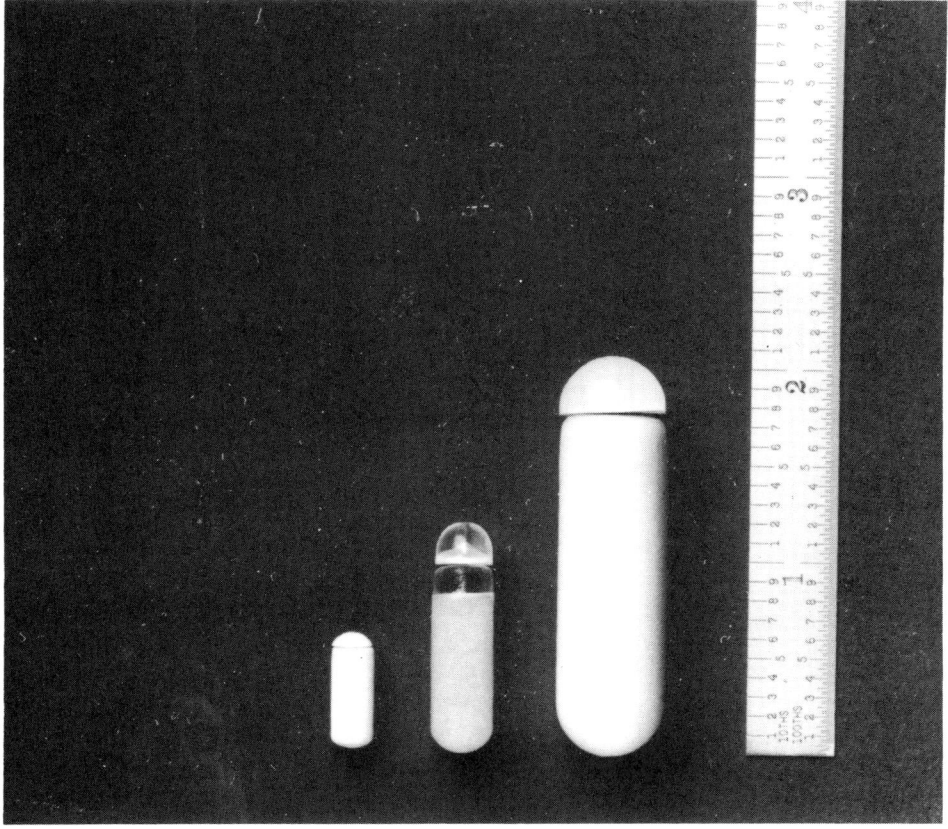

Fig. 1 — Photograph of the three sizes of Alzet® osmotic pump.

(1) 1.7 cm long by 0.6 cm in diameter
(2) 3.0 cm long by 0.7 cm in diameter
(3) 5.1 cm long by 1.4 cm in diameter.

In cross-section, mini-osmotic pumps are composed of three concentric layers (Fig. 2): the drug reservoir, the osmotic sleeve, and the rate-controlling, semiperme-

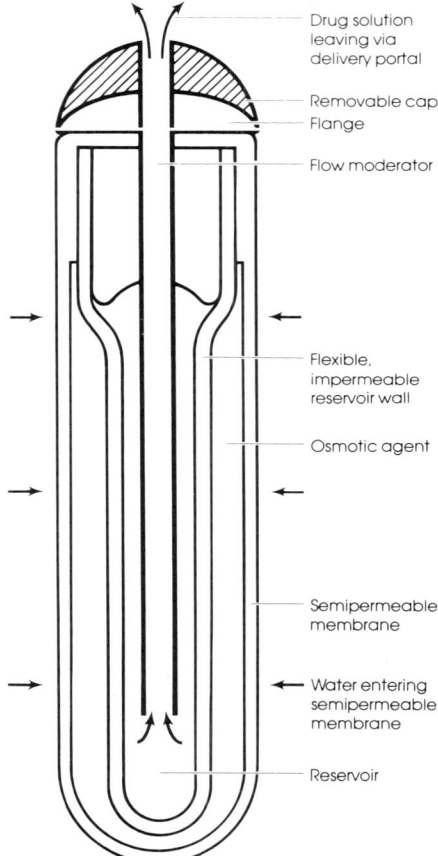

Drug solution leaving via delivery portal

Removable cap
Flange

Flow moderator

Flexible, impermeable reservoir wall

Osmotic agent

Semipermeable membrane

Water entering semipermeable membrane

Reservoir

Fig. 2 — Cross-section of a functioning osmotic pump showing cylindrical reservoir for test solution, layer of osmotic driving agent, and semipermeable outer covering of pump.

able membrane. An additional component, called the flow moderator, a 21 gauge stainless steel tube with a plastic end-cap, is inserted into the body of the osmotic pump after filling. The drug reservoir, the innermost compartment of the pump, is a cylindrical cavity molded from a synthetic elastomer. The reservoir wall is chemically inert to most aqueous drug formulations, dilute acids, bases and alcohols (Table 1).

Table 1 — List of solvents compatible with the reservoir material of Alzet® osmotic pumps

Distilled water
Isotonic NaCl or other salt solution
5% Dextrose in water or NaCL
Ethanol, up to 10% in water
Polyethylene glycol 300, neat or in water
2% Tween in water
Dimethylsulfoxide to 50% in water
Dimethylsulfoxide 50% + 10% ethanol
Propylene glycol, neat or in water
Glycerol
Dilute acids with pH greater than 1.8
Dilute bases with pH less than 14
Rat serum
Bacteriostatic culture media
(1% benzyl alcohol as bacteriostatic)
Artificial cerebrospinal fluid

It is also impermeable, blocking any exchange of material between the drug reservoir contents and the surrounding osmotic sleeve.

Outside the reservoir wall is the osmotic sleeve, a cylinder containing a high concentration of sodium chloride. It is the difference in osmotic pressure between this compartment and the aqueous environment in which the pump is placed that drives the delivery of the test solution. Water enters the sleeve along the osmotic gradient, and in doing so displaces the test soluton from the reservoir of the pump. Consequently, the delivery profile of the pump is independent of the drug formulation dispensed. Drugs of various molecular configurations, including ionized drugs and macromolecules, can be dispensed in a variety of vehicles at zero-order release rates.

The rate at which water enters the osmotic sleeve is regulated by the osmotic permeability of the semipermeable membrane, its dimensions, and the osmotic pressure difference across the membrane. The permeability and osmotic pressure are in turn a function of the ambient temperature. Due to the rigidity of the membrane, imbibed water generates hydrostatic pressure on the flexible reservoir wall, gradually compressing it, and producing a constant flow of its contents up the flow moderator tube and out through the delivery portal in the plastic end-cap. At manufacture, the rate at which water enters the osmotic sleeve and discharges the reservoir's contents is fixed. Pumps are available with a variety of delivery rates between 0.5 and 10 μl per hour and delivery durations between 3 days and 4 weeks (Fig. 3). Different mass delivery rates of test agents are achieved by varying the concentration of agent in the solution which is used to fill the pump.

The researcher fills the reservoir of the mini-osmotic pump with test solution through the delivery portal, using a special filling tube attached to a syringe. In order for the pump to function correctly, all air must be displaced from the reservoir by the

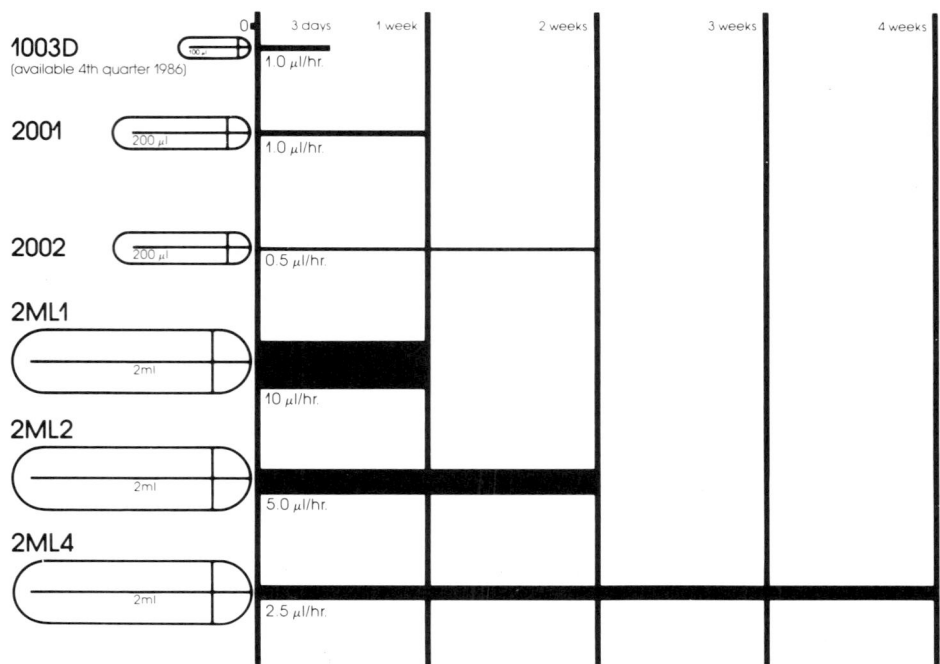

Fig. 3 — Comparison of delivery rates and reservoir capacities of Alzet® osmotic pumps.

test solution. After filling, the flow moderator is inserted into the body of the pump. The flow moderator functions to:

(1) Minimize diffusion of the test agent out of the reservoir, assuring that the osmotic process will control delivery
(2) Minimize the effect on the delivery rate of air accidentally trapped in the reservoir during filling
(3) Prevent accidental spill of the pump contents
(4) Provide a convenient attachment point for a catheter.

The absence of air bubbles in the reservoir can be determined by calculating the weight difference between the unfilled pump and the filled pump with the flow moderator in place.

3.   DELIVERY RATE *In Vivo* and *In Vitro*

Mini-osmotic pumps are designed to deliver at a constant rate by incorporating into the sleeve compartment a mass of osmotic driving agent that suffices to maintain constant osmotic activity in the compartment throughout the life of the pump. Steady-state delivery is reached after an initial transient period arising from: (1) a time-lag for water to enter the osmotic sleeve, (2) equilibration of the temperature and hydrostatic pressure in the system, and (3) relaxation of the semipermeable membrane to temperature and hydrated equilibria.

The constant or zero-order mass delivery rate from the system is given by equation (1).

$$Z = \frac{dV}{dt} \cdot C_d \tag{1}$$

Here C_d represents the concentration of drug formulated by the researcher and dV/dt the volume imbibition rate of water into the osmotic sleeve compartment.

With π_o the osmotic pressure of the osmotic agent, and π_e the osmotic pressure of the pump environment, the volume delivery rate from the system can be written as:

$$\frac{dV}{dt} = K \cdot \frac{A}{h} (\pi_o - \pi_e) \tag{2}$$

In this equation A and h are the membrane area and thickness, respectively, and K is the osmotic permeability coefficient of the membrane.

Fig. 4, an example of the release rate profile for one system, the Model 2002, is typical of the series as a whole. The data indicate that the *in vivo* and *in vitro* volume delivery rates of this Alzet® pump are within 5% of the labelled rate (0.5 μl/h). The *in vivo* delivery rate is obtained with the pump as an implant.

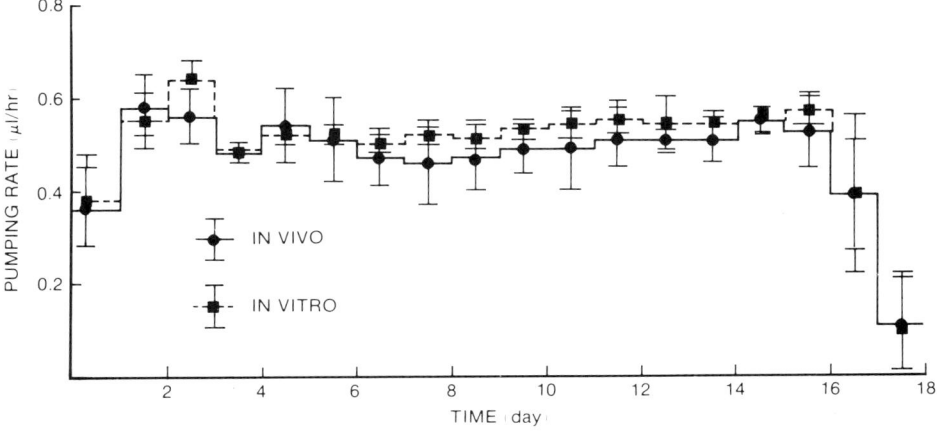

Fig. 4 — Example of delivery rate (μl/h) for Model 2002 Alzet® osmotic pump *in vivo* and *in vitro*. *In vivo* data were derived from subcutaneous implants in nine rats. *In vitro* data were obtained from four mini-osmotic pumps immersed in a 37°C bath of 0.9% saline. As can be seen in the illustration, the *in vivo* and *in vitro* rates are within 5% of each other. The nominal duration of the Model 2002 is 14 days. The nominal delivery rate is 0.5 μl/h.

The *in vivo* and *in vitro* pumping rates of mini-osmotic pumps are specified for 37°C operating conditions. Temperature affects the rate at which water crosses the semipermeable membrane and enters the osmotic sleeve, hence the release rate of the pump is a function of temperature (Fig. 5). The actual pumping rates at temperature T for two models of Alzet® pump are given by equations (3) and (4):

Model 2001: $Q_T = Q_o (0.135 \exp(0.054T) - 0.004\pi + 0.03)$ (3)
Model 2ML1: $Q_T = Q_o (0.141 \exp(0.051T) - 0.007\pi + 0.12)$ (4)

Here Q_o is the specified pumping rate of the pump at 37°C (μl/h), T is the ambient temperature (°C), and π is the osmotic pressure of the pump environment (atm.). Alzet® pumps have infused at a variety of body temperatures from fish at 21°C [2] to chickens at 41°C [3].

4.   MINIATURE OSMOTIC PUMPS AS IMPLANTS

The component materials of the mini-osmotic pump are highly tissue compatible. In accordance with USP standards, the following tests have been performed by the manufacturer for each of the component materials:

(1) Intracutaneous, intraperitoneal and intravenous injections of extracts of the component material derived from extraction with:

    (a) 0.9% Sodium chloride injection
    (b) 5% Ethanol in 0.9% sodium chloride injection
    (c) Polyethylene glycol 400
    (d) Vegetable oil†

(2) Intramuscular implantation of strips of component material.

Tissue and systemic reactions to these tests are compared to the USP-specified negative control. As such, all materials for mini-osmotic pumps pass the USP Class VI Biological Tests for Plastics.† When assembled units are implanted in laboratory animals for the functional lifetime of the system, examination of the implantation site shows no adverse tissue reaction. These procedures assure that manufactured pumps meet strict tissue compatibility criteria.

To date there have been over 1500 publications illustrating the use of osmotic pumps to deliver 600 different compounds (Table 2) in 30 different animal species including rats, mice, cats, cattle, chickens, dogs, fish, frogs, guinea pigs, hamsters, iguana, monkeys, pigs, sheep, and squirrels. Pumps have been used in these species for both systemic administration, by means of a subcutaneous or intraperitoneal implant, or for localized administration via a catheter.

4.1   Mini-osmotic pumps for systemic drug delivery

The pharmacodynamics of both therapeutic effects and side-effects have been found to be dependent on the schedule of administration for drugs with narrow therapeutic indices and short half-lives. During the drug discovery and screening process,

---

† The elastomeric reservoir wall material is not compatible with natural oils, hence extraction with vegetable oil is not performed on this component (Table 1).

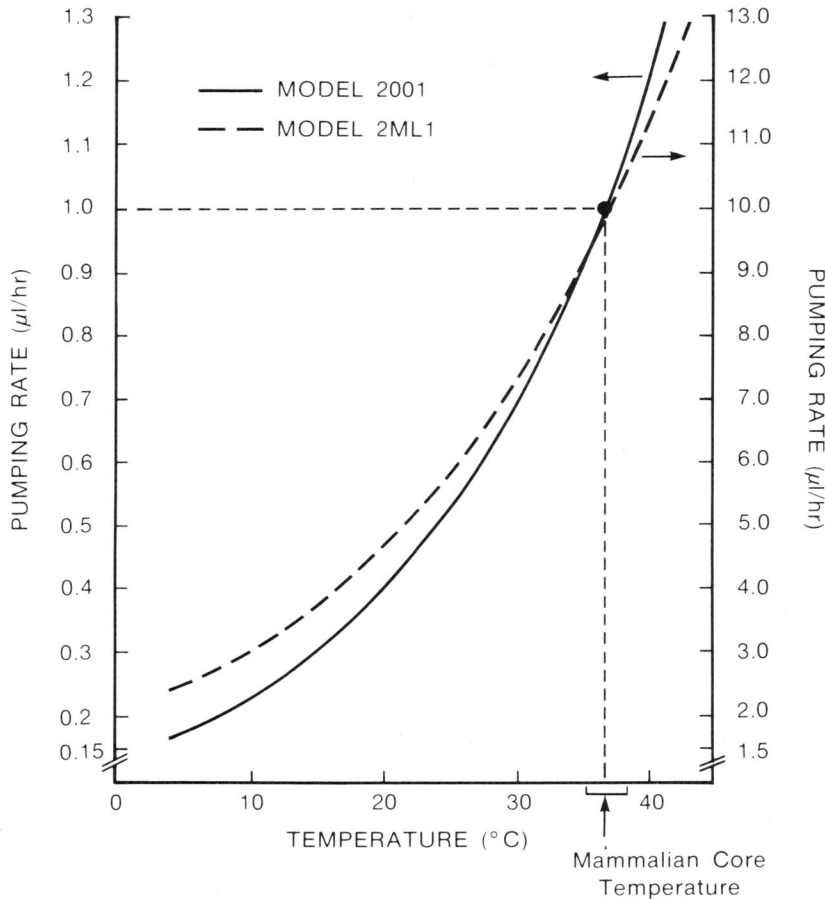

Fig. 5 — Temperature dependence of the delivery rate (μl/h) for Models 2001 and 2ML1 from 4°C to over 40°C in 0.9% saline.

rodents are often used as test species. In these small animals, half-lives of compounds are, as a rule, an order of magnitude shorter than in man [4]. Therefore, conventional drug administration schedules may fail to elicit certain drug effects, or understate others, e.g. toxic effects. For this reason, a protocol which compares the different effects of a given total dose of drug when administered by one or more schedules of injection and by constant infusion has been advocated in preclinical drug screening [5]. Examples of the injection–infusion comparison protocol in the investigation of regimen-dependent pharmacokinetics will be reviewed here.

The work of Nau and his colleagues in Berlin [6,7] exemplifies the value of using osmotic pumps as subcutaneous drug delivery devices in toxicology. Nau studied the effects of the antiepileptic drug valproic acid (VPA) on fetal development in

Table 2 — Classification of agents delivered by Alzet® osmotic pump

Amino acids	Gastrointestinal motility modulators
Anesthetics	Growth factors
Antibiotics	Heavy metals
Antibodies	Lymphokines
Anticancer agents	Metabolites
Anticoagulants	Neurotransmitters
Antiepileptics	Nerve growth factors
Antigens	Nucleosides
Antihypertensives	Nucleotides
Antiparasitic agents	Peptides and peptide hormones
Antiparkinson agents	Prostaglandins
Ascitic fluid	Radio-isotopes
Catecholamines	Renin-angiotensin system hormones and inhibitors
Chelators	Steroids
Cholinergics	Thyroid-related hormones
Central nervous system-acting agents	Toxins
Enzyme inhibitors	Vitamins

pregnant mice. Valproate is eliminated in mice at a much higher rate than in man, resulting in a half-life of less than 1 h (less than 1/10 that of man). A conventional once-daily dosing regimen for man, when given to mice, results in peak plasma concentrations that are seven times higher than the therapeutic level in man, even though doses are weight-adjusted and 24 h average plasma concentrations are equal. This much elevated peak concentration in the mouse might result in exaggerated toxicity of VPA compared to humans. Four hours after each dose, however, drug concentrations in mice have fallen virtually to zero. The resulting drug-free period of 20 h before the next dose does not occur in humans. When daily dosing regimens are studied in the laboratory, such a drug-free interval might be the basis for observations in mice which underestimate the toxicity of VPA in the human.

Nau compared the effects of giving the same total dose by two different administration regimens: a once-daily subcutanesous injection and a constant subcutaneous infusion from an osmotic pump. With constant infusion, an order of magnitude higher total dose was required to produce an incidence of fetal resorptions and exencephaly comparable to that obtained with the once-daily injection regimen. Fetal weight gain was retarded with similar frequency by both regimens. Thus, at a given dose the embryo-toxicity pattern was found to be schedule dependent: intermittent bolus administration produced resorptions, fetal weight retardation, and a high rate of exencephaly, whereas steady-state concentrations produced resorptions and fetal weight retardation, but almost no exencephaly.

This difference in administration regimen results in a shift of the dose–response curves for fetal death and exencephaly to the right when VPA is given by infusion versus by once-daily injection (Fig. 6). A constant infusion of 500 mg/kg per day in mice appears bioequivalent to a conventional regimen of repeated injections in man at the therapeutic dose. In this regimen, the mouse model is significantly free of side-effects while the same dose given by injections results in a high level of resorptions and exencaphaly. Despite the large difference between mouse and man in the half-life of valproate, mini-osmotic pumps can produce plasma concentrations in mice which are bioequivalent to concentrations achieved by conventional dosing in man.

Another pattern of drug dynamics is revealed by the work of Sikic *et al.* [8] on bleomycin. This antineoplastic drug was administered for 1 week to tumour-bearing mice by three different dosing schedules: (1) twice-daily injections; (2) an injection on the first and third day; (3) a continuous infusion by osmotic pump. Over the course of all three schedules the same total dose was administered. Efficacy was measured by reductions in tumor size and toxicity was measured by hydroxyproline content of the lung, an indicator of pulmonary fibrosis. Therapeutic doses given by infusion achieved significantly greater reductions in tumor size than identical doses given by either of the injection schedules. In contrast, at a given dose the infusion regimen resulted in significantly less pulmonary fibrosis than either of the injection schedules.

Thus, bleomycin appears to be a drug where the infusion dose–response curve for one effect (antitumor) is shifted to the left while the infusion dose–response curve for another effect (toxicity) is shifted to the right, relative to the injection dose–response curves. These concomitant shifts have the effect of widening the therapeutic index of bleomycin, the ratio of the dose required for a given therapeutic effect to the dose required for a given toxic effect, when the drug is given by infusion. Bleomycin is thus safer and more effective when given by infusion in this model. Such pharmacodynamic work is drug specific. Constant drug delivery is not *a priori* the superior regimen. For example, it appears that gentamicin and cyclophosphamide are both drugs which are better given by injection than by infusion [9]. It has been advocated that both injection and infusion regimens should be investigated during drug screening programs [5].

4.2 Mini-osmotic pumps for local drug delivery

As stated before, a catheter may be attached to the exit port of an implantable osmotic pump to perfuse a discrete location distant from the site of implantation. In this manner, drug solutions may be delivered into solid tissue or against arterial pressures without measurable reduction of flow with local delivery into tissues, the miniature osmotic pump is capable of changing local drug concentrations around the catheter tip, without influence on the rest of the body. Flows of 0.5 to 1.0 µl per hour appear to be low enough so that hydraulic damage or edema is minimal or absent in the microperfused region [9].

Sendelbeck and Urquhart [10] investigated the spatial distribution of the polar drugs [^{14}C]dopamine hydrochloride (DA), [^{3}H]sodium methotrexate (MTX), and the lipid-soluble drug [^{14}C]antipyrine (AP) during continuous intracerebral microperfusion. Infusion was carried out through a small-gauge stainless steel cannula placed in the diencephalon of a rabbit and attached to a mini-osmotic pump with catheter tubing. After 6 days of continuous infusion, brain tissue was sectioned and

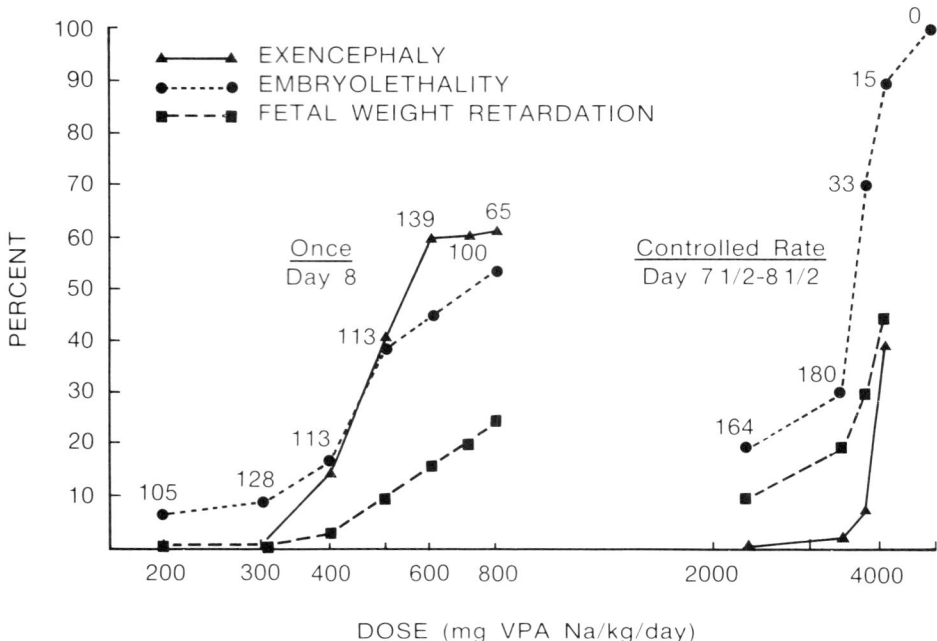

Fig. 6 — Dose–response curves for the embryotoxicity (lethality and fetal weight retardation) and teratogenicity (exencephaly) following single subcutaneous injections of valproic acid (VPA) on day 8 or controlled-rate administration via subcutaneously implanted mini-osmotic pumps between days 7 and 8 of gestation. The exencephaly rates are given as percentage of live fetuses (controls: water-injected, 0%; water-filled mini-osmotic pumps, 1%). The embryolethality was calculated as percentage resorptions per total implantations (controls: water-injected, 8.3%; water-filled mini-osmotic pumps, 12%). The fetal weight retardation is given as the weight reduction in per cent of the weights of the control group (1.18 ± 0.09 g). The numbers of live fetuses examined in each group are given as numerals (From Nau [7].)

the spatial distribution of ^{14}C and ^{3}H was determined relative to the cannula tip location. Tissue concentrations, expressed as a proportion of perfusate concentration, were maximal at the cannula tip and declined dramatically with radial distance from the tip (Fig. 7). Reflecting different physicochemical properties and/or binding and metabolism in brain tissue, each of the drugs perfused had a characteristic and unique distribution pattern (Fig. 7). At any given distance, concentrations of isotopes derived from the polar drugs DA and MTX were two orders of magnitude higher than those derived from the lipid-soluble drug AP. This reflects the exclusion of polar compounds by the blood–brain barrier. Following microperfusion, DA and MTX remain trapped in brain tissue, whereas the more lipid-soluble AP escapes across the blood–brain barrier and is removed by circulation.

From a therapeutic perspective, these results indicate that localized tissue can be exposed to high concentrations of drug directed from a catheter, while drug levels elsewhere remain insignificant. Such targeted administration might maximize local effects and limit side-effects in adjacent tissues or other areas of the body.

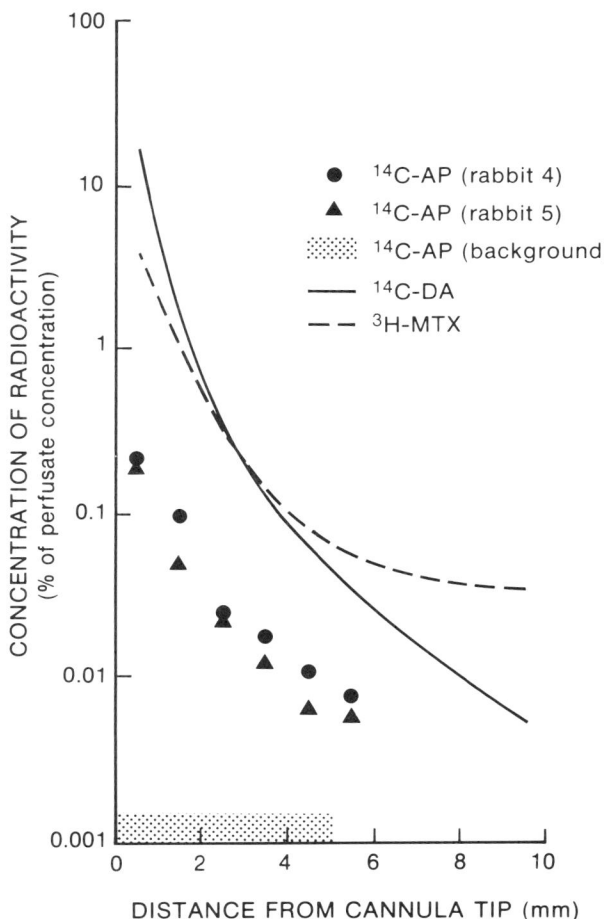

Fig. 7 — The spatial distribution of ¹⁴C in rabbits 4 and 5 after 6 days' microperfusion of [¹⁴C]antipyrine (AP) in the diencephalon. The solid bar shows the range of three background ¹⁴C measurements in the cortex of each rabbit. The spatial distributions of [³H]sodium methotrexate (MTX) and [¹⁴C]dopamine hydrochloride (DA) are the averages from rabbits 1, 2 and 3 plotted here for reference. Note that 'distance from the cannula tip' represents the distance from the cannula tip to the midpoint of 1 mm thick tissue sections. (From Sendelbeck and Urqhuart [10].)

Another example of targeted administration was recently reported in the transplantation literature by Ruers *et al.* [11]. Their work indicates that prednisolone administration to the transplanted kidney is superior to systemic treatment in prolongation of survival time and kidney function. These conclusions were reached by comparing prednisolone administration in rats according to the following schedule:

(a) Continuous intrarenal infusion, via the suprarenal or testicular artery

(b) Continuous systemic infusion delivered intraperitoneally
(c) Continuous systemic infusion delivered intravenously at the jugular vein
(d) Daily intraperitoneal injections.

In dosage regimen (a), prednisolone is administered directly to the kidney from which it is cleared. As a result, systemic concentrations of prednisolone are low when it is administered in this manner. Administration by regimens (b), (c) and (d) results in high systemic concentrations of prednisolone, and lower relative concentrations in the kidney.

At the lowest dose level, continuous intrarenal infusion prolonged graft survival time to a median of 26 days, whereas the same dose given systematically by regimens (b), (c) and (d) resulted in median survival times of 9, 8.5 and 7 days, respectively. At twice the lowest dose level, continuous intraperitoneal infusion increased median survival time (MST) to 16 days, though daily intraperitoneal injections at both two and three times the lowest dose gave an MST of only 8 days (Fig. 8). The MSTs of

Dosage (mg/kg/day)	Daily I.P. Injections		Continuous infusion					
			Intraperitoneal		Intravenous		Intrarenal	
	Survival Time (day)	Median Days	Survival Time (day)	Median Days	Survival Time (day)	Median Days	Survival Time (day)	Median Days
4	7.7.7.7.7 8.8.10.11	7	9.9.9.9 9.10.10.11	9	7.7.7.8 9.15.18	8.8	17.17.18 26.26>50 >50	26*
8	7.7.7.8.8 8.8.32	8	9.9.10.14 18.20.41>50	16**				
12	7.7.7.8 8.10.10	8						

*Wilcoxon rank test for difference between animals treated with intrarenal prednisolone (4 mg/kg body wt/day), continuous i.v. (P<0.05), continuous i.p. (P 0.01), or i.p. bolus injections (P 0.01).
**Wilcoxon rank test for difference between animals treated with continuous i.p. (8 mg/kg body wt/day) and i.p. bolus injections (P<0.01).

Fig. 8 — Survival times (days) of Lewis rats receiving Brown Norway renal allografts after various prednisolone treatments. (From Ruers *et al.* [11].)

untreated and control animals were 8 and 7 days, respectively. Serum urea levels for animals treated with various regimens of prednisolone, an indicator of kidney function, are shown in Fig. 9.

The technique for perfusing prednisolone locally via the suprarenal or testicular artery is shown in Fig. 10. The superiority of locally administered prednisolone in suppressing allograft rejection suggests that renally activated prodrugs of prednisolone or other immunosuppressive agents might be therapeutically attractive.

The longer survival of allografts with continuously infused versus bolus-injected intraperitoneal prednisolone confirms the earlier results of Provoost *et al.* [12] in studies on cardiac allograft survival. Continuously infused prednisolone has greater immunosuppressive action, dose for dose, compared to bolus-injected prednisolone.

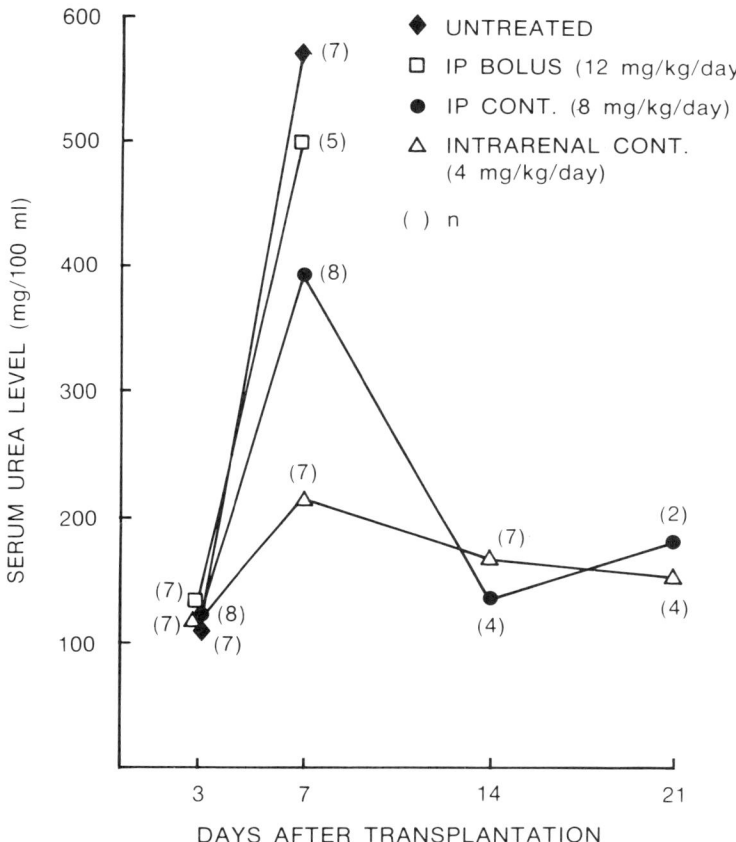

Fig. 9 — Mean serum urea levels in Lewis rats receiving Brown Norway renal allografts. Lewis recipients were untreated or received various prednisolone treatments. The numbers of surviving animals are indicated in the figure. (From Ruers *et al.* [11].)

4.3   Mini-osmotic pumps for patterned drug delivery

Although mini-osmotic pumps operate at a constant rate, they can be readily adapted to deliver drugs according to a time-varying schedule of mass delivery rates. Time-varied drug administration is accomplished by coupling the mini-osmotic pump to a catheter displacement tube containing a predetermined program of sequential drug infusions. The pump is filled with an inert liquid (e.g. Ringer's solution) and the displacement catheter containing the drug sequence can be thermoformed into a tight coil around the pump, forming a compact package that is readily implanted.

For example, if the catheter is loaded with a linear array of segments of drug solution, alternating with segments of an inert, drug-free spacer solution which is immiscible with the drug solutions, a time-based on-off effect is created (Fig. 11). The constant flow from the osmotic pump into one end of the coiled catheter

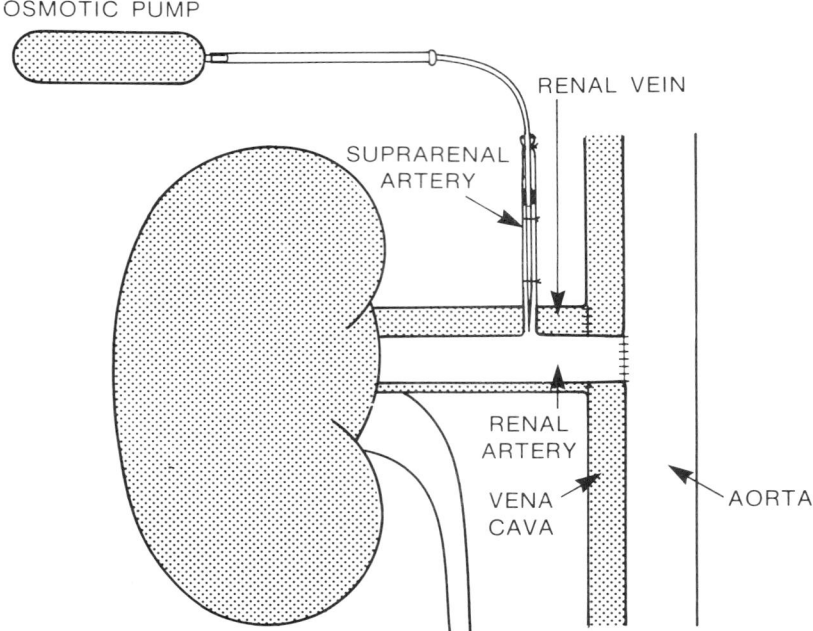

OSMOTIC PUMP

RENAL VEIN

SUPRARENAL
ARTERY

RENAL
ARTERY

VENA
CAVA

AORTA

Fig. 10 — Schematic outline of the experimental model used for drug infusion into the renal artery of a transplanted kidney. A catheter is introduced into the suprarenal (or testicular) artery of the transplanted kidney and connected to an osmotic pump implanted in the abdominal cavity. The osmotic pump delivers the drug in a continuous fashion from day 0 until day 13. (From Ruers *et al.* [11].)

displaces the contents of the coil from the opposite end in a linear, sequential fashion. Thus a linear array of alternating segments of drug solution and drug-free spacer solution in the catheter creates a pulsatile sequence of drug infusions into the animal. Other patterns of administration may be achieved by varying the concentration of drug in the segments (the amplitude of administration) or the length of the drug segments or spacers (the frequency of administration). More complexity is achieved if multiple drugs or multiple drug concentrations are used in the segments.

Adaptation for time-varied administration allows for investigation of the pharmacodynamics of time-varied drug administration patterns and the generation of synthetic circadian rhythms. Cronan *et al.* [13] used this time-varied method of drug administration to mimic the effects of human drug use patterns on rats. Infusion of nicotine with an 8 h on, 16 h off periodicity was used to mimic the normal use pattern of human tobacco smokers.

Lynch *et al.* [14] investigated the artificial induction of circadian melatonin rhythm in pinealectomized rats with this method. A polyethylene catheter was loaded with segments of aqueous melatonin solution accompanied by the dye phenolsulfonphthalein (PSP) alternating with segments of drug-free mineral oil (Fig. 12). The segments were arranged to create a daily cycle of 6 h of melatonin solution

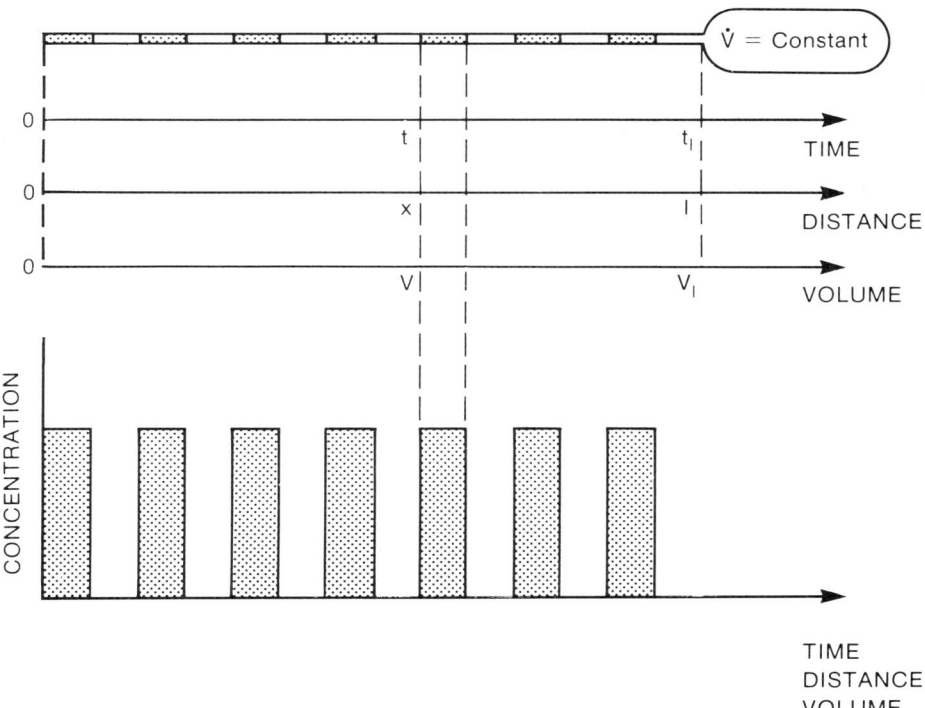

Fig. 11 — Catheter displacement tube filled with a drug program of the on-off type.

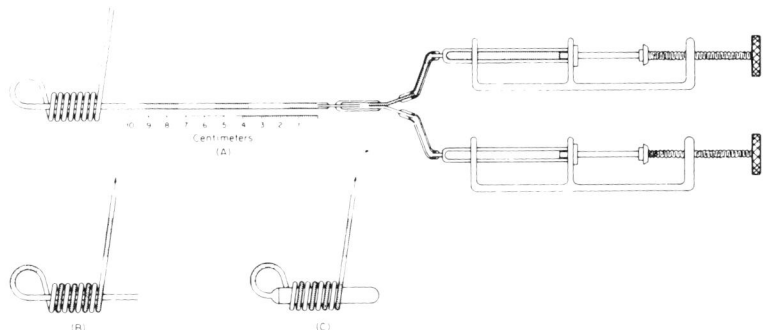

Fig. 12 — Programmed microinfusion apparatus. (A) Individual components of the infusate program are forced from microsyringes, via a manifold, into the straight feeder portion of a thermoformed capillary tubing forming the linearly arrayed program. (B) The program is then driven, with additional vehicle, into the coiled portion of the tubing. (C) The feeder portion of the tubing is cut off, a saline-filled osmotic mini-pump is attached, and the assembly is ready for implantation. (From Lynch *et al.* [14].)

alternating with 18 h of light mineral oil. Urine samples were collected from the infused rats every 6 h for 7 days and analyzed for melatonin and PSP. Because of the uniformity and frequency with which rats produce urine and void, urinary melatonin levels are a good temporal approximation of its renal clearance and blood levels [14]. The results, shown in Fig. 13, show the rhythmic appearance of melatonin and PSP in the urine.

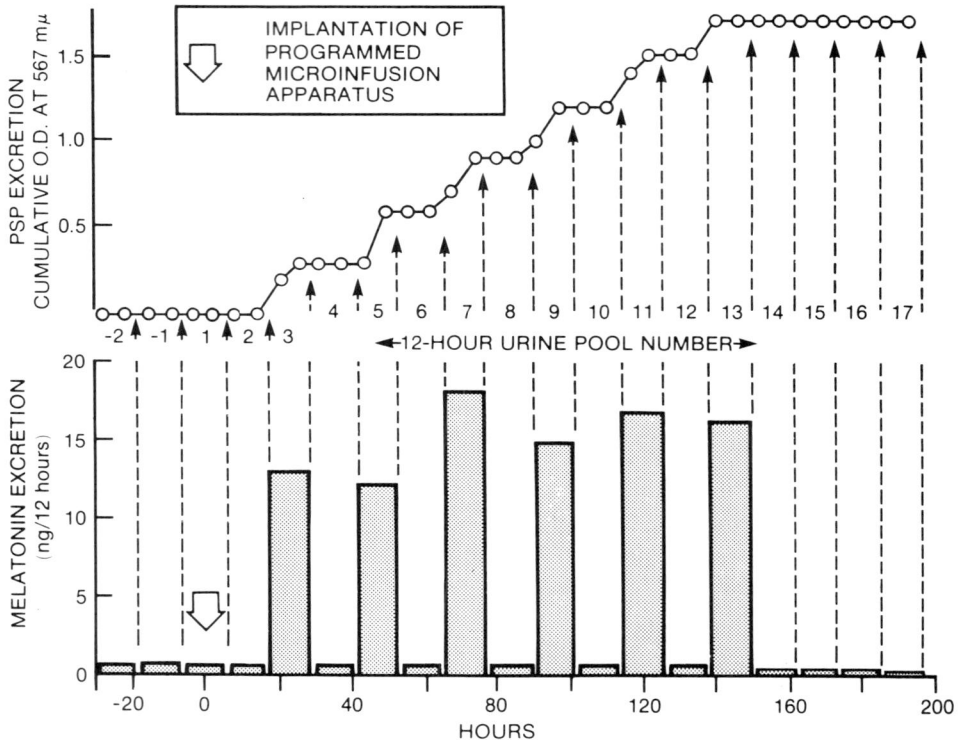

Fig. 13 — Rhythmic infusion of melatonin. A programmed infusate, consisting of 10 µg melatonin in phenolsulfonphthalein (PSP) solution alternating with melatonin-free mineral oil, was implanted in a pinealectomized rat. Urine samples were collected every 6 h and pooled according to the cyclic appearance of PSP, and the melatonin content of the urine samples was measured.

Temporally programmed delivery has also been used in reproductive studies. Lasley and Wing [15] successfully stimulated ovarian function in several exotic female carnivores with pulses of gonadotropin-releasing hormone (GnRH). A clouded leopard, a Temminck's golden cat, and a cheetah were implanted with a pump–coil unit programmed to release a 20-min pulse of GnRH (37.5–1.5 µg) alternating with 4 h of sterile peanut oil. In two of three trials, both at a higher amplitude of administration, estrus was successfully induced. In the case of the cheetah, later mating resulted in successful fertilization and birth (William Lasley, personal communication). Phillips *et al.* [16] achieved similar results with programmed GnRH infusions into female green iguanas. These results suggest that programmed administration may be a promising method of reproducing exotic endangered species in captivity.

5. CONCLUSIONS

Mini-osmotic pumps, although preprogrammed at discrete volumetric rates, allow the researcher freedom in the selection of drug and drug delivery rate. These systems function unattended to make rodent species into bioequivalent models compared to man, despite significant differences between the half-lives of drugs in the two species.

Although osmotic pumps deliver drugs by volume displacement, they deliver at very low flow rates that allow undisturbed targeted tissue or organ perfusion.

Catheter attachments to such pumps can be loaded with varying patterns of drugs for patterned drug delivery. Such systems appear to have unique value for polypeptide drug delivery.

REFERENCES

[1] Theeuwes, F. & Yum, S. I. (1976). Principles of the design and operation of generic osmotic pumps for the delivery of semisolid or liquid drug formulations. *Ann. Biomed. Eng.* **4** (4) 343–353.

[2] Rodrigues, K. T. & Sumpter, J. P. (1984). Effects of background adaptation on the pituitary and plasma concentrations of some pro-opiomelanocortin-related peptides in the rainbow trout (*Salmo gairdneri*). *J. Endocrinol.* **101** 277–284.

[3] Davison, T. F., Freeman, B. M. & Rea, J. (1985). Effects of continuous treatment with synthetic ACTH(1-24) or corticosterone on immature *Gallus domesticus*. *Gen. Comp. Endocrinol.* **59** 416–423.

[4] Nau, H., Trotz, M. & Wegner, C. (1985). Controlled-rate drug administration in testing for toxicity, in particular teratogenicity: towards interspecies bioequivalence. In: Breimer, D. D. & Speiser, P. (eds) *Topics in Pharmaceutical Sciences 1985,* Elsevier Press, New York, pp. 143–157.

[5] Fara, J. & Urquhart, J. (1984). The value of infusion and injection regimens in assessing efficacy and toxicity of drugs. *Trends Pharmacol. Sci.* **5** (1) 21–25.

[6] Nau, H., Zierer, R., Spielmann, H., Neubert, D. & Gansau, Ch. (1981). A new model for embryotoxicity testing: teratogenicity and pharmacokinetics of valproic acid following constant-rate administration in the mouse using human therapeutic drug and metabolite concentrations. *Life Sci.* **29** 2803–2814.

[7] Nau, H. (1985). Teratogenic valproic acid concentrations: infusion by implanted minipumps vs conventional injection regimen in the mouse. *Toxicol. Appl. Pharmacol.* **80** (2) 243–250.

[8] Sikic, B. I., Collins, J. M., Mimnaugh, E. G. & Gram, T. E. (1978). Improved therapeutic index of bleomycin when administered by continuous infusion in mice. *Cancer Treat. Rep.* **62** (12) 2011–2017.

[9] Urquhart, J., Fara, J. & Willis, K. L. (1984). Rate-controlled delivery systems in drug and hormone research. *Ann. Rev. Pharmacol. Toxicol.* **24** 199–236.

[10] Sendelbeck, S. L. & Urquhart, J. (1985). Spatial distribution of dopamine, methotrexate and antipyrine during continuous intracerebral microperfusion. *Brain Res.* **328** 251–258.

[11] Ruers, T. J. M., Buurman, W. A., Smits, J. F. M., van der Linden, C. J., van Dongen, J. J., Struyker-Boudier, H. A. J. & Kootstra, G. (1986). Local treatment of renal allografts, a promising way to reduce the dosage of immuno-suppressve drugs. *Transplantation* **41** (2) 156–161.

[12] Provoost, A. P., de Keyzer, M. H., Kort, W. J. & Wolff, E. D. (1982). Superiority of continuous infusion of prednisolone over daily injections in the prolongation of heart allograft survival in rats. *Transplantation* **34** 221–222.

[13] Cronan, T., Conrad, J. & Bryson, R. (1985). Effects of chronically administered nicotine and saline on motor activity in rats. *Pharmacol. Biochem. Behav.* **22** (5) 897–899.

[14] Lynch, H. J., Rivest, R. W. & Wurtman, R. J. (1980). Artificial induction of melatonin rhythms by programmed microinfusion. *Neuroendocrinol.* **31** 106–111.

[15] Lasley, B. L. & Wing, A. (1983). Stimulating ovarian function in exotic carnivores with pulses of GnRH. *Annu. Proc. Amer. Assoc. Zoo Vet. 1983*, 14–15.

[16] Phillips, J. A., Alexander, N., Karesh, W. B., Millar, R. & Lasley, B. L. (1985). Stimulating male sexual behaviour with repetitive pulses of GnRH in female green iguanas lguana–lguana. *J. Exper. Zool.* **234** 481–484.

8

Implantable pumps for insulin delivery: current clinical status

Perry J. Blackshear, Howard Hughes Medical Institute Laboratories at Duke University, Durham, North Carolina; and the Section of Diabetes and Metabolism, Division of Endocrinology, Metabolism and Genetics, Department of Medicine, Duke University Medical Center, Durham, North Carolina 27710, USA

1 INTRODUCTION

Totally implantable drug delivery systems have many advantages over more conventional forms of drug administration. These include the capability of providing improved rate control for parenteral drug delivery, i.e. for drugs which can only be administered parenterally because they are not absorbed from or are inactivated by the gastrointestinal tract; drugs which have short serum half-lives, and therefore would need to be administered in frequent pulses by conventional administration; and drugs which need to be provided with complex rate control, for example, multiple drugs or multiple infusion rates. In addition, totally implantable drug delivery systems offer the capability of site-specific drug delivery, as shown below. A major advantage is that they decrease the risk of infection which is inevitably associated with a chronic percutaneous access site, and can result not only in local inflammation and abscess formation but septicemia and death. And finally, in certain macroscopic types of delivery systems, the use of drugs is often possible which are commercially available and already approved by regulatory agencies.

Certain of these advantages and others are specific for totally implantable infusion pumps as opposed to, for example, diffusion-controlled and polymeric delivery systems. For example, in many of the infusion pumps under study today, relatively large volumes of relatively dilute drugs can be infused, often using drugs as they are supplied from the manufacturer. In most cases, the drug dose can be readily changed, stopped or alternated with other drugs or a placebo. The drug can be directed into a vascular site or body cavity using the drug delivery cannula, and in most cases, pump refills take the place of device reimplantations. For all of these reasons and more, totally implantable infusion pumps offer some advantages over conventional drug administration for specific uses. In the paragraphs below, I will briefly describe some of the devices currently in use and under study in the United States, describe one device with which I have been associated in some detail, and describe its use as a means of delivering insulin in patients with diabetes mellitus.

2. IMPLANTABLE INFUSION PUMPS

The first device of this type to be built was the relatively simple, vapor pressure-powered device developed by my colleagues and me at the University of Minnesota in 1969–1970, which has since become known as the Infusaid Implantable Infusion Pump, and is manufactured by the company of that name in Norwood, MA. This is a simple device which consists of a titanium disk-shaped cannister and both central and, in some cases, peripheral refill septa for changing the drug in the device. The peripheral septum or auxiliary side port is a useful additive for some clinical indications, and can be used as a means of injecting a bolus of the first drug, a bolus or short infusion of a second drug, a bolus or infusion of radionuclides for organ scanning or contrast agents for angiography, and many other uses. The pump, which we and others have described in detail in many previous publications (see refs [1–7] for reviews), is probably the simplest device of its type available and should be viewed as a first generation of this type of drug delivery device, since it is capable only of providing single rate liquid infusion under most circumstances. However, by far the greatest clinical experience in a variety of indications is with this device, and I will describe its more recent use as an insulin delivery vehicle below. Second- and third-generation implantable infusion pumps which have been developed since that time include a peristaltic pump, originally designed by workers at the University of New Mexico in collaboration with Sandia Laboratories, which utilizes an external controller for variable flow rate control [8]. This device has been used in limited clinical trials as an insulin delivery vehicle over the past several years [9], and newer prototypes are under development for more extensive clinical trials. Another peristaltic device was designed and built by workers at Siemens A. G. in Germany, again with an external rate controller; this has also been used as a means of providing insulin infusion in patients with diabetes, mostly in Europe [10]. Still newer, and probably appropriately called third-generation devices, are those developed by Medtronic, Inc. in Minneapolis [11] and the applied physics laboratory at Johns Hopkins University in collaboration with Pacesetters, Inc. and Parker-Hanafin, Inc. [12]. Both of these are very complex devices with remote programmability and virtually infinitely variable flow rate capabilities. In the case of the Medtronic device, considerable clinical experience has accumulated using this device as a means of providing intra-arterial anticancer drugs, intraspinal preservative-free morphine for patients with intractable cancer pain and antispasticity drugs; in the case of the Johns Hopkins device, extensive animal studies of the device as a means of providing insulin infusion are just now being completed, and clinical trials are expected sometime in the near future.

Let me return to a brief description of the Infusaid implantable infusion pump; details of its design and operating principles can be found in several early papers [1–7]. The device is a disk-shaped titanium cannister divided into two chambers by collapsible welded titanium bellows. The pump's inner chamber contains the drug to be infused or the infusate; the outer chamber contains a vapor–liquid mixture of a fluorocarbon chemical power source. Under the conditions of constant temperature which prevail in the human body under normal circumstances, the vapor–liquid mixture exerts a constant vapor pressure against the pump's inner chamber, thus extruding the drug through a flow-regulating resistance element and a series of filters into the delivery cannula and into a vein, artery or body cavity. During the refill manouver, a special needle is inserted through the skin through the self-sealing refill septum in the center of the pump, and by means of a hand-held injection the new dose of drug is injected into the pump, simultaneously refilling the inner chamber with new drug and condensing the vapor in the outer chamber. Thus, a single operation refills and 'recharges' the pump, allowing continuous functioning with an inexhaustible power source.

For many applications involving central venous infusion or infusions in the head, neck or spine area, the device is implanted under the skin of the anterior chest with the delivery cannula threaded into the appropriate location. This operation is very similar to that involved in a cardiac pacemaker implantation, and can be done by a skilled surgeon in 30–45 min under local anesthesia. By far the biggest use of this pump in the United States is for intra-arterial infusion chemotherapy into the hepatic artery for metastases from colorectal cancer [13–15]; for this indication, the device is generally implanted under the skin of the anterior abdomen under general anesthesia and the delivery cannula is threaded into the hepatic artery via a tributary artery [7]. In both anatomical locations, the pump causes a significant bulge which makes refilling easier but does not appear to interfere significantly with the patients' daily activities, including active sports. For pump refills, the skin over the pump is anesthetized with a bleb of lidocaine, a special needle is inserted through the skin and through the self-sealing septum, the residual fluid within the pump is allowed to fill an empty syringe barrel, and a new syringe with a new supply of drug is injected into the pump, either manually or with a mechanical assist device. Although at a given viscosity of drug solution the fluid flow rate is constant in a given pump, the dose of drug to be delivered can be readily altered by changing the concentration of the drug in the infusate while maintaining constant viscosity.

During its approximately 11 years of clinical use in the USA and in Europe, this infusion pump has been used in a wide variety of clinical indications, and is the first device of its type to be approved by the Food and Drug Administration for certain clinical uses. Examples of these uses include, among the approved uses, intra-arterial, intra-arterial plus intravenous, or intra-arterial or intravenous infusion of FUDR or 5-fluorouracil for metastatic carcinoma. This is an example of an indication where site-specific drug delivery is helpful. The pump has been used to administer heparin into the central venous system for refractory clotting problems that are not responsive to oral anticoagulants. It has also been approved for use in delivering preservative-free morphine into the subdural or intrathecal spinal spaces for intractable pain of malignancy and to deliver localized infusions of chemotherapeutic drugs for a variety of solid tumours. In each case, the delivery cannula can be positioned surgically at the site or sites within the blood vessels or body cavity at which infusion is most advantageous. In addition to the above approved uses of the device, many other drug–device combinations are under study for experimental purposes. Examples of these include the intra-arterial infusion of Adriamycin for treatment of primary liver cancer or hepatoma; direct infusion into the cerebral ventricles of bleomycin for treatment of carcinoma of the brain parenchyma; the intrathecal infusion of other drugs such as codeine for the pain of malignancy; intravenous or intraperitoneal infusion of insulin in the treatment of diabetes, as I will describe in more detail below; the intraventricular infusion or urocholine for Alzheimer's disease; the intravenous infusion of dobutamine for congestive heart failure; and the localized infusion, often with two delivery cannulae, of aminoglyco- side antibiotics in the treatment of refractory localized osteomyelitis. Many of these uses, such as infusion directly into the cerebral ventricles or intrathecal space, are really only practicable using totally implanted delivery systems, since the risk of infection from a percutaneous access site in general is prohibitive.

3. DIABETES MELLITUS

My work with this implantable infusion pump for the past many years has involved its use as a means of providing insulin infusion in patients with diabetes mellitus. This is one of the most common chronic diseases in westernized countries, with prevalence rates approaching 3% in the United States population at the present time, and many extrapolations suggesting that the prevalence rates will be still higher in the succeeding years, especially in the older age group, which comprises most of the patients with adult onset or type II diabetes. In the United States and other westernized countries, approximately 90% of the patients with diabetes have the type II or adult-onset variety, often associated with obesity; 10% or so have type I or juvenile-onset diabetes, for which exogenous insulin administration is mandatory to maintain life over the short term. Although it is commonly assumed by patients and often by their physicians that type II diabetes is a 'mild' form of the disease, numerous studies provide statistical evidence that the long-term complications of the disease are just about as frequent and as devastating in patients with type II diabetes as they are in patients with the type I form of the disease. For example, in data compiled by Pirart and his colleagues [16] and summarized recently by us [5], the prevalence rates of the three major long-term complications of diabetes, retino- pathy, neuropathy and nephropathy, were similar in type I and type II patients as functions of duration of disease, so that by the end of 25 years of diabetes, the prevalence rates of these complications in both groups were approximately 60% for retinopathy, 40% for neuropathy, and 15% for nephropathy. In addition, patients with type II diabetes have increased frequencies of coronoary artery disease and large artery atherosclerosis, leading to increased morbidity and mortality. Finally, the disease is associated with many other medical and social problems leading to patient morbidity and economic loss.

The assumption has been made by most investigators that normalization of glycemic control will be necessary and sufficient to achieve the delay or prevention of the development of these complications. This assumption is based on a large number of animal studies, as well as anecdotal clinical trials. A very large study called the Diabetes Control and Complications Trial supported by the National Institutes of Health in the United States is attempting to change this assumption into fact, but the results will not be available for many years. What is undeniable at the present time is that conventional insulin treatment of patients with both type I and type II diabetes, in general, is not adequate to normalize the blood glucose and thus, I believe, prevent the long-term complications of the disease. A recent example of the failure of conventional therapy is indicated by some data which my colleagues and I compiled at the Massachusetts General Hospital in 1985. Of approximately 200 patients with type II diabetes attending our diabetes clinic, only 23% of patients treated with diet alone, 16% of patients treated with oral agents alone, and 7% of patients treated with insulin had glycosylated hemoglobin values within the normal range. We did not do comparable studies in patients with type I diabetes, but since they are generally more difficult to manage with insulin injections, we assume that the results would be equally dismal. These data suggest that by far the majority of patients with type II diabetes treated in the traditional way are not adequately controlled by whatever treatment modality they are using, and thus are at risk for the long-term complications of diabetes. This is one of the major problems which we have attempted to address using implantable insulin infusion devices.

Our own studies with the Minnesota pump as a means of delivering insulin date back to the early 1970s, when we first attempted to use this device as a means of infusing insulin into dogs with diabetes induced by pancreatectomy. In those days, the thermal stability of insulin was a major problem which prevented successful use of this device as an insulin delivery vehicle. However, in the mid 1970s, with the development of neutral regular insulin solutions which were stable at 37°C, we believed that clinical use of this device as a means of providing insulin infusion would be just around the corner. However, it rapidly became clear that insulin precipitated within the devices, preventing effective drug delivery after 20–60 days of infusion in the diabetic animals [17]. This phenomenon has been seen by many investigators attempting to use implantable devices as means of delivering insulin infusions [18], and is probably due to a combination of factors which lead to insulin precipitation or the formation of insoluble insulin fibrils in a process known as heat fibrillation. Examples of factors which lead to insulin precipitation include: acidification of the neutral insulin to the isoelectric point of the protein, which is approximately pH 5.8; chelation of the zinc which is naturally included in the zinc insulin hexamer, which is the way insulin exists in solution; excess divalent cation; heat fibrillation, which is the formation of insoluble insulin fibrils due to one or more stresses such as heat, shear, or agitation; and finally, insulin has the propensity to form soluble, presumably less active, polymers and oligomers, in some cases in opposite circumstances from those which promote formation of the insulin fibrils. All of these factors have led to difficulties in the formulation of insulin/pump combinations which can provide effective insulin delivery. Thus, although we were able to infuse insulin successfully for relatively short periods of time in the late 1970s in diabetic animals, including variable rate infusions with mealtime insulin boluses [19], we were never able to sustain these constant infusions long enough for human clinical use.

However, early in the 1980s we hit upon the solution of using high concentrations of glycerol to stabilize the insulin in these pumps. Glycerol was chosen because of its well-known ability to prevent denaturation of proteins which occurs after subjecting the proteins to a variety of stresses [20]. In our earliest studies, glycerol appeared to prevent the formation of the insulin aggregates which clogged pumps and delivery cannulae and prevented flow in animals and some patients with diabetes; however, it soon became apparent that the insulin was losing potency in the drug delivery devices at 37°C, even though it would remain in solution. We discovered that this was due to the glycerol-induced formation of soluble insulin oligomers or polymers, which seemed to have lower biological activity [21]. Various buffering solutions were used in an attempt to combat the formation of oligomers with relatively modest success [21]. This gradual insulin inactivation by glycerol remained a minor problem with the device in its earliest clinical uses as an insulin delivery vehicle, with decreases in potency of 10–15% over the course of a refill cycle being acceptable for the degree of diabetes control achieved by the device. However, not only was the loss of potency worrisome, but there was also the possibility that the insulin oligomers could prove antigenic in themselves or could inhibit the binding of native insulin to its receptors within the body. Very recently, T. D. Rohde and his colleagues at the University of Minnesota have found that purification of the glycerol itself by use of several column fractionation steps could remove apparent impurities from even the most pure commercially available glycerol. Purified glycerol with insulin has now been used in animal studies where it has provided superior glycemic control and superior insulin potency to the commercially available glycerol solutions in use before; in addition, as assessed by polyacrylamide gel electrophoresis under non-reducing conditions, the purified glycerol does not promote the formation of insulin polymers and oligomers, which reflected its gradual inactivation at 37°C [22]. Thus, although the glycerol/ insulin solution is somewhat unwieldy because of its extreme viscosity, it appears that the use of purified glycerol in combination with neutral regular insulin might be a feasible insulin formulation for use in this device for long-term infusions; clinical studies of this combination are now underway. It should be noted that glycerol has a long history of intravenous use for a variety of indications including cerebral edema [23–26]; the amount of glycerol to be delivered intravenously or intraperitoneally when used as an insulin adjunct is much lower than the amount of glycerol formed in a typical day by adipose tissue lipolysis.

There have been several recent studies of this device as a means of providing continuous, intravenous or interperitoneal insulin infusion in patients with both type II and type I diabetes. The first report was by Buchwald *et al.* [27], which demonstrated feasibility in a single patient. A later report by the same group [28] showed that very reasonable glycemic control could be achieved with infusions up to 9 months in patients with type II diabetes. Irsigler and his colleagues, using the interperitoneal route, used the device as a means of providing long-term insulin infusions in patients with both type I and type II diabetes; they have accumulated by far the largest clinical experience to date with this device [29, 30]. Our own group at the Massachusetts General Hospital infused intravenous insulin for more than 4 years as of this writing in two patients with adult-onset or type II diabetes [31]. Their glycemic control during this period has been excellent and no complications or significant hypoglycemic episodes have ensued. On the basis of this encouraging result, we have embarked upon a larger cross-over study, comparing basal insulin delivery by this means with two types of conventional insulin therapy, which we judged to be the most common forms of insulin therapy in type II patients used in the United States today. These were single daily injections of lente or NPH insulin and a single daily injection of ultralente insulin. Although not all of the data have been analyzed, our preliminary data suggest that the control achieved by carefully monitored single daily injections of lente insulin is very similar to that achieved by continuous, basal rate intravenous insulin infusions when the same patients were crossed over and used as their own controls. However, the ambient insulin concentration and the risk of hypoglycemic episodes appeared to be somewhat lower in the patients receiving pump therapy. Completion of the study and the final data analysis will determine whether these points can be substantiated. A final group of patients in whom this device has been particularly useful is a rare group of patients suffering from a poorly understood syndrome of resistance to subcutaneously injected insulin. Buchwald and his colleagues have recently published their results with a series of such patients [32]; there are other anecdotal reports in the literature, including our own unpublished data on a single patient with this syndrome. The provision of intravenous insulin infusions using this device in these patients has radically altered their lives in many cases, from lives of total invalidism in which they spent most of their time in the hospital with ketoacidosis or on intravenous insulin infusions, to lives resembling those of normal type I or type II diabetic patients with few, if any, returns to the hospital.

Although I believe that it is fair to say that this device has been shown to function appropriately as a means of providing continuous, basal rate insulin infusions in patients with type I and type II diabetes, and that the use of the purified glycerol–insulin combination should substantially improve upon this record, there are several problems with its use as an insulin delivery vehicle. One obvious problem is that the device in its current formulation is only capable of providing basal rate infusions, which might be appropriate for some type II patients but which are certainly likely to be inappropriate for most patients with type I diabetes, for whom bolus injections of insulin at mealtime and possibly at other times would be indicated. Major design modifications will have to be made in this device for this type of infusion to be possible; this has already been done in the case of some of the second- and third-generation devices mentioned above, and it may be that they will prove more suitable for use in the insulin infusion indication. Another problem is that, even for type II patients, there is no convincing evidence that continuous infusion therapy of this kind provides superior glycemic control over conventional therapy, or provides equivalent therapy with substantial decreases in complication, frequency, hypoglycemic episodes or other problems. Finally, the patients who have been included in the various experimental trials of the device have all been willing volunteers; it remains to be seen whether this type of drug delivery might be considered too radical for use in the general population.

An interesting study which addresses this last point to some extent is a recent survey of attitudes of patients undergoing implantable infusion pump-mediated insulin therapy conducted by Meize-Grochowski [33]. She studied 61 patients from three centers, both type I and type II diabetic subjects, in which 57 received extensive questionnaires and 23 were subjected to in-depth interviews. The results of her study are quite illuminating, and I will summarize some of the interesting points here. First, although in reality the patients had no control over the amount of insulin which they received, more than 75% of the patients felt that they had more control over their diabetes with the pump than before the pump. Seventy per cent felt that the pump had no impact on their social life and 65% felt that it had no impact on their relationships with others or with their jobs and no patients complained of interference with sexual activity. Many patients reported positive aspects of the implantable pump therapy including more freedom in life-style reported by 47% of the patients, improvement in their blood glucose control reported by 38% of the patients, and many other positive aspects. The negative aspects of having an implanted pump were somewhat surprising to those of us involved in these studies. By far the most commonly cited negative aspect was the inconvenience of the clinic appointments for the pump refills, an aspect which was complained about by fully 47% of the respondents. All other negative aspects each comprised less than 10% of the patients' complaints. The patients also expressed a number of fears about having an implantable insulin pump, fears which seemed to be appropriate under the circumstances, including fear of catheter occlusion, pump malfunction, surgery to replace or remove the pump, nocturnal hypoglycemic reactions, sudden release of all insulin, air embolism, or in one case, the inability to detect incipient breast cancer under the pump. The most revealing statistics to me, were that 87% of the patients felt that their overall health was improved with the pump, and fully 100% said that they would do it again, knowing what they now know about the pump and about the research program. Again, these are studies on willing, normal volunteers, but may give some indication as to the acceptability of this type of therapy in the normal population.

4.   THE FUTURE

Based on our experience with these devices as implantable insulin delivery vehicles, I believe that these or related devices may well be in widespread clinical use within the next 10 or 20 years. This implies the availability of devices which can provide not only basal rate insulin infusion but bolus or square-wave infusions of higher insulin delivery rates at mealtime. Obviously, it would be highly desirable to combine such an insulin delivery device with a totally implanted glucose sensor, and thus achieve what has been the 'Holy Grail' for researchers in this field, the development of a completely close-loop implantable artificial beta cell. Although sensor development has been under study for more than 15 or 20 years, there is still no sensor, to my knowledge, which is ready for combination with one of these insulin delivery devices to make a completely closed-loop artificial beta cell. Several serious problems in sensor technology, including electrode drift and problems with standardization in a totally implanted device, as well as changes in sensor function with overgrowth of tissue cells, have made this an extremely difficult problem to solve. In addition, it is possible that within the next 10, 20 or 30 years, many types of diabetes will be treated with various therapies which are now considered experimental. For example, recent advances in the immunotherapy of recent-onset type I diabetes suggest the possibility that appropriate immunological modifications might prevent the development of the full-fledged diabetes syndrome by preventing the permanent damage to the beta cells which occurs due to this apparently autoimmune insult. Similarly, recent advances in the molecular biology of the insulin gene and studies of its tissue-specific expression suggest that it might be possible to consider gene transplantation in patients with type I diabetes, who have few or no functioning beta cells. In type II diabetes, much remains to be learned about the primary defect and how it might best be treated. The simple expedient of preventing obesity in susceptible patients would reduce to a huge extent the percentage of the population which has type II diabetes. Since this group has some of its own endogenous insulin secretion, it may be that this will become the most appropriate population for implanted insulin infusion systems, with the timing rather than the amount of insulin restored by this artificial means. Whatever the eventual outcome it seems clear that the next 10 to 20 years will be an active time for research into insulin delivery devices of all kinds, and their clinical evaluation.

ACKNOWLEDGEMENTS

I thank my many colleagues for their contributions to the work described here, especially T. D. Rohde and A. R. Meize-Grochowski for providing me with unpublished data, and I thank Lessie Detwiler for typing the manuscript.

REFERENCES

[1] Blackshear, P. J., Dorman, F. D., Blackshear, P. L., Jr., Varco, R. L. & Buchwald, H. (1972). The design and initial testing of an implantable infusion pump. *Surgery, Gynecology & Obstetrics* **134** 51–56.

[2] Blackshear, P. J., Rohde, T. D., Varco, R. L. & Buchwald, H. (1975). One year of continuous heparinization in the dog using a totally implantable infusion pump. *Surgery, Gynecology & Obstetrics* **141** 176–186.

[3] Blackshear, P. J., Rohde, T. D., Prosl, F. & Buchwald, H. (1979). The implantable infusion pump: a new concept in drug delivery. *Med. Prog. Technol.* **6** 149–161.

[4] Blackshear, P. J. (1979). Implantable drug-delivery systems. *Sci. Am.* **241** 66–73.

[5] Blackshear, P. J. & Rohde, T. D. (1984). Artificial devices for insulin infusion in the treatment of patients with diabetes mellitus. In: Bruck S. D. (ed.) *Controlled Drug Delivery*, Vol. II, CRC Press, Inc., Boca Raton, pp. 111–147.

[6] Blackshear, P. J. (1985). Implantable infusion pumps: clinical applications. In: Colowick, S. P. & Kaplan, N. O. (eds) *Methods in Enzymology,* vol. 112, Academic Press, New York, pp. 520–530.

[7] Blackshear, P. J., Wigness, B. D., Roussell, A. M. & Cohen, A. M. (1985). Implantable infusion pumps: practical aspects. In: Colowick, S. P. & Kaplan, N. O. (eds) *Methods in Enzymology,* vol. 112, Academic Press, New York, pp. 530–545.

[8] Carlson, G. A., Love, J. t., Urenda, R. S., *et al.* (1981). Development of an artificial beta cell suitable for animal implantation. *Trans. Am. Soc. Artif. Intern. Organs* **26** 523–526.

[9] Schade, D. S., Eaton, R. P., Edwards, W. S., *et al.* (1982). A remotely programmable insulin delivery system: successful short-term implantation in man. *JAMA* **247** 1848–1853.

[10] Selam, J. L., Slingenmeyer, A., Chaptal, P. A., Franetzki, M., Prestele, K. & Mirouze, J. (1982). Total implantation of a remotely controlled insulin mini-pump in a human insulin-dependent diabetic. *Artif. Organs* **6** 315–319.

[11] Comben, R., Bartelt, K., Elsberry, D., *et al.* (1983). Experimental and clinical

studies using medtronics programmable implantable drug administration device. *Artif. Organs* **7A** 107.

[12] Fischell, R. E., Radford, W. E., Hogrefe, A. F., *et al.* (1983) . A programmable implantable system (PIMS) for the treatment of diabetes. *Artif. Organs* **7A** 82.

[13] Buchwald, H., Grage, T. B., Vassilopoulos, P. R., Rohde, T. D., Varco, R. L. & Blackshear, P. J. (1980). Intra-arterial infusion chemotherapy for hepatic carcinoma using a totally implantable infusion pump. *Cancer* **45** 866–869.

[14] Enzminger, W., Niederhuber, J., Dakhil, S., Thrall, J. & Wheeler, R. (1981). Totally implanted drug delivery system for hepatic arterial chemotherapy. *Cancer Treat. Rep.* **65** 393–400.

[15] Cohen, A. M., Woods, W. C., Greenfield, A., Waltman, A., Dedrick, C., & Blackshear, P. J. (1980). Transbrachial hepatic arterial chemotherapy using an implantable infusion pump. *Dis. Colon. Rectum* **23** 223–227.

[16] Pirart, J. (1978). Diabetes mellitus and its degenerative complications: a prospective study of 440 patients observed between 1947 and 1973. *Diabetes Care* **1** 168–188, 253–263.

[17] Blackshear, P. J., Rupp, W. M., Rohde, T. D. & Buchwald, H. (1983). A totally implantable constant rate insulin infusion device: preliminary studies in Type II diabetic subjects. In: Brunnetti, P., Alberti, K. G. M. M., Albisser, A. M., Heff, K. D. & Mussin Benedetti, M. (eds) *Artificial Systems for Insulin Delivery,* Raven Press, New York, pp. 131–139.

[18] Lougheed, W. D., Woulfe-Flanagan, H., Clement, J. R. & Albisser, A. M. (1980). Insulin aggregation in artificial delivery systems. *Diabetologia* **19** 1–9.

[19] Blackshear, P. J., Rohde, T. D., Grotting, J. C., Dorman, F. D., Perkins, R. P., Varco, R. L. & Buchwald, H. (1979). Control of blood glucose in experimental diabetes by means of a totally implantable insulin infusion device. *Diabetes* **28** 634–639.

[20] Back, J. F., Oakenfull, D. & Smith, M. B. (1979). Increased thermal stability of proteins in the presence of sugars and polyols. *Biochemistry* **18** 5191–5196.

[21] Blackshear, P. J., Rohde, T. D., Palmer, J. L., Wigness, B. D., Rupp, W. M. & Buchwald, H. (1983). Glycerol prevents insulin precipitation and interruption of flow in an implantable insulin infusion pump. *Diabetes Care* **6** 387–392.

[22] Blackshear, P. J., Robbins, D. C., Rohde, T. D., Langer, R. S., Moses, A. C. & Massey, E. H. (1986). Insulin replacement: current concepts. Proceedings of the 32nd Annual Meeting of American Society for Artificial Organs, Inc., Anaheim, CA, May, 1986. *ASAIO Trans.* (in press).

[23] Mathew, N. T., Rivera, V. M., Meyer, J. S., Charney, J. Z. & Hartmann, A. (1972). Double-blind evaluation of glycerol therapy in acute cerebral infarction. *Lancet* **2** 1327–1330.

[24] Meyer, J. J., Fukuuchi, Y., Shimazu, K., Ohnchi, T. & Ericsson, A. D. (1972). Effect of intravenous infusion of glycerol in hemispheric blood flow and metabolism in patients with acute cerebral infarction. *Stroke* **3** 168–180.

[25] Sloviter, H. A. (1958). Effects of the intravenous administration of glycerol solutions to animals and man. *J. Clin. Invest.* **37** 619–626.

[26] Tourtellotte, W. W., Reinglass, J. L. & Newkirk, T. A. (1972). Cerbral

dehydration action of glycerol. 1. Historical aspects with emphasis on the toxicity and intravenous administration. *Clin. Pharmacol. Ther.* **13** 159–171.

[27] Buchwald, H., Barbosa, J., Varco, R. L., Rohde, T. D., Rupp, W. M., Schwartz, R. A., Goldenberg, F. J., Rublein, T. G. & Blackshear, P. J. (1981). Treatment of type II diabetic patients by a totally implantable insulin infusion device. *Lancet* **1** 1233–1235.

[28] Rupp, W. M., Barbosa, J., Blackshear, P. J., McCarthy, H. B., Rohde, T. D., Goldenberg, F. J., Rubelin, T. G., Dorman, F. D. & Buchwald, H. (1982). Implantable insulin pump therapy in type II diabetics. *N. Engl. J. Med.* **307** 265–270.

[29] Irsigler, K., Kritz, H., Hagmueller, G., Najemnik, C. & Lovett, R. (1983). Implanted constant basal rate infusions systems for Type I diabetic patients. In: Irsigler, K., Kritz, H. & Lovett, R. (eds) *Diabetes Treatment with Implantable Insulin Infusion Systems,* Urban & Schwarzenberg, Vienna, Austria, 52–63.

[30] Najemnik, C., Kritz, H. & Irsigler, K. (1983). Improvement of diabetic neuropathy in Type I patients after six months of treatment with insulin infusion devices. In: Irsigler, K., Kirtz, H. & Lovett, R. (eds) *Diabetes Treatment with Implantable Insulin Infusion Systems,* Urban & Schwarzenberg, Austria, Vienna pp. 184–193.

[31] Blackshear, P. J., Shulman, G. I., Roussell, A. M., Nathan, D. M., Minaker, K. L., Rowe, J. W., Robbins, D. C. & Cohen, A. M. (1985). Metabolic response to three years of continuous basal rate intravenous insulin infusion in Type II diabetic patients. *J. Clin. Endocrinol. & Metab.* **61** 753–760.

[32] Buchwald, H., Chute, E. P., Goldenberg, F. J., Hitchbock, C. R., Hoogwerf, B. F., Barbosa, J. J., Rupp, W. M. & Rohde, T. D. (1985). Implantable infusion pump management of insulin resistant diabetes mellitus. *Ann. Surg.* **202** 278–282.

[33] Meize-Grochowski, A. R. (1986). Psycho-social aspects of implantable insulin pump therapy in diabetic individuals. PhD Thesis, University of Texas-Austin.

9

Technological advances in oral drug delivery

D. Ganderton, Chelsea Department of Pharmacy, King's College London (KQC), Chelsea Campus, Manresa Road, London SW3 6LX

1. INTRODUCTION

Unlike all other systems described in this volume, control of the delivery of drugs by the oral route has a long history which began with the introduction of the 'Spansule' in 1952. It has enjoyed great commercial success with sales of products reaching almost $700 million during 1984 in the USA alone. Although potassium supplements, xanthines, non-analgesic cold remedies and medicines for cardiac arrhythmias are major product areas, the fragmentation of the market is exemplifed by the 80 or so products licensed in Great Britain and listed in Table 1.

The developed nature of this market ensures that a formal regulatory response will meet further innovations. Guidelines are now well established which largely define the performance criteria of new products. Furthermore, hostility to much new product development exists and a recent statement in *Drug and Therapeutics Bulletin* [1] dismissed sustained-release formulations of antidepressives, antihistamines, benzodiazepines, glyceryl trinitrate, isosorbide dinitrate, phenobarbitone, phenothiazine, pyridoxine and other vitamins as unnecessary. Elsewhere, it has been argued that many other products are superfluous because slow elimination confers long action or a wide therapeutic index permits a suitable dosage interval with conventional products. Thus, perhaps only one chemical entity in ten or fifteen is a logical candidate for refined oral presentation. This, then, is the technical climate in which the innovator must work.

The result is that much invention is orthodox and dull. A British patent published on 26 March 1986 to the Nikken Chemical Company of Japan [2] describes a simple mixture of theophylline and ethylcellulose, the ratio of which is varied to systematically modulate release from a compact. It exemplifies the extensive efforts within the pharmaceutical industry on minor variants of disintegrating or non-disintegrating matrices and on drug reservoirs enclosed by a constraining boundary, the principles of which are well established and need not be further discussed here. Occasionally, however, the scientific or patent literature decribes truly novel devices and, like

Table 1 — List of sustained-release products on British market

Acetazolamide	Isosorbide dinitrate
Aloin	Isosorbide mononitrate
Aminophylline	Isoxsuprine
Amitriptyline	
Ascorbic acid	Ketoprofen
Aspirin	
Azatadine maleate	Levamphetamine
Belladonna alkaloids	Levodopa
	Lithium carbonate
Benzhexol	Lithium citrate
Brompheniramine	Metoprolol
Bufyline	
Butmetanide	Mexiletine
Butriptyline	Morphine sulphate
Carbenoxolone	Nicotinyl alcohol
Chlorpheniramine	Noscapine
Clioquinol	
Cyclopenthiazide potassium	Orphenadrine
Dexamphetamine	Papaverine hydrochloride
Diazepam	Pentaerythritol tetranitrate
Dibenzepin	Pheniramine
Diclofenac	Phenolphthalein
Dicyclomine	Phentermine
Diethylpropion	Phenylephrine hydrochloride
Dimethindine	Phenylpropanolamine hydrochloride
Diphenylpyraline	Pindolol
Disopyramide	Propranolol
Doxylamine	Potassium chloride
	Procainamide
Enzymes, various	Prochlorperazine
Ephedrine hydroxychloride	Pyridoxine hydrochloride
Ferrous glycine sulphate	Quinidine bisulphate
Ferrous sulphate	
Frusemide	Reserpine
Glyceryl trinitrate	Salbutamol
	Sodium chloride
Hydrochlorothiazide	
Hyoscyamine sulphate	Terbutaline
	Tetracycline
Indomethacin	Theophylline
Isoetharine	Theophyllinate, choline
Isoprenaline	Trifluoperazine
Isopropamide iodide	
	Vitamins, various

other delivery systems, they can be analysed in terms of three criteria: the site, the duration and the intensity of drug action.

Relatively few inventions address the first criterion by releasing drugs at a specific site. These are either designed to give a local effect in a particular part of the gut, such as carbenoxalone in the treatment of duodenal ulcer, or select a particular part of the gut for transfer to the systemic circulation. This is exemplified by enteric coating.

Rather more devices seek to modify the intensity of effect, either as an increase facilitated by a carrier which raises the rate or extent of absorption or as a decrease brought about by the erection of a barrier to drug release and absorption. These barriers reduce peak blood levels and associated side-effects without unduly decreasing the amount absorbed. However, if future developments can be judged from an extrapolation of current activity, the devices meeting the third criterion and extending the duration of drug action will continue to dominate the field.

2.   TARGETING OF DRUGS IN THE GASTROINTESTINAL TRACT

Gastrointestinal motility — a vigorous and variable phenomenon — presents a major impediment to the invention of residential devices necessary for site-specific drug release. This is most easily overcome in the large intestine where conditions are most predictable and quiescent. The scintigraphic studies carried out by Hardy et al. [3] to measure the transit of single and multiparticulate devices to the colon showed that drugs should be retained in the product for 5 h followed by a release period of 10 h. Such devices might have advantages in the treatment of ulcerative colitis, Crohn's disease or cancer of the colon. A patent assigned to Roussel-UCLAF [4] describes a colonic delivery device which consists of a conventional core containing an active ingredient, such as 5-amino salicylic acid, which bears two coats. The inner coat consists of a plasticized film resistant to neutral and alkaline conditions. Ethyl cellulose is preferred and through the film a significant proportion of microcrystalline cellulose is dispersed. A conventional enteric coat, such as cellulose acid phthalate is then applied. In use, the rise in pH strips the outer film during passage through the small intestine but when colonic bacteria degrade the cellulose component of the inner layer, the film is disrupted and the contents released to the colon. It is clear that other enzymatic characteristics of this heavily colonized region could also be used.

More recently, Alza's osmotic devices have been adapted for colonic delivery [5]. By dipping the conventional form in a slurry of ethylene-vinyl acetate copolymer containing the salt of a fatty acid, a surfactant or a salt such as sodium chloride, a laminate around the core is produced. A further enteric layer of shellac may also be applied. The osmotic function of the device is depressed until the water-soluble elements leach from the polyolefin barrier and its aqueous permeability is increased. By this time, the device should be in the colon.

Targeting delivery to the stomach is technically more difficult due to the power of gastric movement during both the digestive and interdigestive phases. Buoyancy, dimensional change, mucosal adhesives, drugs such as propantheline and fatty excipients have all been suggested as methods of ensuring gastric retention of small devices. The carcinogenic nature of nitrosamines derived from the interaction of nitrates in food with secondary or tertiary amines in both food and drugs has prompted the delivery of N-nitroso-blocking agents to the stomach. This is the objective of a patent assigned to Roche Products Inc. [6]. Ascorbic acid and a-tocopherol, which are effective in aqueous and lipid phases respectively, are introduced into a dry hydrogel compressing in the form of a tablet. This consists of carboxymethylcellulose, hydroxypropylmethylcellulose and carboxypolymethylene. This 'hydrodynamically balanced system' is the subject of earlier patents and derives its effect from hydration and swelling of the outer layers which entrap significant quantities of air and confer a density on the partly wetted compact which is less than that of gastric fluid. This buoyancy is claimed to greatly extend the residence time in the stomach, allowing its active principles to diffuse into the gastric milieu and prevent the formation of nitrosamines.

Change of dimension is combined with buoyancy in an invention asssigned to the 3M company [7] and illustrated in Fig. 1. Drug and selected water-soluble

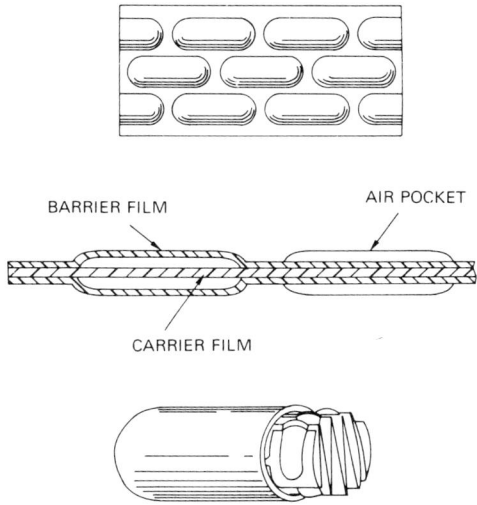

Fig. 1 — A gastric retention device employing buoyancy and dimensional change.

excipients are incorporated into a carrier film of, for example, ethylcellulose. A water-permeable barrier film is applied to each side in a way which entraps air pockets at regular intervals. This gives the device an effective specific gravity of 0.65. An appropriate length of this complex laminate is folded and encapsulated. Following ingestion, the device unfolds and floats, releasing its contents at a rate determnined by the permeability of both carrier and barrier films. Experiments with beagle dogs showed an average extension of gastric retention time from 2.5 to 6.5 h. Individual results were, however, somewhat variable.

The conversion of a small flaccid device into an enlarged, comparatively rigid unit the shape of a doughnut is represented in Fig. 2. It is one application of an invention which places dessicated hydrogel particles in an envelope [8]. In this form, the device can be easily swallowed. Subsequently, the volumetric changes to the hydrogel caused by absorption of gastric fluids create a volumetric change which exactly matches the capacity of the envelope. The configuration leads to retention in the stomach. Drugs can be incorporated and their rate of release modulated by the properties of the hydrogel and of the envelope. No information on eventual discharge from the stomach is given.

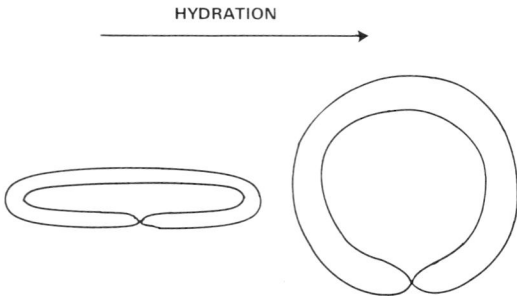

Fig. 2 — Dimensional changes in an envelope containing a hydrogel.

In appraising these inventions, the principles of the colonic delivery systems seem practicable. Those quoted employ either bacterial degradation in the colon or gastrointestinal transit time. Variation in both factors may confer variability on effectiveness and future innovation may well be devised which ensure predictable and catastrophic break-up when arrival in the colon is more certain.

Many of the inventions applied to gastric residence time appear to produce only modest and variable increases. Greater effects, such as might follow a major change in dimensions after ingestion, obviously carry a toxicological risk which is never addressed in patent disclosures. However, since the principle is also of value in controlling the intensity and duration of drug action, it will continue to attract the inventor. He must find a principle in which consistency defeats the motility of the stomach without creating a hazard to the patient.

3.   MODULATING THE INTENSITY OF DRUG ACTION

Reducing peak blood levels and any concomitant side-effects by slowing the rate of absorption is a legitimate objective of refined dosage forms. However, the large therapeutic indices which characterize most drugs diminish its importance. Existing technology should be capable of accommodating any future new drug for which, like theophylline and quinidine, wanted and unwanted effects are narrowly seaprated. In any event, such technical manipulation is likely to be also associated with increasing the duration of effect, an issue discussed in the next section.

Of far greater importance is the reduced efficiency of many drugs because they are slowly or incompletely absorbed. If this is due to low solubility, adjuvants can sometimes be used to create and maintain a microenvironment which favours high concentrations in solution. For example, the solibility of dipyridamole decreases markedly with increase in pH so that undissolved material leaving the stomach is unlikely to be absorbed. However, the inclusion of fumaric acid in a ratio of 10 moles of acid to 1 mole of drug and a proportion of sodium starch glycollate gives a tablet which dissolves satisfactorily over a pH range 1–7 [9]. The sodium starch glycollate controls the size and wet strength of the aggregates into which the tablet disintegrates. The high acid content in the aggregate maintains conditions conducive to dissolution even though the pH of the intestinal milieu may be high.

If the hydrophilic, polar nature of the molecule limits absorption, the intrinsic permeability of the absorbing membrane can be modified. T. Higuchi [10] included sodium salicylate, sodium-5-methoxysalicylate or related compounds in a series of macrolide antibiotic formulae. The amount of adjuvant was varied from 50 to 750 mg depending on the drug, the objective being to exceed a concentration of 0.01% at the site of absorption. Studies in beagles showed that the addition of 300 mg of sodium-5-methoxysalicylate to enteric capsules containing an equal amount of gentamycin sulphate increased absorption of the latter from 9 to 30%.

Whatever the impediment to absorption, increase in gastric residence time should reduce its influence. The retentive mechanisms referred to in the preceding section have been widely applied in this respect. For example, Roche's 'hydrodynamically balanced system' is used in a formula containing riboflavine and a mixture of hydrocolloids [11]. The influence of delayed transit on absorption over a 24 h period is given in Table 2. A comparable dose of riboflavine is included in formulations

Table 2 — Absorption of riboflavine from a 'hydrodynamically balanced system' (HBS)

Time interval	Riboflavine excreted (mg)	
(h)	Control	HBS
0–2	2.03	0.98
2–4	2.11	1.79
4–6	0.84	1.14
6–8	0.47	1.14
8–12	0.84	3.23
12–24	0.38	1.86
	6.87	10.14
Per cent of administered dose	44	67.5

described by Groning and Heun [12]. Triethanolamine myristate (165 mg) in a layered tablet was used to delay gastric emptying, an event monitored by the simultaneous administration of a pH-telemetering device. Of the natural fatty materials, myristic acid is one of the most effective in slowing discharge from the stomach [13] and, in this case, the triethanolamine salt was used to improve dispersibility. The results are shown in Fig. 3 and, although comparison with the 'hydrodynamically balanced system' is difficult to make, both devices appear to increase bioavailability by about 50%.

Longer, Ch'Ng and Robinson [14] have shown that mucosal adhesives may provide a powerful mechanism for increasing drug absorption. Preferring polymers which interact with the mucin-epithelial surface by non-covalent mechanisms, they selected polycarbophil on the basis of earlier studies [15] which showed that polyanionic polymers showed greater adhesion than their natural or cationic

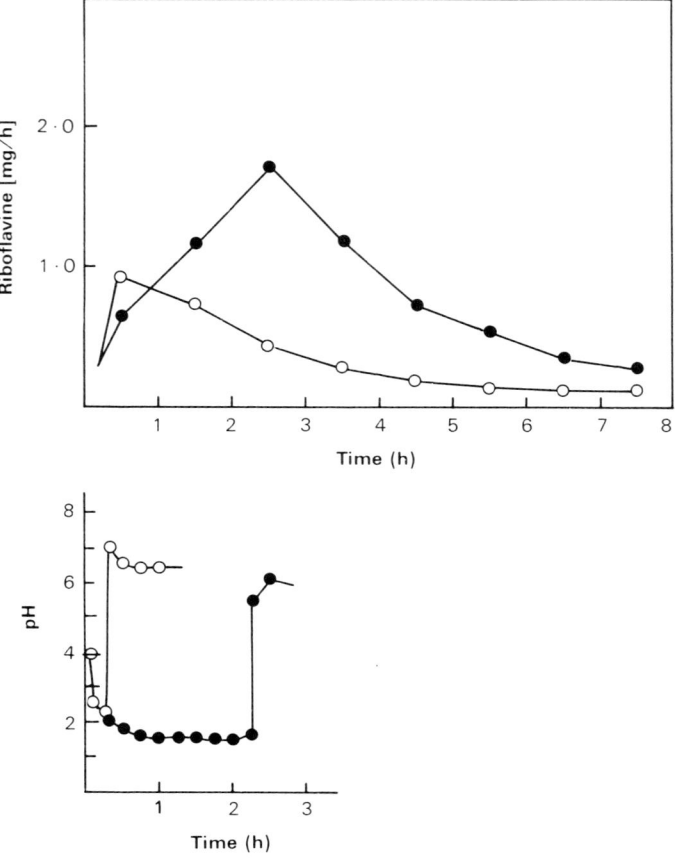

Fig. 3 — Excretion and gastric residence time in a patient administered a pH-telemetering capsule and tablet with (●) and without (○) triethanolamine myristate.

counterparts. Chlorothizide, chosen because of its poor, dose-dependent bioavailability, was incorporated into albumin beads prepared by dispersion and cross-linking with glutaraldehyde. The drug loading was about 30%. These beads were mixed with polycarbophil of the same particle size to give a drug:adjuvant ratio of 1:7, encapsulated and surgically administered to rats. Controls were prepared in which pure albumin beads replaced the polycarbophil. The disposition of the beads in the gastrointetinal tract after 6 h is shown in Fig. 4, indicating that 90% of the beads from the polycarbophil formulation remained in the stomach. This produced a massive increase in bioavailability as drug diffused from the beads and passed to absorptive regions lower in the tract. As shown in Fig. 5, peak blood levels increased from $1.0\,\mu g$ ml^{-1} to almost $1.8\,\mu g\,ml^{-1}$ and high levels are sustained for 30 h following administration.

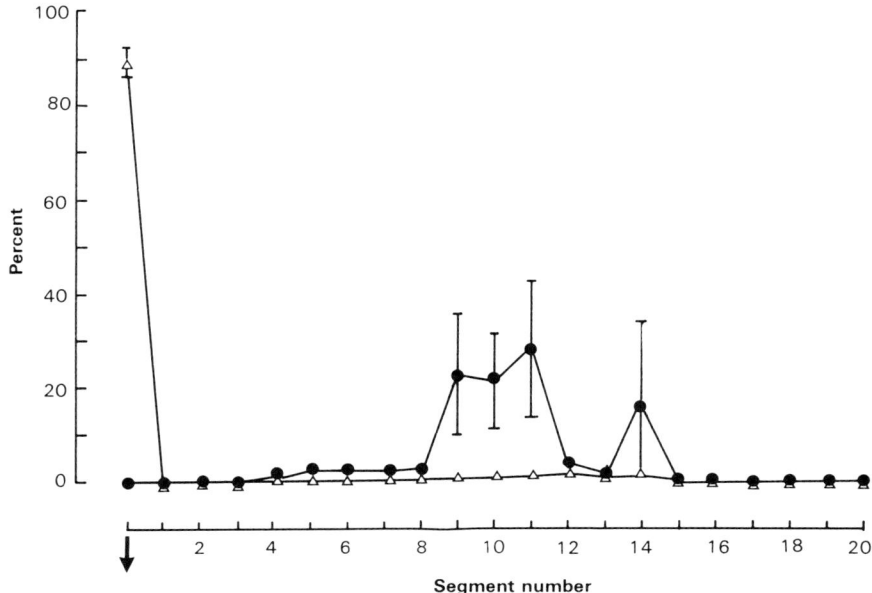

Fig. 4 — Distribution of albumin beds in the rat small intestine after 6 h with ($\triangle$) and without ($\bullet$) bioadhesive.

Poor absorption is a characteristic of many important drugs. Enhancement has, therefore, attracted much invention in the form of specific adjuvants which increase solubility and gut permeability or decrease gut transit time. There are not, as yet, sufficient data to assess whether or not these principles can be generalized. The enhancement must be significant or confusion will arise from the introduction of bioequivalent formulations which contain marginally different amounts of active principle. Thus the invention should at least double bioavailability. Even better, the invention should confer total availability, thus providing consistent effects and even an option to extend duration of action by further manipulation. These advantages should be gained without excessive amounts of the adjuvant and, of course, without toxic hazard. Such objectives are still far from realization but the nature of the commercial prize will ensure continuing efforts to refine and extend today's inventions.

4. EXTENDING THE DURATION OF DRUG ACTION

Simpler dosage regimes and better patient compliance are well-established benefits of dosage forms which define a drug's absorptive phase. Ideally, the rate of absorption should be constant with abrupt termination at the end of the dosage interval. An invariant blood level is the result. The recent study by Summers *et al.* [16] shows the extent to which four sustained-release preparations approach this

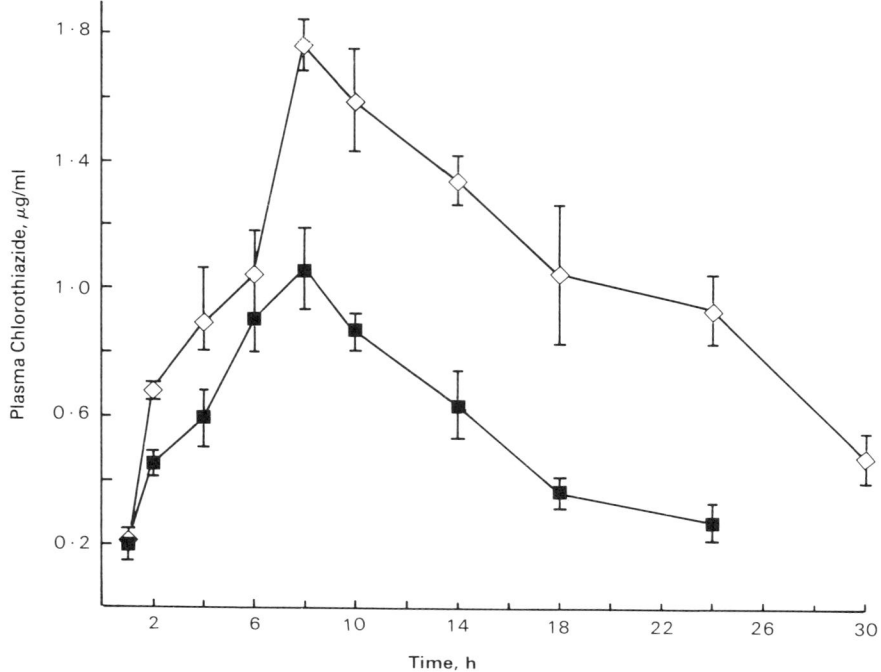

Fig. 5 — Plasma concentration of chlorothiazide in rats dosed with albumin beads with (◇) and without (■) bioadhesive.

ideal. For example, the data in Fig. 6 show that the release pattern of the mixture of fast and slow components of 'Theo-dur' leads to a period of between 3 and 6 h after administration in which virtually no drug is absorbed. Three of the four products release drug quickly in the early phases and then tail off at the end of the dosage period.

Decrease in release rate is fundamental to the exhaustion of dosage forms which embed drug in matrices or entrap them in reservoirs. Recent patents disclose attempts to overcome the drawback. For example, Merrell Dow [17] describe a tablet in which layers of decreasing concentrations are compressed on to a core. The concentration, D_L, in any one of a 'multitude of enveloping concentric layers' is given by the equation

$$D_L = D_T (R_D/R_T)$$

where R_T is the total radius, R_D is the radius of the layer in question and D_T is the total drug concentration. In practice, up to four layers can be applied by conventional press coating. Non-uniform distributon also characterizes a Ciba-Geigy invention [18] in which a conventional hydrogel containing the active agent is selectively extracted with a volatile solvent. Patent exemplification gives a 50%

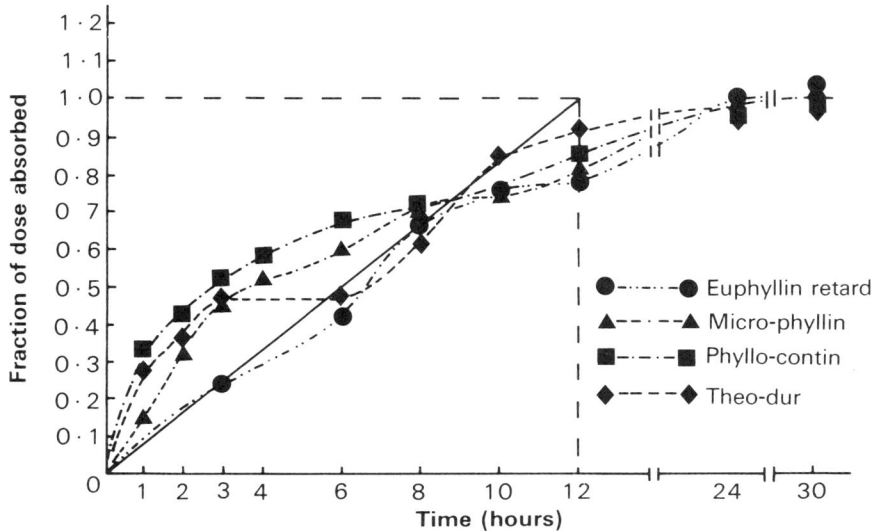

Fig. 6 — The absorption of theophylline from four commercial products.

dispersion of oxprenolol in a hydroxyarylacrylate or vinylpryrrolidone polymer. Extraction with ethanol/water modifies the drug distribution to that given in Fig. 7. As the degree of extraction increases, the release pattern in subsequent use becomes more linear and, at a drug loading of 35% closely approaches zero-order kinetics (Fig. 8).

Presentation of very high doses in sustained-release formulation poses a different problem for the product designer, who must minimize the size of his product knowing that a high drug adjuvant ratio may disturb his chosen method of control. A generalized solution is to deposit the small amount of adjuvant with great precision. For example, a dissolution barrier may be deposited on individual crystals by a microencapsulation technique. This has been chosen for methyl-dopa [19]. The drug was suspended with ethyl cellulose in cyclohexane, heated and cooled to deposit the polymer at a level of 10% by weight. The mixture was then filtered, dried and compressed with a small amount of microcrystalline cellulose. However, the complexity of this process is in great contrast to Syntex's naproxen formulation [20] in which a simple mixture of drug, hydroxypropylmethycellulose (4–9%) and lubricant (0.1–0.2%) is compressed. The tablets have a consistent release pattern suitable for once-a-day treatment. Even simpler is Mead Johnson's tablet, which contains 99.6% theophylline [21]. The lubricated drug is compressed to form a thin slab-like tablet which maintains a fairly constant surface during dissolution. A clever use of differential compression using sloping punches is another simple technique [22]. The tablet's differential disintegration is used to control the release of its contents.

These simpler examples are an alternative inventive strategy. Rather than refine

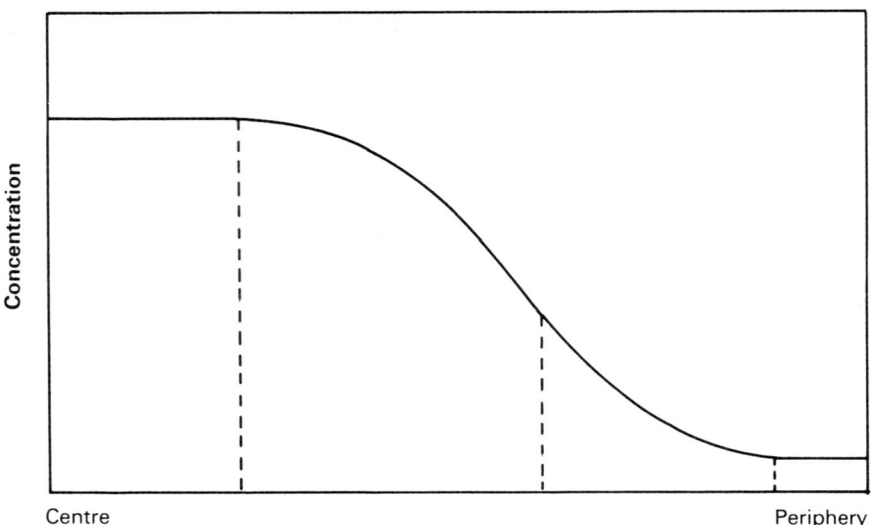

Fig. 7 — Distribution of oxprenolol in a partially extracted matrix.

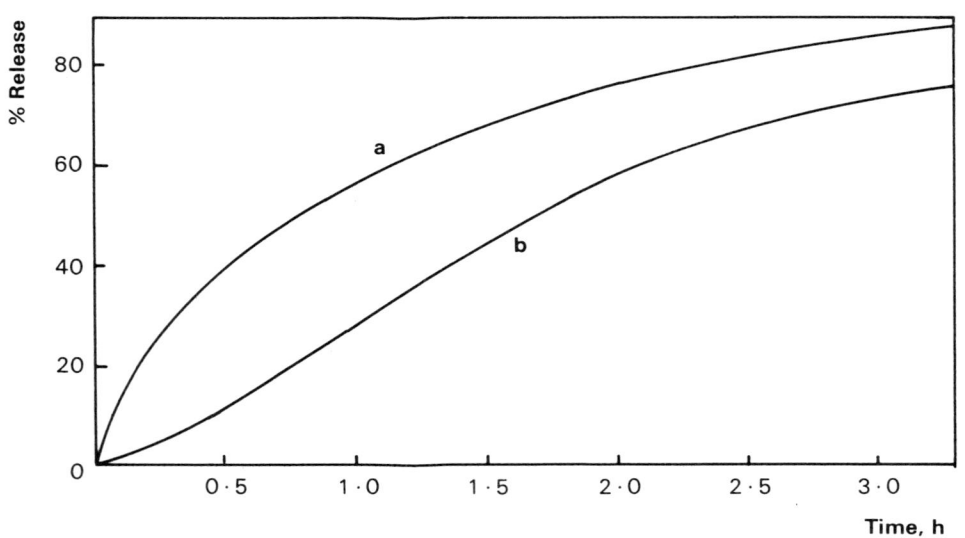

Fig. 8 — Release of oxprenolol from an unextracted matrix (a) and a partially extracted matrix (b). (a) contains 50% drug and (b) 37%.

structures and release rates, they generate simple, cheap formulae which can be manufactured by conventional processes. This is typified by tablets which contain hydrocolloids and fatty components prepared by solvent formulation and compression. The release pattern is determined by a complex pattern of swelling and erosion but, as the example [23] in Table 3 shows, very satisfactory results seem possible. A

Table 3 — The properties of a quinidine tablet formulated with hydrogenated cotton seed oil and carboxy-polymethylene

Disintegration at pH 1.2–1.4

Time (h)	0	1	2	3		
Weight remaining (mg)	414.3	409.6	405.3	395.5		
Standard deviation	1.86	2.3	2.6	4.3		
% Loss	0	1.13	2.2	4.8		

Dissolution USP apparatus II, 50 rpm, pH 7.5

Time (h)	1	2	3	4	5	6
% Dissolved	22.7	31.0	42.7	53.5	63.0	74.5
Standard deviation	2.6	1.4	2.2	1.9	2.6	1.9

similar formula [24] is claimed to accomodate from 10 to 90% drug, which may have a solubility of any value between 1:5 and 1:1000 and yet still give a constant-release pattern of any chosen value.

Whether the device used is simple or highly refined, its period of usefulness will be limited by intestinal motility, which will remove it from absorptive regions. Unless a drug is freely absorbed from the colon, this will normally limit the dosage interval to 12 h. There is, however, advantage in once-a-day dosage and the mechanisms for increasing gastric residence time already discussed find application in the respect. A doubling of the dosage interval would seem to be within the capability of one of a combination of these factors but, as yet, this has not been realized.

An alternative is to maintain the device in the mouth to allow a constituent to be dissolved, swallowed and absorbed. Using *in vitro* models, Gurney *et al.* [25] have undertaken fundamental studies on the bioadhesion of gels to the oral activity. Gels containing polyethylene, gelatin and sodium carboxymethyl-cellulose were refined as the basis for system-releasing febuverine, a local anaesthetic. For systemic administration such studies could prove invaluable in the design of small, secure and impalpable devices which must be retained in the mouth for long periods.

It has been assumed to this point that constant-release rates are required during the extended period. Whilst this is so for many situations, there are some for which a drug pulse at some point in time could be an advantage. The efficiency of some hormones, antibiotics, anthelmintics and cytotoxic agents might increase if blood levels were systematically varied within an extended period of release. The 'Alza' osmotic device has been recently adapted for this purpose [24] by including an adjuvant which depresses the solubility of its active component. For example, the saturation solubility of salbutamol hemisulphate is reduced from 275 mg ml^{-1} in water to 16 mg ml^{-1} in saturated sodium chloride solution. If sodium chloride is included in the device in relatively small quantities, the initial release of salbutamol will be reduced. However, once the salt is exhausted, the solubility and release rate of the salbutamol will rise to give the pulse shown in Fig. 9.

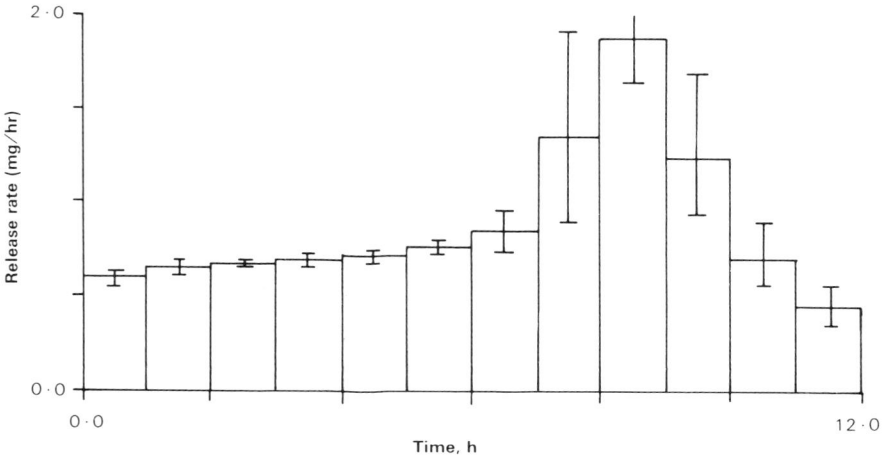

Fig. 9 — Pulsed release from an osmotic device containing salbutamol hemisulphate.

Control of duration of effect has been the most important influence on the design of refined oral dosage forms. Although much effort has been expended on extending the period to 24 h, no general solution to this challenge has been found. True invention is now needed. The imposition of drug pulse during the release period, exemplified in Alza's invention, is an exciting concept. It needs refinement with regard to the timing and intensity of the pulse and the ideal system might well consist of a matrix, a membrane or some other containment which can be made to fail at some predetermined time. However, such an invention would find wide application throughout the field of drug delivery. Finally, we may continue to read of formulation refinements which lie within existing achievement. These will only be justified by the simplicity and consistency which they bring and there is little place for some of the over-elaborate devices already described.

REFERENCES

[1] Anon. (1984). Oral sustained release products — pro's and con's. *Drug and Therapeutics Bulletin* **22**, 57–60.

[2] British patent 2,165,555A. 26 March 1986.

[3] Hardy, J. G., Wilson, C. G. & Wood, E. (1985). Drug delviery to the proximal colon. *J. Pharm. Pharmacol.* **37**, 874–877.

[4] US Patent 4,432,966. 21 February 1984.

[5] British Patents 2,166,051A and 2,166,052A. 30 April 1986.

[6] British Patent 2,097,676A. 28 April 1982.

[7] European Patent 90,560. 18 March 1983.

[8] British Patent 2,144,051. 27 February 1983.

[9] European Patent 121,901. 17 October 1984.

[10] US Patent 4,459,295. 10 July 1984.

[11] US Patent 4,167,558. 21 November 1978.

[12] Groning, R. & Heun, G. (1984). Oral dosage froms with controlled gastro-intestinal transit. *Drug. Dev. Industr. Pharm.* **10** 527–539.

[13] Palin, K. J. (1985). Lipids and oral drug delivery. *Pharm. Int.* **6** 272–275.

[14] Longer, M. A., Ch'Ng, H. S. & Robinson, J. R. (1985). Bioadhesive polymers as platforms for oral-controlled drug delviery: oral delivery to chlorothiazide. *J. Pharm. Sci.* **74**, 406–411.

[15] Park, K. & Robinson, J. R. (1984). Bioadhesive polymers as platforms for oral-controlled drug delivery: method to study bioadhesion. *Int. J. Pharm.* **19**, 107–127.

[16] Summers, R. S., Summers, B. & Rawnsley, S. (1986). The bioavailability, absorption characteristics and formulation of four commercially-available controlled release theophylline products. *Int. J. Pharm.* **30** 83–88.

[17] European Patent 111,144. 20 June 1984.

[18] European Patent 164,311. 11 December 1985.

[19] International Patent PCT WO 84/02843. 2 August 1984.

[20] British Patent 2,141,338. 19 December 1984.

[21] US Patent 4,547,358. 15 October 1985.

[22] European Patent 126, 453. 28 October 1984.

[23] US Patent 4,522,804. 11 June 1985.

[24] European Patent 131,485. 16 January 1985.

[25] Gurney, R., Meyer, J.-M. & Peppas, N. A. (1984). Modelling of sustained release of water soluble drugs from porous hydrophobic polymers. *Biomaterials* **5** 336–340.

10

Evaluation of the gastrointestinal transit and release characteristics of drugs

S. S. Davis, Department of Pharmacy, University of Nottingham, University Park, Nottingham NG7 2RD, UK

1. INTRODUCTION

The gastrointestinal tract is usually the preferred site of absorption for most therapeutic agents as seen from the standpoints of convenience of administration, patient compliance and cost. The majority of oral dosage forms comprise tablets and capsules and these are often provided as instant release systems designed to disintegrate rapidly in the stomach. The dissolved drug substance is expected to be absorbed from the small intestine. The efficiency of these processes of release and uptake is dependent upon the physicochemical charcteristics of the drug (e.g. solubility, stability in acid and alkaline environments, permeability through (gastrointestinal) membranes) as well as physiological variables such as gastrointestinal transit. Recently Ho and others [1] have attempted to quantify these factors with their so-called 'reserve length concept'. Briefly, the approach has been to consider the distance a dispersed drug would have to pass down the small intestine before the total available dose was absorbed. Their mathematical analysis has shown that the more efficient the dissolution and absorption processes, the greater the reserve length. Whether the small intestine alone should be taken as the predominant absorption site is debatable. The opinions presented in the literature would suggest that absorption of drugs from the large bowel is poor and erratic. However, recent studies conducted on beta-blockers indicate that the large intestine may have a more significant contribution to total absorption than hitherto realized [2].

Controlled-release (modified-release) dosage forms are growing in popularity. These more sophisticated systems can be used as a means of altering the pharmacokinetic behaviour of drugs in order to provide twice- or once-a-day dosage. Other applications include enteric coatings for the protection of drugs from degradation within the gastrointestinal tract or the protection of the stomach from the irritating effects of the drug, and the delivery of drugs to so-called absorption windows or specific targets within the gastrointestinal tract, particularly the colon [3, 4].

Much about the performance of a system can be learned from *in vitro* release studies using conventional and modified dissolution methods; however, an essential stage in development must be subsequent evaluation *in vivo*. At Nottingham we have used the non-invasive technique of gamma-scintigraphy to follow the gastrointestinal transit and release characteristics of a variety of pharmaceutical dosage forms in human subjects. Such studies not only provide insight into the fate of dosage form and its integrity, but also allow correlation to be made between the position of a system in the gastrointestinal tract and resultant pharmacokinetic profiles.

2. *IN VIVO* EVALUATION OF PHARMACEUTICAL DOSAGE FORMS

Table 1 lists some of the methods that can be employed to evaluate the *in vivo*

Table 1 — Methods for the evaluation of the fate of orally administered dosage forms

Radiology (X-ray)
Endoscopy
Radiotelemetry
Epigastric impedance
Gamma-scintigraphy
Deconvolution of pharmacokinetic data

performance of orally administer dosage forms. The majority of these techniques can be considered as direct and either invasive or non-invasive approaches. The deconvolution of pharmacokinetic data represents an indirect means of obtaining information on the performance of an administered dosage form [5]. Gastroscopy is a direct and invasive technique largely restricted to studies on the performance of dosage forms in the stomach [6]. Radio-telemetry using pH-measuring capsules (Heidelberg capsule) can be used to provide information on gastric emptying but not on subsequent intestinal transit [7, 8]. Radiological (X-ray) studies can provide information on the transit of dosage forms throughout the gastrointestinal tract and also yield useful details of anatomical features [9–11]. Nevertheless they suffer from three major disadvantages: exposure of subjects to the repeated risk of taking serial X-rays, the necessity of modifying the physical state of a dosage form in order to make it radio-opaque, and the fact that the information obtained cannot be easily quantified. In contrast, gamma-scintigraphy is a much safer technique than X-ray (a typical scintigraphic investigation lasting 1 day usually exposes the subject to a total dose of radioactivity equivalent to a quarter of an abdominal X-ray). Furthermore, the recorded information stored on computer can be manipulated and quantified to provide numerical estimates of gastric emptying, intestinal transit, etc. [12–14]. Pharmaceutical dosage forms can be labelled with a minute quantity of active material, such that the physical properties of the final product are not altered in any significant way [15–17].

During the past 5 years we have used the technique of gamma-scintigraphy to evaluate the gastrointestinal transit behaviour of a variety of dosage forms in over 200 human subjects [18]. We have studied the effects of a variety of physiological, pharmaceutical, pharmacological and pathological factors and have also examined the possible relation between the position of dosage forms in the gastrointestinal tract and derived pharmacokinetic profiles [19–25]. In these studies the drugs investigated have included aspirin, naproxen, indomethacin, isosorbide-5-nitrate, acyclovir, oxprenolol, theophylline, tiaprofenic acid. Numerical deconvolution of blood level data [5] has allowed comparison of *in vivo* and *in vitro* release profiles and for the absorption characteristics of different regions of the gastrointestinal tract to be quantitifed. In some cases the movement of the dosage form from the small to large intestine (where the gastrointestinal mucosa is much less permeable) is heralded by a change in absorption rate. In other cases no apparent change in the absorption of the drug is observed as it passes through the different regions of the gastrointestinal tract, indicating that the rate-limiting factor is always the controlled-release system.

3.   METHODOLOGY

Non-invasive scintigraphic studies can be conducted in human subjects by labelling a pharmaceutical dosage form with a suitable gama-emitting radionuclide. Radionuclides approved for use in man include technetium-99m (half-life 6 h), iodine-123 (half-life 13 h), indium-111 (half-life 67 h) and indium-113m (half-life 1.7 h), all of which have suitable energy levels for imaging using a conventional gamma camera. In most instances it is neither possible or sensible to label a drug molecule [15]; instead a pharmaceutical formulation can be labelled in a number of alternative ways. A marker material, labelled with a suitable radionuclide, can be used as a model compound and to mirror the behaviour of the drug. Extensive *in vivo* and *in vitro* tests are conducted to show that the release of this marker is indeed very similar to that of the drug in question [19]. These non-absorbable marker materials usually comprise various chelating agents (DTPA, HIDA, etc.). The HIDA materials are available as different analogues (ethyl, butyl) with increasing lipophilicity and can be used to match a variety of drug substances. The *in vitro* and *in vivo* release of these radiolabelled markers from different matrix tablet formulations, through processes of diffusion and erosion, has been reported [19]. *In vivo* it is possible to discern easily the undisintegrated matrix and to quantify the remaining activity. For a pellet formulation it is not possible to follow the release of a marker using conventional scintigraphic equipment, since released activity in close proximity to the pellets cannot be distinguished from the pellets themselves.

A marker material can be incorporated into the dosage form as a small quantity (10 mg) of labelled excipient (for example in ion-exchange resin powdered or as microspheres). The chosen material can be arranged to remain with the intact single unit or be released through a process of erosion and/or disintegration. If so desired it is possible to label a matrix formulation with two different labels that give information concurrently on the two processes of diffusion and erosion, provided the chosen radionuclides have different energy states that can be measured simultaneously with the gamma camera. A total non-releasing marker can be employed to ascertain the position of a dosage form within the gastro-intestinal tract. This process is normally essential for pellet systems. Here a label can be incorporated either using an ion exchange mechanism or by coating labelled cores [24, 26].

The scintigraphic method provides various strategies for determining the position of a dosage form within the gastro-intestinal tract and/or to follow its integrity or the release of the labelled marker. As a consequence the technique is ideal as a means of answering questions about a formulation, but it is not necessarily a suitable technique for answering questions about the fate of the drug substance. It is therefore an adjunct to pharmacokinetic investigations rather than a replacement. Indeed, objective information about the release and absorption of an administered drug can be gained by making conventional pharmacokinetic measurements followed by numerical deconvolution of derived data.

Fig. 1 shows some typical scintigraphic pictures obained for single-unit and pellet dosage forms. With a dispersible pellet system it is possible to distinguish quite easily certain anatomical features such as the stomach and the large intestine. For the case of a single-unit dosage form, anatomical features can be identified through the release of marker or by the concomitant administration of a simple solution labelled with a different radionuclide [19].

4. STUDIES ON PHYSIOLOGICAL FACTORS

It is well known in gastroenterology that the motility of the gastrointestinal tract can be influenced by a large number of factors, the most important being the intake of food [12]. The fed stomach behaves in a very different way to the fasted stomach and such a difference can have an important bearing on the gastro-intestinal transit of dosage forms [27]. In the fed state contractions in the antrum of the stomach mix and grind digestible material. Periodically, waves of activity move solid material to the distal antrum. The pylorus contracts and liquids and suspended materials smaller than about 5 mm in size can pass through the pylorus into the duodenum. Larger sized material is returned (retropelled) to the body of the stomach where it undergoes a further process of mixing and grinding. This process continues until the stomach is empty of food. This process is controlled by a variety of subtle feedback mechanisms that operate through sensors in the duodenum, that apparently can detect not only the presence of acids, carbohydrates and differences in osmolarity, but also specific factors like the amino acid tryptophan. Non-disintegrating, indigestible objects larger than about 5 mm in size cannot normally leave the stomach while it remains in the fed mode and consequently are retained.

In the fasted state, or after the digestive phase has been completed, the stomach has a specific mechanism that clears undigested material into the small intestine. This is known as the migrating myoelectric complex (MMC) and has at least four phases [28]. In one important phase, the third phase (sometimes called the 'housekeeper wave'), which occurs about every 2 h, a series of rapid contractions causes undigestible material to be swept through the open pylorus, down the small intestine to the ileocaecal junction. Therefore, on physiological grounds it is to be expected that a liquid, pellet formulation, or disintegrating tablet will be emptied from the stomach

(a)

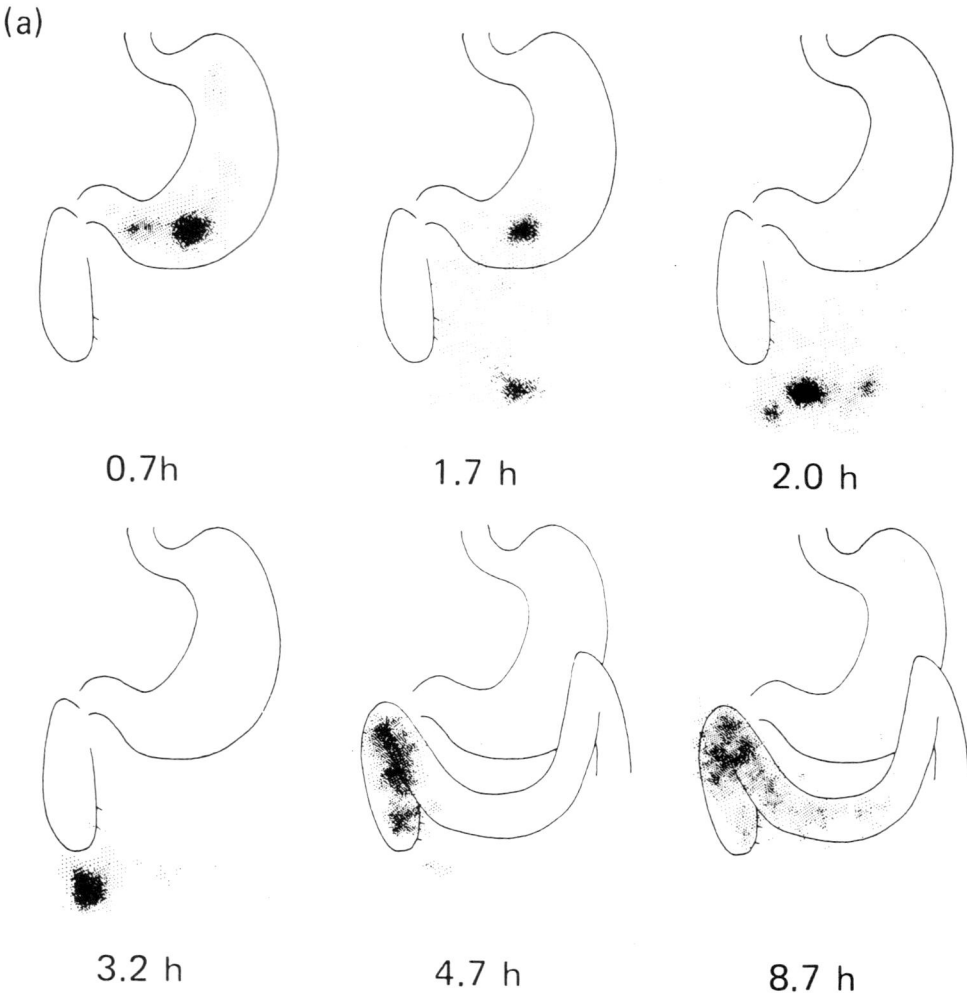

Fig. 1a — Scintigraphic images showing the gastrointestinal transit of pharmaceutical dosage forms administered after a light breakfast. (a) Pellets.

even while it is in the digestive mode. In contrast, a non-disintegrating single unit administered to a fed stomach or any dosage form administered to a fasted stomach will be cleared through the action of the MMC [29]. These differences in emptying behaviour for single- and multiple-unit dosage forms and the importance of the fed state are well illustrated in Fig. 2 and Table 2. In the fasted mode both single units and pellets are emptied quite rapidly and the pellets can even empty as a bolus rather than as a spreading system [24]. On a lightly fed stomach single units will be delayed, but pellets can empty, the rate of emptying for the latter and their spreading in the small intestine depending on the quantity of food. A heavy breakfast will result in a

(b)

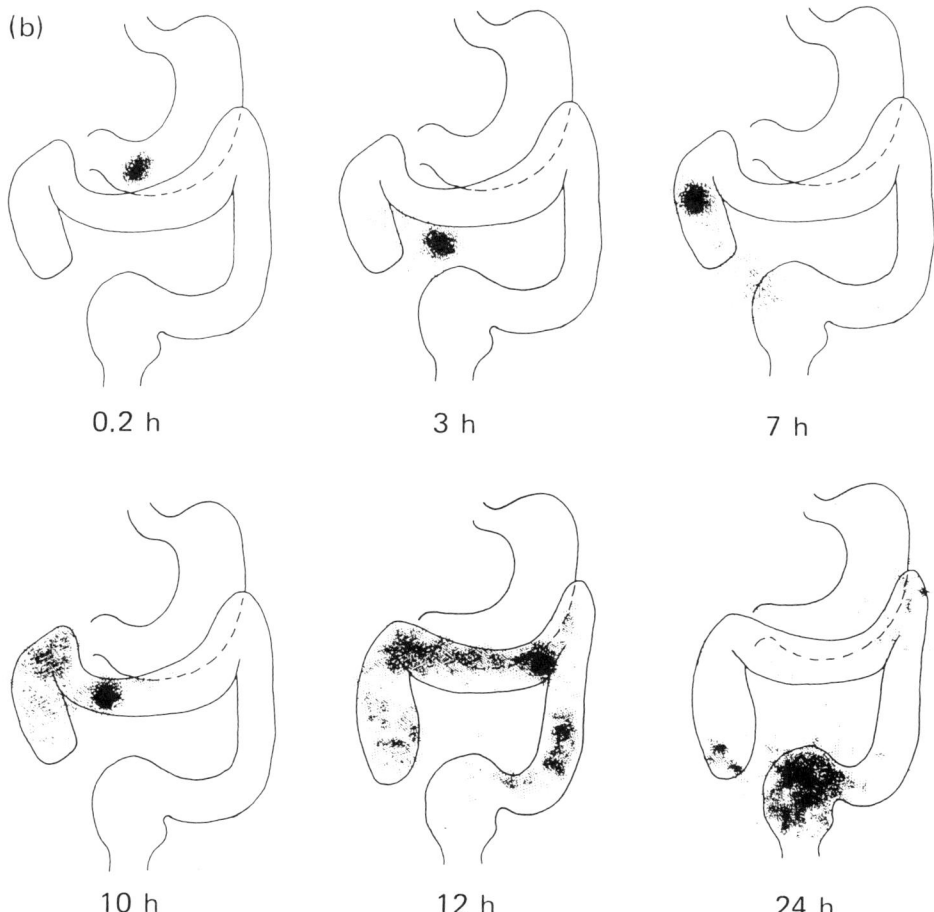

Fig. 1b — Scintigraphic images showing the gastrointestinal transit of pharmaceutical dosage forms administered after a light breakfast. (b) Matrix tablet.

slow steady emptying of pellets from the stomach with a large amount of spreading of the dosage form [20, 21]. Single units administered to a heavily fed stomach will remain in the stomach so long as it is in the digestive mode. Thus, if subjects (or patients) are fed continuously during the day then the dosage form will not be able to empty until the fasted state has been re-established [8].

The dependence of gastric emptying on the nature of the dosage form, and more particularly food intake, can have an important bearing upon the rational design of controlled-release dosage forms. For the case where a drug is absorbed only from the small intestine, or has an 'absorption window' in the duodenum, the delivering system could well be past the absorption site after a short period of time if it is given on a fasted stomach. In contrast a single-unit dosage form (and to a much lesser extent a multiparticle system) given with food, will be retained within the stomach so

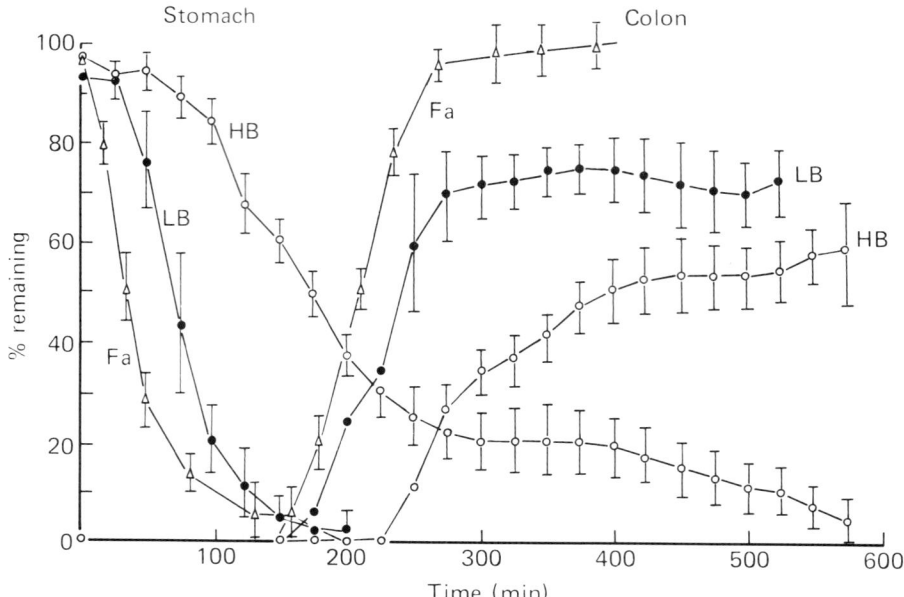

Fig. 2 — The effect of fed state on the gastrointestinal transit of a pellet formulation. Fa=fasted; LB=light breakfast; HB=heavy breakfast.

that released drug in solution (or as fine particles) will have the opportunity of accessing the absorption site for an extended period of time.

A great benefit would accrue if it was possible to gain control over gastric emptying profiles through pharmaceutical means. For this reason we have studied the effect of dosage form density to include heavy pellets and floating tablets and the use of putative mucoadhesive materials [31, 32]. Unfortunately, as yet we have not found any advantages for these various systems when administered to fasted and (in some cases) fed subjects (Fig. 3).

While gastric emptying is highly variable, especially with regard to the nature of the dosage form and food intake, the time of transit of dosage forms in the small intestine is very much more reproducible. We have shown recently, in a detailed compilation of our studies, that solutions, pellets and single units administered to fasted, lightly fed and heavily fed stomachs, have a surprisingly constant small intestinal transit time [18]. This is normally of the order of only 3 h with a standard deviation of about 1 h. These results have a direct bearing on the rational design of controlled-release dosage forms, especially for systems intended for drugs that are only well absorbed within the confines of the small intestine. It is quite possible for a dosage form to be emptied rapidly from the (fasted) stomach and to be in the colon (near non-absorptive surfaces) in less than 4 h. In this situation, the rationale for once-a-day therapy and perhaps even twice-a-day therapy may be questioned.

In other recent studies we have investigated the effects of a range of additional (physiological) factors on the gastrointestinal transit of pharmaceutical systems, for

Table 2 — Gastrointestinal transit times (h) of single units (naproxen matrix tablets): the effect of food and age [30]

Subject	Old Fasted (G1)	Fed (G2)	Subject	Young Fasted (G3)	Fed (G4)
Gastric emptying					
1	0.4	2.8	7	0.7	9.0
2	1.5	0.8	8	0.5	1.8
3	0.6	4.6	9	1.2	2.1
4	1.6	3.6	10	0.4	2.1
5	0.7	6.6	11	0.4	1.4
6	0.4	1.7	12	0.7	3.3
Mean	0.86	3.3		0.64	3.0
SEM	0.22	0.83		0.12	1.2
Median	0.65	3.2		0.57	2.1
Small intestinal transit					
1	1.6	2.7	7	2.1	2.3
2	3.5	5.7	8	4.6	4.4
3	4.4	3.4	9	3.9	5.1
4	1.2	1.6	10	1.9	2.6
5	2.7	4.0	11	3.9	3.3
6	6.2	2.8	12	1.6	1.3
Mean	3.3	3.4		3.0	3.2
SEM	0.74	0.56		0.50	0.56
Median	3.1	3.1		3.0	3.0

example the age of subjects, the effects of exercise, time of administration of the dosage form, bed rest, body position. Few of these factors altered gastric emptying or small intestinal transit times significantly, and even if they did so, the effects were of little consequence in relation to the clinical use of oral dosage forms. Limited studies on pathological conditions such as constipation and diarrhoea, although indicating obvious differences in transit in the large bowel, have once again served to show that small intestinal transit time is largely independent of processes controlling input and output. These findings are largely in agreement with simiar investigations conducted on the gastrointestinal transit of foods in liquid or solid form [33–41].

Data on the transit of a tablet through different regions of the gastrointestinal tract are given in Fig. 4. These show clearly that a dosage form has a relatively short transit time within the small intestine as compared with the much longer transit times in the large bowel, particularly the descending colon. Interestingly, if pellet formultions and single units are administered simultaneously these seem to have a similar transit to the ileocaecal sphincter but thereafter single units have a faster transit time than multiple-unit systems [42].

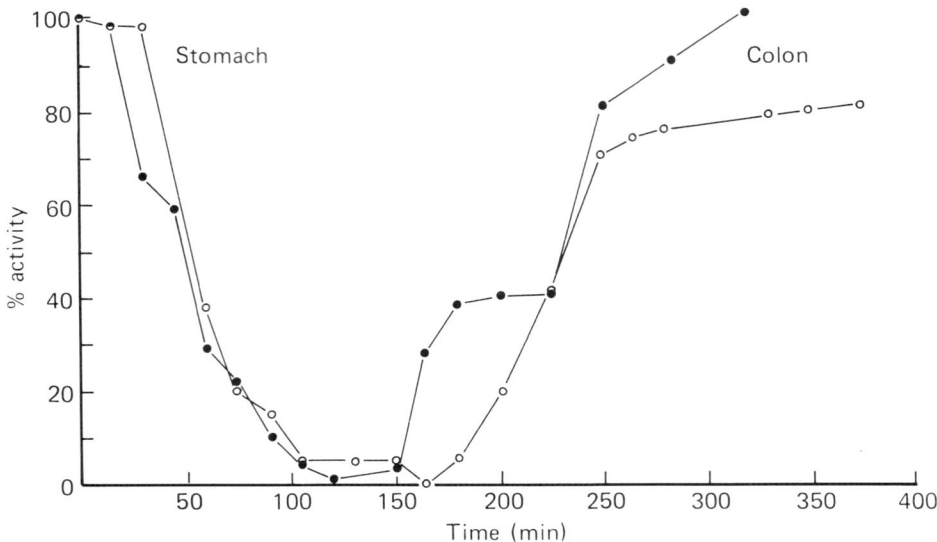

Fig. 3 — The evaluation of a putative mucoadhesive agent (polycarbophyll) by scintigraphy. (○) Control pellets; (●) with added bioadhesive.

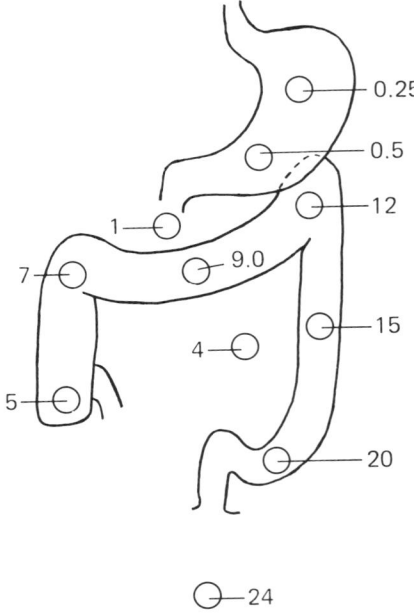

Fig. 4 — The gastrointestinal transit time (h) of a non-disintegrating tablet administered to a fasted subject.

Our measured values for total transit (mouth to anus) would confirm literature observations that this is of the order of 24 h or longer, depending upon diet, but we have found in a normal, healthy, fasted, young subject a total transit time as short as 6 h after administration of a single unit. The literature suggests that such low values are not particularly uncommon [43] and again our results have implications for the design and administration of dosage forms intended for once- or twice-daily therapy.

5. DRUG RELEASE STUDIES

The release of a drug and the labelled marker from a pharmaceutical matrix system and pellet system *in vitro* can be studied by conventional dissolution experiments. It is possible to evaluate the *in vivo* release of the drug through deconvolution of pharmacokinetic data, provided that release rather than absorption is the rate-determining parameter [5]. With matrix systems containing a labelled marker material it is also possible to measure *in vivo* release of the maker directly in a non-invasive way using scintigraphy [19]. Excellent correlation has been obtained between *in vitro* and *in vivo* release profiles for matrix systems, where little variation in release with changes in pH and agitation conditions is to be expected (Fig. 5).

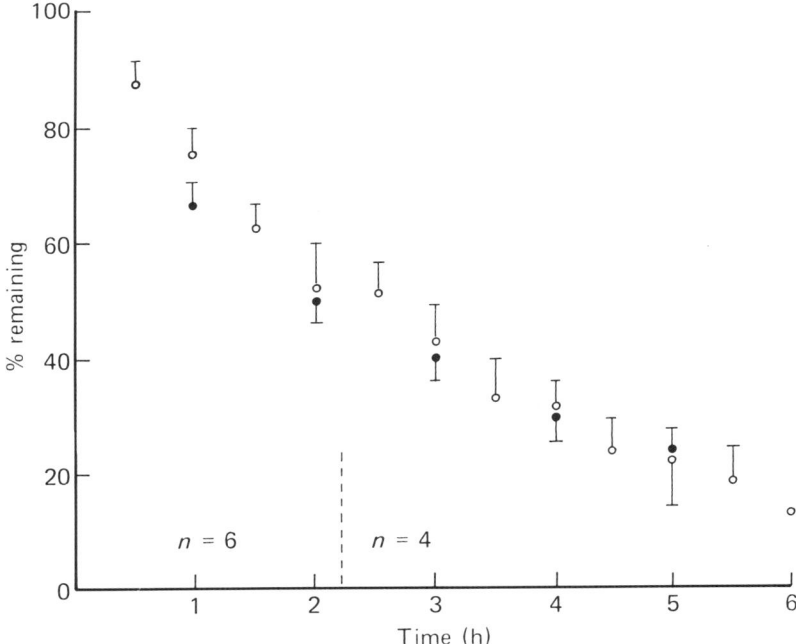

Fig. 5—The *in vitro* and *in vivo* release of a labelled marker (99m-technetium E-HIDA) from a matrix tablet. (●) *In vitro* (*n*=5); (○) *in vivo* (*n*=6 or 4).

As already discussed, it is normal practice in our scintigraphic investigations with dosage forms containing active drug, to collect blood samples and to measure blood level–time profiles. In this way it is possible to relate position to the absorption characteristics of the gastrointestinal tract and to evaluate important differences for anatomical sites (e.g. colon versus small intestine) as well as to map out so-called absorption windows. The data shown in Fig. 6 for a controlled-release isosorbide

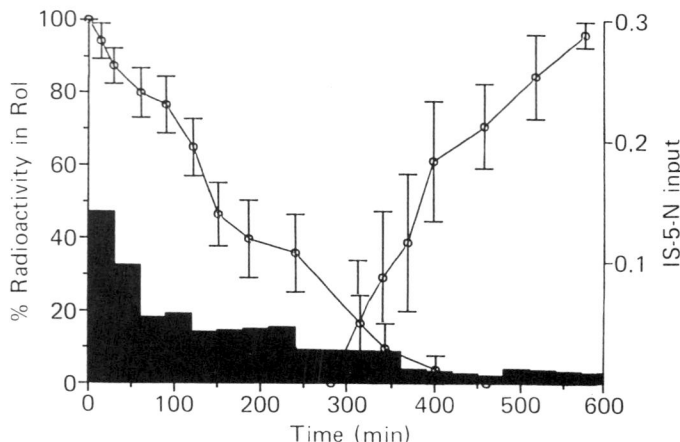

Fig. 6 — Relationship between the gastrointestinal transit of pellets containing isosorbide-5-nitrate (15-5-N) and drug input as obtained by deconvolution analysis.

formulation illustrate the good absorption of this compound in the small intestine and the poorer absorption that results when the dosage form moves into the colon. Such a pellet formulation will have a non-zero-order release profile and in early studies on candidate drugs it is preferable to use devices that can provide a well-defined input function.

The Alza Corporation in California supply osmotic pumps (Osmet) that can release a solution or suspension of a test drug over various time periods [22]. The devices work on an osmotic pumping mechanism and they can be modified to provide delayed and even pulse release characteristics [44]. When the contents of such modules are labelled with a small quantity of a gamma-emitting marker, it is possible not only to ascertain the position of the module within the gastrointestinal tract, but also to measure the pumping characteristics of the dosage form *in vivo* [22]. It is possible to have pumps that will start releasing the drug immediately or to have pumps that will release activity when they reach the colon. This is achieved through a built-in delay to the pumping mechanism and exploitation of the well-defined small intestinal transit time mentioned above. Pharmacokinetic data obtained with the osmotic pumping system are shown in Fig. 7 [45]. Here it is demonstrated that when the dosage form is administered with food, good correlation is found between the *in vivo* data (as obtained by deconvolution analysis) and the *in vitro* release rate. This indicates that the device is controlling drug input and thereby the bioavailability. If, however, the product is given on a fasted stomach, so that it can empty rapidly from

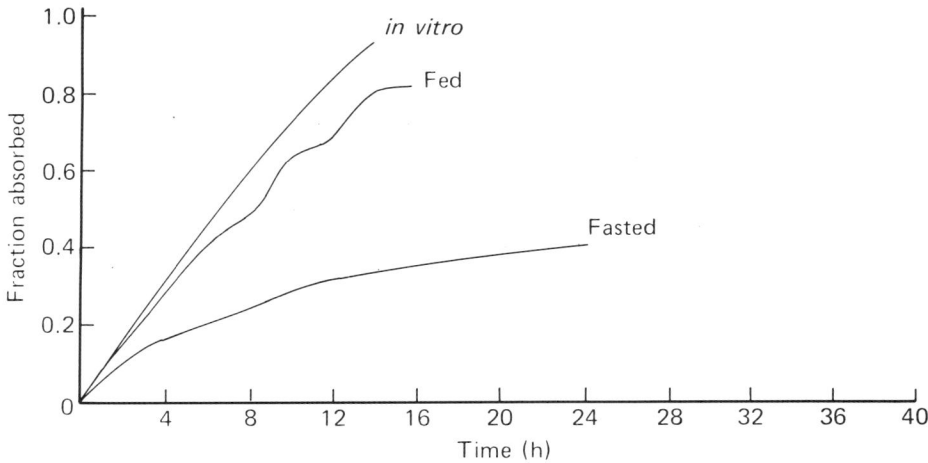

Fig. 7 — The effect of food on the correlation between drug input data derived by *in vitro* and *in vivo* (deconvolution) methods. The drug was administered in an osmotic pump (Osmet).

the stomach and thence move quickly to the colon, a different picture results. The test drug is not well absorbed from the colon and consequently absorption from the colon rather than release from the pump becomes rate limiting. A poor correlation between *in vivo* and *in vitro* release data is found.

6.   TARGETING WITH THE GASTROINTESTINAL TRACT

So far, much of what has been described relates to controlled-release dosage forms intended to give steady-state sustained blood levels for more effective drug therapy. The scintigraphic method can also be used to evaluate dosage forms that have been designed to release a drug in designated areas of the gastrointestinal tract. A simple example is an enteric coating that should ensure that the drug will be released when it reaches the small intestine [3]. More specific targets for delivery within the small intestine include the duodenum, for the preferential absorption of peptides and proteins by exploiting known facilitated transport mechanisms for dipeptides and tripeptides, and the delivery of antigens and allergens to the M-cells residing in the Peyer's Patch regions [46]. Similarly, there is growing interest in the specific delivery of drugs to the colon [4, 42, 47], either for local treatment such as that of ulcerative colitis and irritable bowel syndrome, or for the systemic delivery of compounds that are normally not well absorbed from the gastrointestinal tract by exploitation of the long residence time in the colon. Here one has in mind the products of biotechnology, and interesting studies conducted in the rat model by Muranishi and others in Japan have demonstrated that it is possible to modify the absorption characteristics of the colon using a variety of absorption enhancers including mixed micelles [48]. Clearly for such applications sophisticated delivery systems will need to be developed that will allow site-specific delivery of not only the drug, but also the absorption enhancer. Scintigraphic measurements could prove to be invaluable for the evaluation of these novel systems in human subjects.

REFERENCES

[1] Ho, N. F. H., Merkle, H. P. & Higuchi, W. I. (1983). Quantitative, mechanistic and physiological realistic approach to the biopharmaceutical design of oral drug delivery systems. *Drug Development and Industrial Pharmacy* **9** 1111–1184.

[2] Antonin, K.-H., Bieck, P., Scheurlen, M., Jedrychowski, M. & Malchow, H. (1985). Oxprenolol absorption in man after single bolus dosing into two segments of the colon compared with that after oral dosing. *Br J. Clin. Pharmac.* **19** 137S–142S.

[3] Bogentoft, C., Alpsten, M. & Ekenved, G. (1984). Absorption of acetylsalicylic acid from enteric-coated tablets in relation to gastric emptying and *in vivo* disintegration. *J. Pharm. Pharmacol.* **36** 350–351.

[4] Bogentoft, C., Eskilsson, C., Jonsson, U. E., Lagerstrom, P. O., Lovgren, K. & Rosen, L. (1983). Delivery of drugs to the colon by means of a new microencapsulated oral dosage form. *Acta Pharm. Suec.* **20** 311–314.

[5] Langenbucher, F. & Mysicka, J. (1985). *In vitro* and *in vivo* deconvolution assessment of drug release kinetics from oxprenolol Oros preparations. *Br. J. Clin. Pharmac.* **19** 151S–162S.

[6] Hey, H., Matzenm, P., Thorup Anderson, J., Didriksen, E. & Nielsen, B. (1979). A gastroscopic and pharmacological study of the distintegration time and absorption of pivampicillin capsules and tables. *Br. J. Clin. Pharmac.* **8** 237–242.

[7] Dressman, J. B. & Amidon, G. L. (1984). Radiotelemetric method for evaluating entgeric coatings *in vivo*. *J. Pharm. Sci.* **73** 935–938.

[8] Mojaverian, P., Ferguson, R. K., Vlasses, P. H., Rocci, M. L. Jr., Oren, A., Fix, J. A., Caldwell, L. J. & Gardner, C. (1985). Estimation of gastric residence time of the Heidelberg capsule in humans: effect of varying food composition. *Gastroenterol.* **89** 392–397.

[9] Bertrand, J., Metman, E.-H., Danquechin Dorval, E., Rouleau, Ph., D'Hueppe, A., Itti, R. & Philippe, L. (1980). Etude du temps d'evacuation gastrique de repas normaux au moyen de granules radio-opaques, applications cliniques et validation. *Gastroenterol. Clin. Biol.* **4** 770–776.

[10] Galeone, M., Nizzola, L., Cacioli, D. & Moise, G. (1981) *In vivo* demonstration of delivery mechanisms from sustained release pellets. *Curr. Ther. Research* **29** 217–234.

[11] Jian, R., Assael, T., Grall, Y., Romary, D., Jobin, G., Valleur, P., Dhamlincourt, A.-M. & Bernier, J.-J. (1983). Etude comparee de la vidange gastrique de solides digestibles et non degradables chez l'homme normal et l'ulcereux duodenal. *Gastroenterol. Clin. Biol.* **7** 272–276.

[12] Minami, H. & McCallum, R. W. (1984). The physiology and pathophysiology of gastric emptying in humans. *Gastroenterol.* **86** 1592–1610.

[13] Caride, V. J., Prokop, E. K., Troncale, F. J., Buddoura, W., Winchenbach, K.

& McCallum, R. W. (1984). Scintigraphic determination of small intestinal transit time: comparison with hydrogen breath technique. *Gastroenterol.* **86** 714–720.

[14] Jian, R., Najean, Y. & Bernier, J. J. (1984). Measurement of intestinal progression of a meal and its residues in normal subjects and patients with functional diarrhoea by a dual isotope technique. *Gut* **25** 728–731.

[15] Digenis, G. (1982). The utilisation of short-lived radionuclides in the assessment of formulation and *in vivo* deposition of drugs. In: Wilson, C. G., Hardy, J. G., Frier, M. & Davis, S. S. (eds) *Radionuclide Imaging in Drug Research,* Croom Helm, London, pp. 103–143.

[16] Davis, S. S. (1983). The use of scintigraphic methods for the evaluation of drug dosage forms in the gastrointestinal tract. In: Breimer, D. D. & Speiser, P. (eds) *Topics in Pharmaceutical Sciences,* Elsevier, Amsterdam, pp. 205–215.

[17] Fell, J. T. & Digenis, G. A. (1984). Imaging and behaviour of solid oral dosage forms *in vivo*. *Int. J. Pharm.* **22** 1–15.

[18] Davis, S. S., Fara, J. & Hardy, J. G. (1986). The intestinal transit of pharmaceutical dosage forms. *Gut* (in press).

[19] Daly, P. B., Davis, S. S., Frier, M., Hardy, J. G., Kennerley, J. W. & Wilson, C. G. (1982). Scintigraphic assessment of the *in vivo* dissolution rate of a sustained release tablet. *Int. J. Pharmaceut.* **10** 17–24.

[20] Davis, S. S., Hardy, J. G., Taylor, M. J., Whalley, D. R. & Wilson, C. G. (1984). A comparative study of the gastrointestinal transit of a pellet and a tablet formulation. *Int. J. Pharmaceut.* **21** 167–177.

[21] Davis, S. S., Hardy, J. G., Stockwell, A., Taylor, M. J., Whalley, D. R. & Wilson, C. G. (1984). The effect of food on the gastrointestinal transit of pellets and an osmotic device (Osmet). *Int. J. Pharmaceut.* **21** 331–340.

[22] Davis, S. S., Hardy, J. G., Taylor, M. J., Stockwell, A. & Wilson, C. G. (1984). The *in vivo* evaluation of an osmotic device (Osmet) using gamma scintigraphy. *J. Pharm. Pharmac.* **36** 740–742.

[23] Wilson, C. G., Parr, G. D., Kennerley, J. W., Taylor, M. J., Davis, S. S., Hardy, J. G. & Rees, J. A. (1984). Pharmacokinetics and *in vivo* scintigraphic monitoring of a sustained release acetylsalicylic acid formulation. *Int. J. Pharm.* **18** 1–8.

[24] Christensen, F. N., Davis, S. S., Hardy, J. G., Taylor, M. J., Whalley, D. R. & Wilson, C. G. (1985). The use of gamma scintigraphy to follow the gastrointestinal transit of pharmaceutical formulations. *J. Pharm. Pharmac.* **37** 91–95.

[25] Bechgaard, H., Christensen, F. N., Davis, S. S., Hardy, J. G., Taylor, M. J., Whalley, D. R. & Wilson, C. G. (1985). Gastrointestinal transit of pellet systems in ileostomy subjects and the effect of density. *J. Pharm. Pharmacol.* **37** 718–721.

[26] Boertz, A., Cawello, W., Cordes, G., Davis, S. S., Fischer, W. & Sandrock, K. (1986). Gastrointestinal transit investigation and the *in vivo* drug release of isosorbide-5-nitrate. In preparation.

[27] Kelly, K. A. (1981). Motility of the stomach and gastrodudenal junction. In: Johnson, L. R. (ed.) *Physciology of the Gastrointerestinal Tract,* vol. 1, Raven Press, New York, pp. 393–410.

[28] Szurszewski, J. H. (1969). A migrating electric complex of the canine small

intestine. *Am. J. Physiol.* **217** 1757–1763.

[29] Park, H. M., Chernish, S. M., Rosenek, B. D., Brunelle, R. L., Hargrove, B. & Wellman, H. N. (1984). Gastric emptying of enteric-coated tablets. *Digestive Dis. and Sci.* **29** 207–212.

[30] Davis, S. S., Hardy, J. G., Wilson, C. G., Feely, L. C. & Palin, K. J. (1986). The gastrointestinal transit of a controlled release naproxen tablet formulation. *Int. J. Pharm.* (in press).

[31] Davis, S. S., Stockwell, A., Taylor, M. J., Hardy, J. G., Whalley, D. R., Wilson, C. G., Bechgaard, H. & Christensen, F. N. (1986). The effect of density on the gastrointestinal transit time of single and multiple unit dosage forms. *Pharm. Res.* (in press).

[32] Khosla, R. & Davis, S. S. (1986). The effect of polycarbophil on the gastric emptying of pellets. *J. Pharm. Pharmacol.* (submitted).

[33] Read, N. W., Miles, C. A., Fisher, D., Holgate, A. M., Kime, N. D., Mitchell, M. A., Reeve, A. M., Roche, T. B. & Walker, M. (1980). Transit of a meal through the stomach, small intestine and colon in normal subjects and its role in the pathogenesis of diarrhoea. *Gastroenterol.* **79** 1276–1282.

[34] Cammack, J., Read, N. W., Cann, P. A., Greenwood, B. & Holgate, A. M. (1982). Effect of prolonged exercise on the passage of a solid meal through the stomach and small intestine. *Gut* **23** 957–961.

[35] Holt, S., Reid, J., Taylor, T. V., Tothill, P. & Heading, R. C. (1982). Gastric emptying of solids in man. *Gut* **23** 292–296.

[36] Kerlin, P. & Phillips, S. (1983). Differential transit of liquids and solid residue through the human ileum. *Am. J. Physiol.* **245** G38–G43.

[37] Moore, J. G., Tweedy, C., Christian, P. E. & Datz, F. L. (1983). Effect of age on gastric emptying of liquid-solid meals in man. *Digestive Dis. and Sci.* **28** 340–344.

[38] Horowitz, M., Maddern, G. J., Chatterton, B. E., Collins, P. J., Harding, P. E. & Shearman, D. J. C. (1984). Changes in gastric emptying rates with age. *Clin. Sci.* **67** 213–218.

[39] Malagelada, J. R., Robertson, J. S., Brown, M. L., Remington, M., Duenes, J. A., Thomforde, G. M. & Carryer, P. W. (1984). Intestinal transit of solid and liquid components of a meal in health. *Gastroenterol.* **87** 1255–1263.

[40] Kupfer, R. M., Heppell, M., Haggith, J. W. & Bateman, D. N. (1985). Gastric emptying and small bowel transit rate in the elderly. *J. Am. Geriatr. Soc.,* **33**, 340.

[41] Narducci, F., Bassotti, G., Granata, M. T., Pelli, M. A., Gaburri, M., Palumbo, R. & Morelli, A. (1986). Colonic motility and gastric emptying in patients with irritable bowel syndrome. Effect of pretreatment with ocylonium bromide. *Digestive Dis. and Sci.* **31** 241–246.

[42] Hardy, J. G., Wilson, C. G. & Wood, E. (1985) Drug delivery to the proximal colon. *J. Pharm. Pharmacol.* **37** 874–877.

[43] John, V. A., Shotton, P. A., Moppert, J. & Theobald, W. (1985). Gastrointestinal transit of Oros drug delivery sytems in healthy volunteers: a short report. *Br. J. Clin. Pharmac.* **19** 203S–206S.

[44] Eckenhoff, B. & Yum, S. I. (1981). The osmotic pump: novel research tool for optimising drug regimens. *Biomaterials* **2** 89–97.

[45] Dressman, J. (1986). Paper presented to conference on *Oral Control Release Dosage Forms,* Arden House, New York.

[46] O'Hagan, D., Palin, K. J. & Davis, S. S. (1986). The absorption of macromolecules from the gastrointestnal tract. *CRC Critical Reviews in Therapeutic Carrier Systems* (in press).

[47] Davis, S. S. (1985). The use of scintigraphic methods for the evaluation of novel delivery systems. In: Borchardt, R. T., Repta, A. J. and Stella, V. J. (eds) *Directed Drug Delivery: A Multidisciplineary Problem* Humana Press, New Jersey, p. 319–340.

[48] Muranishi, S. (1986). The rectal and lymphatic delivery of proteins and peptides. In: Davis, S. S., Illum, L. & Tomlinson, E. (eds) *Advanced Drug Delivery Systems for Peptides and Proteins,* Plenum, New York (in press).

11

Mucoadhesive polymers in drug delivery systems

Graham Hunt, Patrick Kearney and **Ian W. Kellaway**, The Welsh School of Pharmacy, University of Wales Institute of Science and Technology, P.O. Box 13, Cardiff CF1 3XF, UK

1. INTRODUCTION

Bioadhesive polymers have been employed in both surgery and dentistry for many years. Such polymers include the well-documented 'super glues', the esters of α-cyanoacrylates [1,2], which have found applications ranging from repair of osteochondral fractures to capping extraction wounds in dentistry. Other synthetic bone glue candidates [3,4] have included polyurethanes, epoxy resins, acrylates and polystyrene. Often the mechanism of bonding involves the formation of covalent bonds with the target tissue to provide a permanent or semipermanent linkage.

In the development of oral controlled-release dosage forms, considerable benefits may ensue from the use of bioadhesive polymers providing relatively short-term adhesion between the drug delivery system and the mucus or epithelial cell surface of the gastrointestinal (GI) tract. Bonding will therefore involve secondary forces such as hydrogen bonds or London–van der Waals forces. Mucoadhesives may therefore be regarded as a specific class of bioadhesives. Polymer candidates would need to be non-toxic and non-absorbable, adhere rapidly to wet tissues and release the incorporated drug in a controlled manner. Further refinements would seek to achieve specificity as to the site of adherence within the GI tract.

One of the principal objectives of oral controlled drug delivery is to achieve once-a-day dosing, which reduces patient non-compliance and generally improves drug therapy. The vagaries of the GI transit profile therefore present a challenge to the design of such delivery systems. Although transit times of 8–10 h from mouth to colon may be regarded as normal in humans, nevertheless considerable variations are known to exist. Most of this variation occurs in the gastric emptying of dosage forms, which is influenced by both form type and diet [5]. Small intestinal transport appears less dependent on such factors [6]. It is for this reason that control of the gastric emptying of dosage forms by mucoadhesive formulations is an attractive proposition.

The ability to localize a drug delivery system in a selected region of the tract would, in general, lead to improved bioavailability; more especially for drugs exhibiting narrow windows of absorption or instability in certain sectors of the tract. Intimate contact with the target absorption membrane should lead to optimization of both the extent and rate of drug absorption. Alternative mechanisms for the control of GI transit of the dosage form, for example through manipulation of particle size and density [7], together with the use of fibrous materials, have not, in the main, been successful.

This paper will attempt to review the development of mucoadhesive polymers, from a consideration of the target tissue, polymer characteristics, *in vitro* testing techniques and the limited amount of *in vivo* evaluation reported to date.

2. CHARACTERISTICS OF THE TARGET TISSUE

There are two ways a material may adhere to a mucosal surface, either by binding to the tissue itself or by associating with the mucus coat which is intimately associated with the tissue surface. The characteristics of these surfaces are quite different and the distinction ought to be emphasized.

2.1 The mucus layer

The stomach mucosa is the primary target in the development of a mucoadhesive-based sustained/retarded-release action as gastric retention will be the main mechanism in delaying the rapid absorption which occurs once a formulation reaches the specialized absorbtive areas of the small intestine. Throughout the GI tract the mucosal surface is comprised of columnar epithelial cells, the morphology of which changes as the tract is descended. In the stomach there are specific mucus-secreting glands in the cardiac and pyloric regions [8], which serve to coat incoming food boli and hence reduce the possible abrasive action. Mucus cells are also found in the necks and depths of the acid-secreting gastric pits where they form a protective buffer zone around the stream of acid. The mucus coating over the rest of the stomach surface is maintained by the surface columnar epithelial cells and secretion is stimulated by mechanical and chemical irritation [9]. The mucus layer also serves to protect the gastric epithelium from the action of secreted acid and proteolytic enzymes [10]. The layer is usually continuous but can be disrupted under the action of certain irritant substances and an ineffective mucus layer is usually associated with conditions of gastric ulceration [11].

In the small intestine the Brunner's glands of the duodenum supply a copious mucus secretion to protect against the high acid content of the chyme released from the stomach. Mucus throughout the rest of the GI tract is provided by the goblet cells, which represent an increasing fraction of the total epithelial surface towards the colon. They constituted 30% by volume of the mucosa in the upper small intenstine, 40% in the lower small intestine and 55% in the colon [12]. Mucus is stored in granules in the apical supra-nuclear half of these cells, which causes them to distend into the characteristic 'goblet' shape. As with the surface cells of the gastric mucosa, irritation can cause these cells to discharge the granules *en masse*, though basal secretion is low [13].

The mucus coating is present throughout the whole GI tract where it functions as both a protective layer and a lubricant. To serve this dual function the mucus gel has particular physical characteristics, the most important of which is its viscoelasticity. This property enables it to act as a mechanical barrier, yet to flow under the influence of peristalsis. Thus a mucus gel can exist in reasonable layer thicknesses before it begins to flow under its own weight [14] and layer thicknesses of up to 600 μm have been measured on human gastric mucosa [15]. As it is secreted by the surface cells, it is intimately associated with the mucosal membrane and is quite tenacious. In this respect mucus is itself an excellent mucoadhesive and it must be borne in mind that any mucoadhesive bond can only be as strong as the mucus–mucosa interaction. Even a material which binds irreversibly to the surface molecules of the mucus gel will be dissociated from the mucosa if the underlying mucus becomes detached or is sheared from the surface by the peristaltic action of the gut.

The particular physical properties of mucus derive from its primary component which is a large glycoprotein or 'mucin' [16]. This large molecule is built up from a fundamental subunit of molecular weight 500000, which consists of a protein backbone some 800 amino acids long, rich in serine, threonine and proline. Most of the hydroxy residues are *O*-glycosidically linked to oligosaccharide side chains, which are composed of a combination of *N*-acetylgalactosamine, *N*-acetylglucosamine, galactose, fucose or *N*-acetylneuraminic acid residues and may be up to 18 residues in length [17]. This results in a stiffened glycosylated unit which resembles a 'bottle-brush' structure and is about 200 nm long. Four such subunits are associated via disulphide bonds to a globular type protein moiety of some 70000 molecular weight [18], although the actual physical arrangement of these structures is under debate [10, 19]. The primary structure which interacts to form the mucus gel is thus a species of about 2 million molecular weight. In addition to the large protein unit, non-covalently-linked protein is associated with the glycoprotein taken directly from the mucosa and constitutes some 15% of the total protein measured [20].

The viscosity of mucin solutions increases with increasing concentration and rises asymptotically at around 20 mg/ml [21]. This is the gel threshold and mucus, as secreted, usually contains between 3 and 5% glycoprotein [16]. The nature of the interactions of the glycoprotein molecules in the gel is unknown but must arise from a combination of hydrogen bonds, van der Waals forces and physical entanglement, with mechanical spectroscopy showing the gel to be a weakly cross-linked structure [22]. Charged groups can only have a limited influence on the interaction, as removal of the terminal *N*-acetyl neuraminic acid residues produces no measurable effect on the physical properties of the resulting gels [23]. However, the glycosylation of the subunits and the polymeric structure of the whole mucin are essential for the viscous and gel-forming properties.

2.2   Adhesion of solid material

The mucus gel is 95% water so any surface which is wettable could form an intimate contact with the gel. Particles which are small enough to be buried in the surface of the mucus (<600 μm) will be securely held due to the relatively high storage modulus (elasticity) of the gel. However, as mucus is continually secreted, such particles will be pushed further from the mucosal surface to a point where they are sheared away, either under the weight of the gel itself, or due to mechanical abrasion of the luminal contents. Larger particles for which there is a favourable interfacial interaction with the mucus gel may, nevertheless, be pulled from the mucosal surface due to their weight alone or because they are more easily dislodged by the peristaltic action of the mucosa. One method of prolonging mucosal association and stasis would be to use a hydrophilic polymer in a dry powder or granule form which, after embedding in the mucus, would slowly hydrate and take up water at the expense of the mucus gel. This would compensate for the continuing secretion by increasing the elasticity or storage modulus of the gel, thereby enabling a more substantial layer to exist on the mucosa.

2.3 Adhesion of agents in solution

Although mucus gels present only a limited barrier to small molecules [24] due to the low microviscosity of the interstices [25], the diffusion of macromolecules is more severely restricted [10] because of physical obstruction. Thus, molecularly dispersed polymers could interact with the mucus gel at the surface via a combination of secondary bonds, although diffusional resistance of the mucus gel would prevent a total mixing of mucin and polymer on the mucosa which may bring about a stiffening or strengthening of the mucus gel such as that observed under selected conditions *in vitro* [26]. However, a limited degree of chain interpenetration at the adhesive–mucus interface would be essential for effective mucoadhesion.

The most effective mucoadhesives are linear or lightly cross-linked polymers which differ considerably in structure to the mucus glycoprotein molecules. Consequently, it is unlikely that they adhere to the gel through interactions similar to the mucin–mucin interaction which is so important in the gel structure. Interestingly, one common factor in the effective mucoadhesives is the presence of carboxylate groups [27] which have no significant role in the purely mucin–mucin interaction. Likely points of interaction for these polymers is the oligosaccharide side chains on the mucin which are aligned normal to the linear axis of the protein backbone of the glycosylated subunit. If penetration of this glycosylated coat is a prerequisite in the formation of a viable interaction, then the 'free ends' of the interacting polymers need be no more than several monomer units long. However, as there seems to be a relation between the molecular weight of a polymer and its supposed mucoadhesive properties [28], it could be that interdigitation between the whole mucin subunits (~200 nm) is of greater relevance in the polymer–mucin interaction. The polymers considered to date are not of a nature which may be considered to interact with the hydrophobic regions of the glycoprotein such as the globular protein unit or the numerous esterified fatty acid residues [29].

2.4 The tissue surface

The apical membrane of the surface epithelial cells which is exposed to the lumen has a typical lipoidal bilamella structure, but integrated into the membrane and extending into the luminal space are filamentous structures composed of glycolipids and glycoproteins which form the glycocalyx or 'brush border' [30]. These glycoproteins, which contain polysaccharide moieties (mucopolysaccharides), are to be distinguished from the mucus glycoproteins (mucins) which form the mucus layer, as they differ markedly in their chemistry and physical properties. It will only be via association with the glycocalyx that a true tissue adhesion will be achieved. However, to form a viable bond with the tissue the overlying layer of mucus must first be penetrated, Heavy, or dense particles may have sufficient force to penetrate the elastic gel but for the reasons discussed above, this will not be the case for material which is molecularly dispersed. Small latex particles penetrate into the intravillous space quite rapidly although larger particles such as yeast cells penetrate less readily [31]. The passive penetration of bacteria-sized particles is very slow but, for bacteria such as *Vibrio cholerae*, this is increased if they are motile and are guided by chemotactic stimuli. Also, firm fixation of these organsims to the cell surface is achieved via certain bacterial adhesions which promote a specific lectin-type bond with the sugar components of the glycocalyx [31]. Non-specific electrostatic and hydrophobic interactions may play a part in initiating the binding process. Synthetic polymeric materials will not have the specificity required to form such enzyme–substrate type bonds but secondary interactions and physical entanglement with the filaments of the glycocalyx are possibilities.

The area available for adhesion must also be considered. In addition to the roughness brought about due to the indentations of the gastric pits, the microvilli at the luminal face of the columnar epithelial cells serve to further increase surface irregularity. The base of these microvilli is about 1 μm from the tips so the only readily accessible membrane areas are the tips of the microvilli themselves. Conditions are even less favourable in the small intestine where the presence of villi and Kerckring folds serves to render the majority of the tissue surface even more remote from the lumen. This would severely reduce the scope for a polymer–tissue bond. However, as the membrane surfaces of the epithelial cells are rarely exposed directly to the luminal contents, the interface with the lumen will be formed mainly by the surface mucus coating and direct interaction with the membrane surface must be of secondary importance in the assessment of potential mucoadhesive materials.

3. MUCOADHESIVE POLYMERS

The development of mucoadhesive polymers may be traced back as far as 1947 when gum tragacanth and dental adhesive powders were combined to form a vehicle for applying penicillin to the oral mucosa [32]. An improvement in this system resulted when carboxymethyl cellulose (CMC) and petrolatum were combined to form the vehicle [33]. The development of Orahesive followed, leading to trials of Orabase in 1959 [34]. Orahesive is a mixture of finely ground sodium carboxymethyl cellulose (SCMC), pectin and gelatin, and Orabase a blend of SCMC, pectin and gelatin, in a polyethylene/mineral oil base. However, after trials [35] it was considered that dry polymer powders would form better mucoadhesive agents, since such formulations would be capable of absorbing a greater amount of water and hence adhere more strongly to the tissue substrate than when blended with the hydrophobic carrier. A further development was the blending of SCMC with poly(isobutylene) (PIB) and laminating this mixture onto a polyethylene sheet. This system benefited from both wet surface adhesion (due to the SCMC) and dry surface adhesion (due to the PIB), with the added bonus of being protected from physical interference, e.g. from the tongue, by the polyethylene sheet backing.

An extensive range of such systems, whereby a water-soluble polymer and PIB (60/40) are blended together and laminated with a polyethylene film, was tested by Chen and Cyr [35]. This study yielded results in terms of 'excellent'. 'satisfactory', 'fair' or 'poor' mucosa adhesives, according to the duration of application force required, and ease of dislodgement thereafter of test discs applied to the oral mucosa. The polymers identified as exhibiting the best adhesion were sodium alginate, SCMC (high molecular weight), Guar gum (high concentration), hydroxyethylcellulose (HEC), Karya gum (high concentration), methylcellulose (MeC) (low molecular weight), polyethylene glycol (PEG) (high molecular weight), Retene, and tragacanth. However, there was no further classification in terms of *in vivo* adhesive strength, between these materials. *In vitro* lap-shear tests were carried out on some of the above, and all gave very similar results, except MeC, which gave lower values.

A number of polymers had therefore been identified as possessing mucoadhesive properties, and a number of patents cover formulations of such materials. Acrylic polymers were soon identified as useful mucoadhesive materials and the early 1980s saw a plethora of patents (Japanese patent numbers 80 118, 413; 80 118, 414; 58 109, 059; 59 232, 552; 59 232, 553; 60 05, 159; 60 05, 160; 60 116, 630; 60 116, 631; 60 237, 018) where hydroxypropylcellulose (HPC) or MeC and poly(acrylic acid) (PAA) were blended together to form mucoadhesive preparations. By far the most-studied mucoadhesive polymers through the 1980s have been PAA, HPC and SCMC. Some polymers used have been standard pharmaceutical materials such as MeC, HEC and sodium alginate, and others have been specifically synthesized to achieved optimal results, such as 2-ethylhexyl acrylate–lauryl methacrylate–vinyl stearate copolymer (Japanese patent 60 04,125), and isooctyl acrylate–methoxy poly(ethylene oxide) acrylate–acrylic acid copolymer (World patent 84 03, 837). It is interesting to note that a recent Japanese patent (61 30, 517) is for a product which utilizes tacky rubber compounds and mucoadhesive celluloses (CMC, HEP, HPC, etc.) blended together to obtain a product which may be applied to dry or wet tissues, the same principle studied earlier by Chen and Cyr [35].

The work of Chen and Cyr [35], together with other work by Park and Robinson [36] and Smart *et al.* [28], entailed the investigation of a range of polymers of varying molecular character and appeared to arrive at similar conclusions as to the molecular characteristics required for mucoadhesion. The properties exhibited by such a molecule are detailed by Peppas and Buri [27], and may be summarized thus:

(a) Strong H-bonding groups (—OH, —COOH)
(b) Strong anionic charges
(c) Sufficient flexibility to penetrate the mucus network or tissue crevices
(d) Surface tension characteristics suitable for wetting mucus/mucosal tissue surfaces
(e) High molecular weight.

Obviously some of these are inter-related, for example the presence of —COOH groups and strong anionic charges, but this also brings into account other factors such as pH of the environment. Also, for good adhesion through any kind of secondary bonding (H-bonding, ionic bonding, van der Waals forces), the adhesive material must wet the surface (classical adhesion theory), hence these factors are inter-related. Table 1 lists, in order of decreasing mucoadhesive ability, the major polymers studied by Smart *et al.* [28] and is similar to the results of Chen and Cyr [35] and Park and Robinson [36].

If these polymers are considered in the light of the criteria listed above, it is possible to identify certain factors that would appear to be main contributors to the mucoadhesive properties of the materials. Fig. 1 shows the structures of the polymers in Table 1 and a comparison of their chemical and structural features allows establishment of the aforementioned contributory factors.

In accordance with the theory that secondary bond formation is the principal source of mucoadhesion, those polymers with carboxyl groups present are all, without exception, mucoadhesive. The carboxyl group in its unionized form is capable of strong H-bond formation, and in its ionized form also able to intract electrostatically. However, the functional groups on the polymer backbone should not be in such close proximity that they interfere with each other (e.g. by intramole-cular H-bonding). As the carboxyl concentration along a polymer chain decreases, for example in moving from sodium alginate to Karya gum to gelatin, the mucoadhe-sive strength also decreases.

The effect of other secondary bond-forming groups (e.g. hydroxyl, ether oxygen, amine) on the mucoadhesive properties of the polymers above is not as definite as for the carboxyl group. The cellulosic polymers have an abundance of hydroxyl and ether groups along their length, yet the mucoadhesion exhibited bears little relation-ship to this, since the cellulose derivatives are found throughout Table 1. Further variation in the possible rank order of the cellulosics is introduced by varying the degree of substitution of the polymer.

Another important feature of mucoadhesive molecules is believed to be the ability to form physical bonds principally by entanglement with the substrate molecules. This would appear to be demonstrated by polyethylene oxide (PEO), a linear flexible molecule with minimal secondary bond-forming capacity. Yet at high molecular weights this molecule exhibits a mucoadhesive strength comparable to MeC and sodium alginate whose secondary bond-formation ability is far greater. The reason for this could be that the segmental mobility of PEO is extremely high, the ether linkages make for a very flexible backbone, and hence interpenetration into substrate networks is deep and relatively rapid. The effective depth is, however, limited by molecular chain length (i.e. molecular weight) since a short-chain molecule can form fewer entanglements and penetrate to a lesser degree than a larger molecule. This can be illustrated by reference to PEO (molecular weight 60000) and PEG (molecular weight 6000) in Table 1. Primarily the intimacy of interaction between the adhesive and mucus or mucosal tissue is a surface tension phenomenon; hence the lower the contact angle between the adhesive and the mucus/mucosa the better the chances of interaction of the two molecular systems.

The ideal mucoadhesive would arise from a combination of various carefully balanced properties. It must be a polymer of high molecular weight to maximize adhesion through entanglements and van der Waals forces. The segmental mobility of the polymer chain should be high to facilitate rapid and deep penetration into the substrate. The repeating unit of the polymer should contain carboxyl groups and

Table 1 — Rank order of mucoadhesive force for various polymers [37]

Test polymer	Mean % adhesive force	Standard deviation
Sodium carboxymethyl cellulose	192.4	12.0
Poly(acrylic acid)	185.0	10.3
Tragacanth	154.4	7.5
Poly(methyl vinylether co-maleic anhydride)	147.7	9.7
Poly(ethylene oxide)	128.6	4.0
Methylcellulose	128.0	2.4
Sodium alignate	126.2	12.0
Hydroxypropylmethylcellulose	125.2	16.7
Karya gum	125.2	4.8
Methylethylcellulose	117.4	4.2
Soluble starch	117.2	3.1
Gelatin	115.8	5.6
Pectin	100.0	2.4
Poly(vinyl pyrrolidone)	97.6	3.9
Poly(ethylene glycol)	96.0	7.6
Poly(vinyl alcohol)	94.8	4.4
Poly(hydroxyethylmethacrylate)	88.4	2.3
Hydroxypropylcellulose	87.1	13.3

other secondary bond-forming groups, principally primary hydroxyl groups and short-chain ethers. This would ensure the potential for adhesion via as many modes as possible.

4. *IN VITRO* TEST METHODS

A number of methods have been employed in an attempt to measure the bioadhesion exhibited by polymers, with some techniques designed specifically for the measurement of mucoadhesion. The methods used to determine the mucoadhesive ability of polymers have measured tensile strength, the closely related peel strength, or a chemical interaction. Chen and Cyr [35] used lap-shear and bending tensile tests to study mucoadhesive formulation. In this method a carriage of weights was attached via a pulley to a strip of plastic bearing the mucoadhesive polymer. The polymer had previously been pressed onto a sample of wet dialysing cellophane, and the time taken for a load of 250 g to separate the two materials was measured. A similar procedure using a Chatillon strain gauge was also employed. Peel tests were also carried out, again using a Chatillon strain gauge, on oral mucosa and teeth, and showed similar results to those obtained *in vitro*. The duration of adhesion was also

POLYMER	STRUCTURE

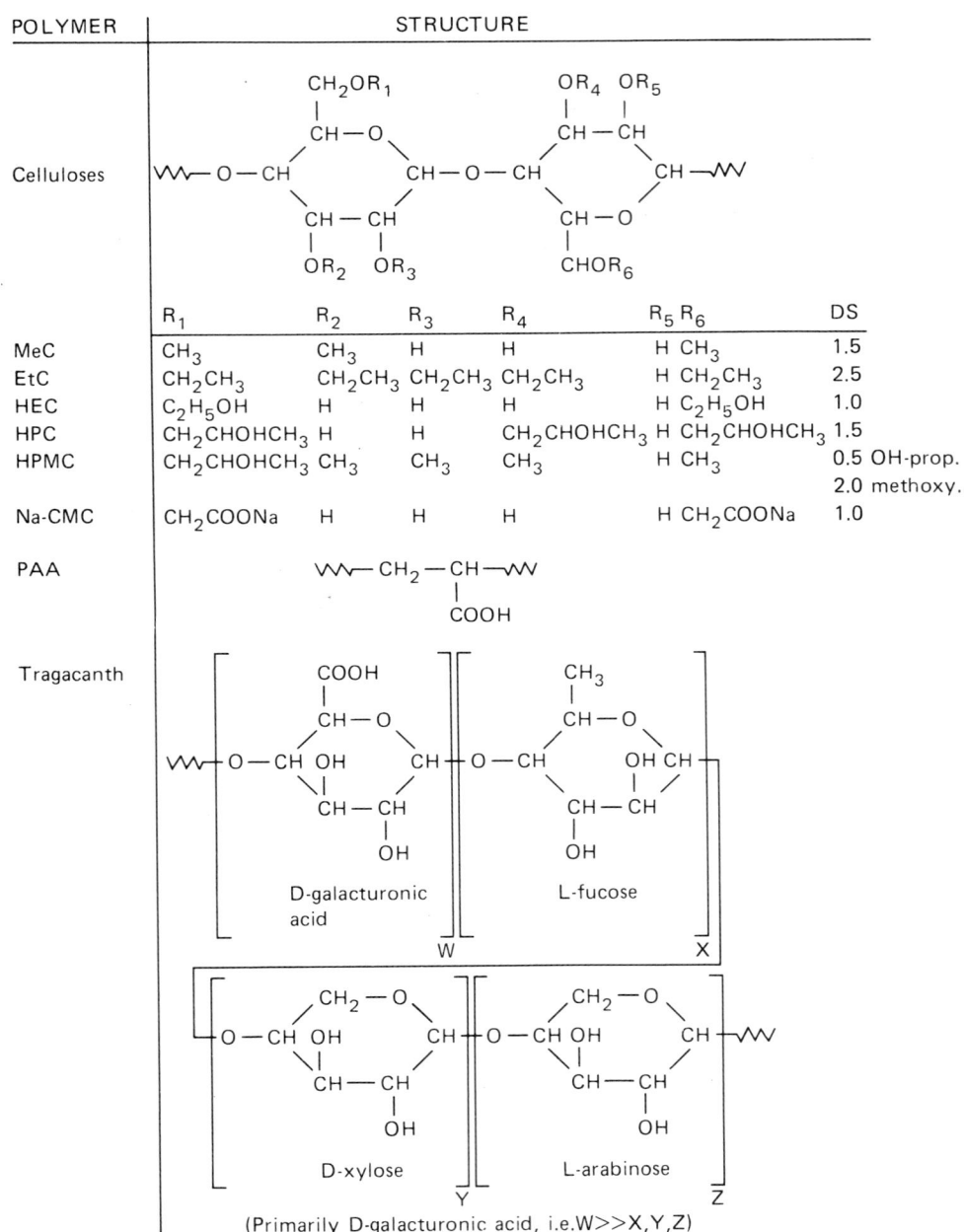

	R₁	R₂	R₃	R₄	R₅ R₆	DS
	R_1	R_2	R_3	R_4	R_5 R_6	DS
MeC	CH_3	CH_3	H	H	H CH_3	1.5
EtC	CH_2CH_3	CH_2CH_3	CH_2CH_3	CH_2CH_3	H CH_2CH_3	2.5
HEC	C_2H_5OH	H	H	H	H C_2H_5OH	1.0
HPC	$CH_2CHOHCH_3$	H	H	$CH_2CHOHCH_3$	H $CH_2CHOHCH_3$	1.5
HPMC	$CH_2CHOHCH_3$	CH_3	CH_3	CH_3	H CH_3	0.5 OH-prop. 2.0 methoxy.
Na-CMC	CH_2COONa	H	H	H	H CH_2COONa	1.0

(Primarily D-galacturonic acid, i.e.W>>X,Y,Z)

Fig. 1 — *Continued on next page.*

p(MWEcoMA)

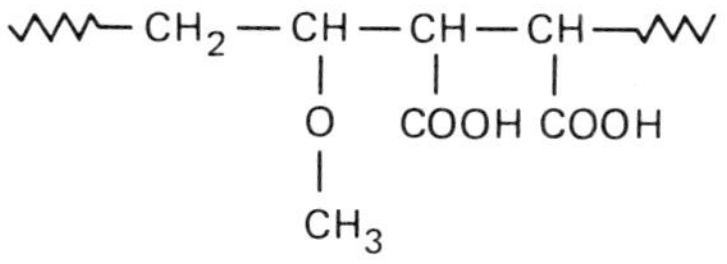

$$\text{\small \Large\wwww} - CH_2 - CH - CH - CH - \text{\small \Large\wwww}$$

O   COOH COOH

CH₃

PEO

$$\text{\Large\wwww} - CH_2 - CH_2 - O - \text{\Large\wwww}$$

Na-Alginate

2 components;

i)

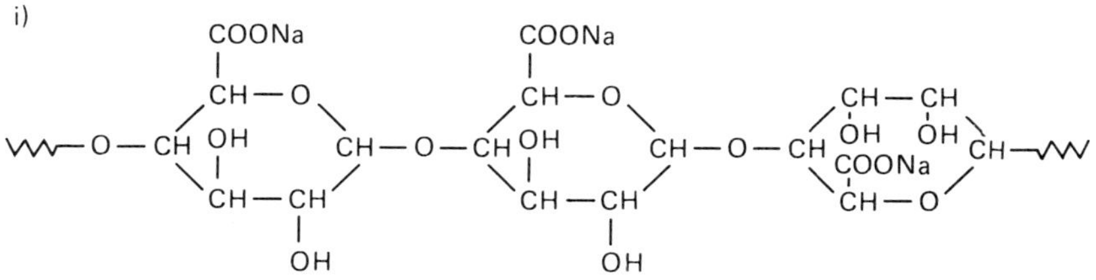

ii)

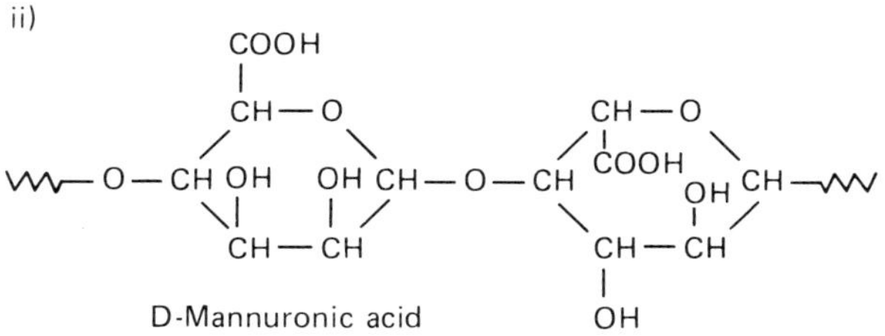

D-Mannuronic acid

L-Glucronic acid (Ratio 60:40)

Karya gum

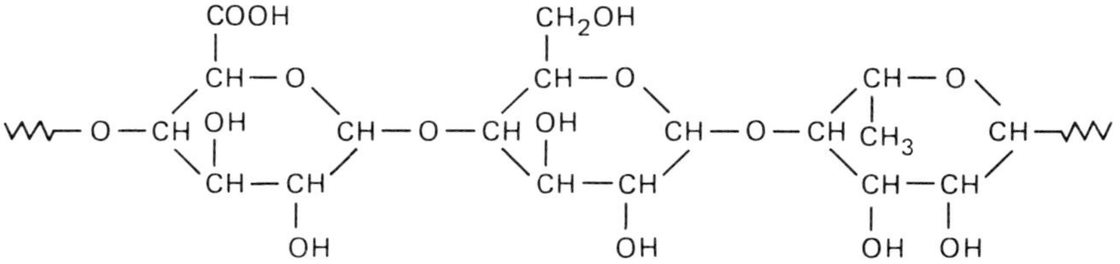

D-galacturonic
acid

D-galactose

L-rhamnose

(Ratio 43:14:15)

Starch

2 components:

i) Amylose,

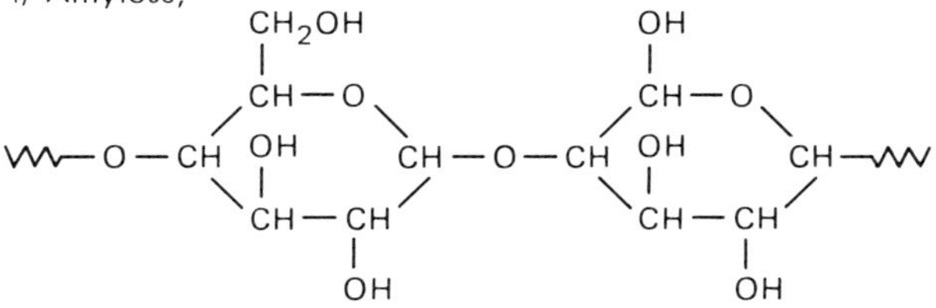

Fig. 1 — *Continued on next page.*

ii) Amylopectin,

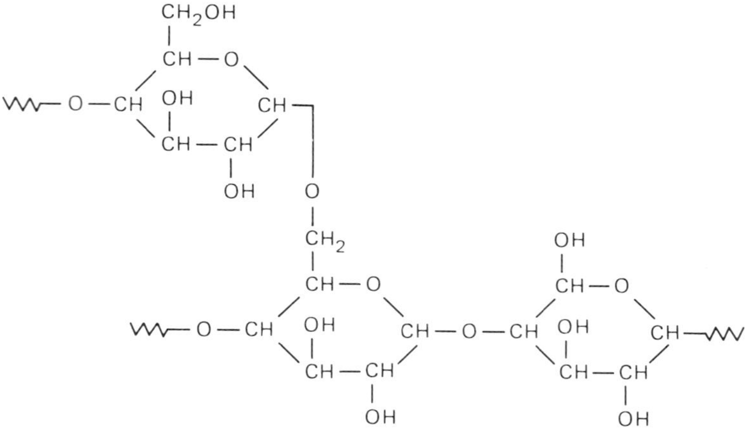

Gelatin | General formula for amino acid:

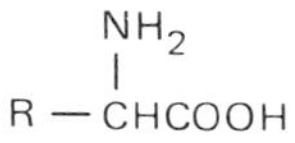

$$\underset{\underset{R-CHCOOH}{|}}{NH_2}$$

Amino acid	R	% abundance
Glycine	H—	27
Proline	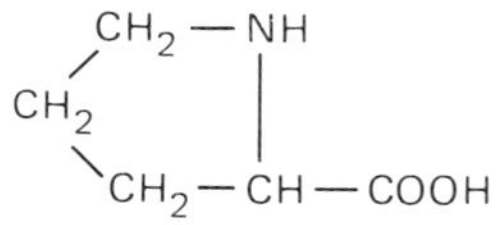 (ring structure)	16
Hydroxyproline	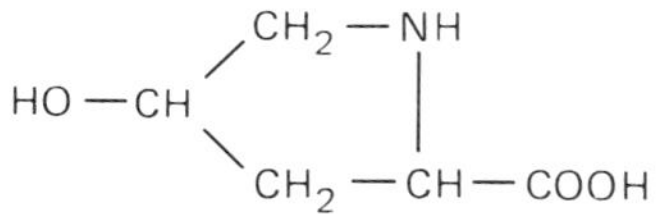 (ring structure)	15
Glutamic acid	$HO\overset{O}{\overset{\|}{C}}CH_2CH_2$ —	11
Alanine	CH_3 —	10

Arginine, Aspartic acid, Leucine, Isoleucine, Lysine,   <2
Serine, Threonine, Phenylamine, Valine, Tyrosine,
Histidine, Hydroxylysine, Methionine,

Fig. 1 — *Continued on next page.*

Pectin

3 components:

i) Galacturonan (methyl ester)

ii) Poly(arabinofuranose)

iii) Galactan

PVP

PVA

p(HEMA)

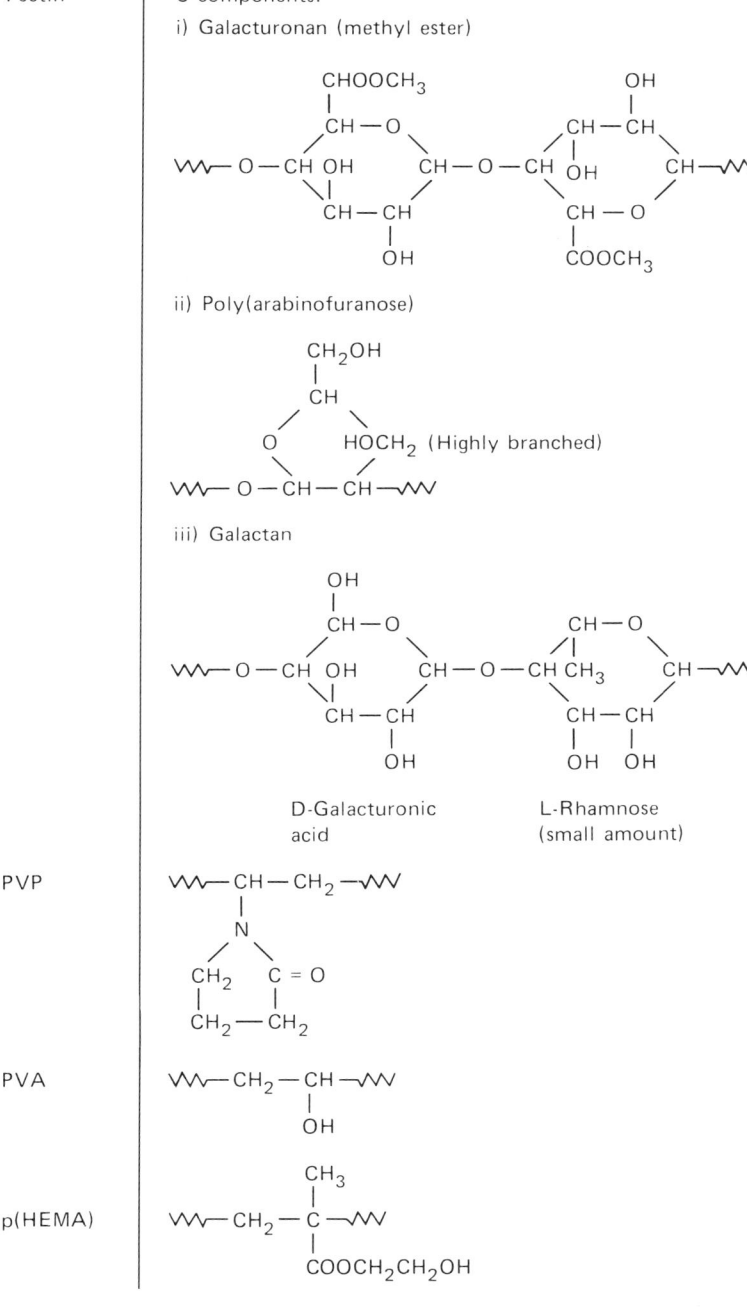

Fig. 1 — Structures of mucoadhesive polymers.

measured, and for the Orahesive bandage the effect of the force applied, water avilable for hydration, and hydration time were studied.

Gurny *et al*. [38] used a tensometer to separate two Plexiglass (polymethylmeth-acrylate, PMMA) discs separated by a mixture of mucoadhesive polymer SCMC, polyethylene gel, and hydrolysed gelatin. While this method gives useful information about the concentration of mucoadhesive polymer required for optimal adhesion, it is nevertheless measuring the cohesive forces of the polymer system and/or the strength of the mucoadhesive system/PMMA bond, rather than any interaction with mucus. Furthermore, since there is little similarity between PMMA and mucus, there is no indication that the optimal formulation according to this method will be the same as that for use with mucus or mucosa substrates.

Smart *et al*. [28] used a microforce balance as the measuring unit for an apparatus based on the Wilhelmy plate method of measuring surface tension. In this procedure a thin glass plate coated with polymer is dipped into a preparation of purified glycoprotein, and removed slowly at a constant rate. The force exerted on the glass plate by interaction with the glycoprotein preparation is measured by the microforce balance and compared to that for the same, clean, glass plate before and after each test, this method was used to characterize a range of polymers (Table 1), and although tedious it gives reproducible results. No correction is made in this technique for variations in contact angle and therefore the results, in addition to measuring adhesion, contain a component due to wetting effects.

Another tensile test method is being developed by the authors (Fig. 2) for use

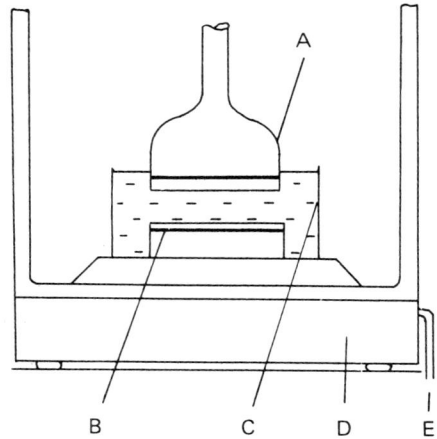

Fig. 2 — Mucoadhesion measurement apparatus. A, Test material; B, mucus/ mucosal tissue substrate; C, cell; D, Balance; E, data output to computer.

with cross-linked hydrogels that are not readily amenable to other forms of analysis, e.g. Wilhelmy plate, lap-shear tests, etc. This method involves the separation of the test material, A, from a mucus or mucosal tissue substrate, B. The cell, C, is placed on a sensitive analytical balance, D, equipped with a data output, E, to a computer for subsequent analysis. This procedure has the advantage of being rapid, simple to operate, and capable of analysing any form of mucoadhesive candidates. However, it currently lacks adequate reproducibility due mainly to the variable nature of the tissues and mucus used, and the inability to ensure complete contact between the gel and mucus/mucosa.

Park and Robinson [36] developed a procedure whereby the strength of interaction between a cellular surface (e.g. epithelial cells) and mucoadhesive polymers could be gauged by measuring the change in the fluorescence properties of a probe molecule present in the lipid cell wall. This method provides information on the fundamental characteristics of the interaction between mucoadhesive polymers and cell surface molecules. It is prone to very different errors and variabilities from those of the procedure previously described. Errors arise from the effect that the polymer has on the probe itself (rather than the cell wall), and non-bonding effects that some polymers have on the cells causing misinterpretation of the results. However, many such variables may be eliminated by further experiments with the probe and the polymer alone, when this becomes a reproducible procedure for measuring cell/polymer interactions. Park and Robinson [39] developed a system based on a tensiometer and employing swollen mucoadhesive polymer and fresh rabbit stomach mucosa. This apparatus was used to compare various formulations of polyacrylic acid polymers with pHEMA, Amberlite resin, and gelatin.

Mikos and Peppas [40] have recently introduced a method of measuring mucoadhesion whereby a small bioadhesive particle is place on a mucus bed and humid air blown over the surface of the mucus. A camera records the rate of progress of the particle across the mucus bed, and mathematical analysis allows estimation of the bioadhesive component of the drag experienced by the particle. This method may represent more closely the conditions encountered *in vivo*. It suffers, though, in its presented form from an absence of fluid simulating a body fluid such as saliva, gastric juices, etc., which will confer different surface and interfacial tension properties to the system from those of humid air.

5.   *IN VIVO* STUDIES

To date, most research activities have concentrated on the development of animal models to investigate the *in vivo* performance of putative mucoadhesives.

In our laboratories [37], the mouse was selected as the test animal and an Amberlite resin (IRA-400Cl) milled and sieved to provide a $9 \pm 3.6 \ \mu$m diameter fraction served as model particles which were readily surface labelled with ^{99m}Tc. Adsorbed monolayers of the polymers SCMC (P75) and Carbopol 934P were deposited on the labelled particle surface and the stability of such films was confirmed at the stomach pH of the mice by monitoring the electrophoretic mobility of particles exposed to a range of acidic solutions. After overnight fasting, the mice received an oral administration of 0.1 ml of a 10% suspension containing 10% sucrose. After 1 h the mice were sacrificed and the GI tract from stomach to rectum was removed and the positional radioactivity determined by a gamma counter. Fig. 3 illustrates the distribution of activity observed in five mice for the polymer-free resin. The activity is concentrated in two areas: residual stomach activity and the activity

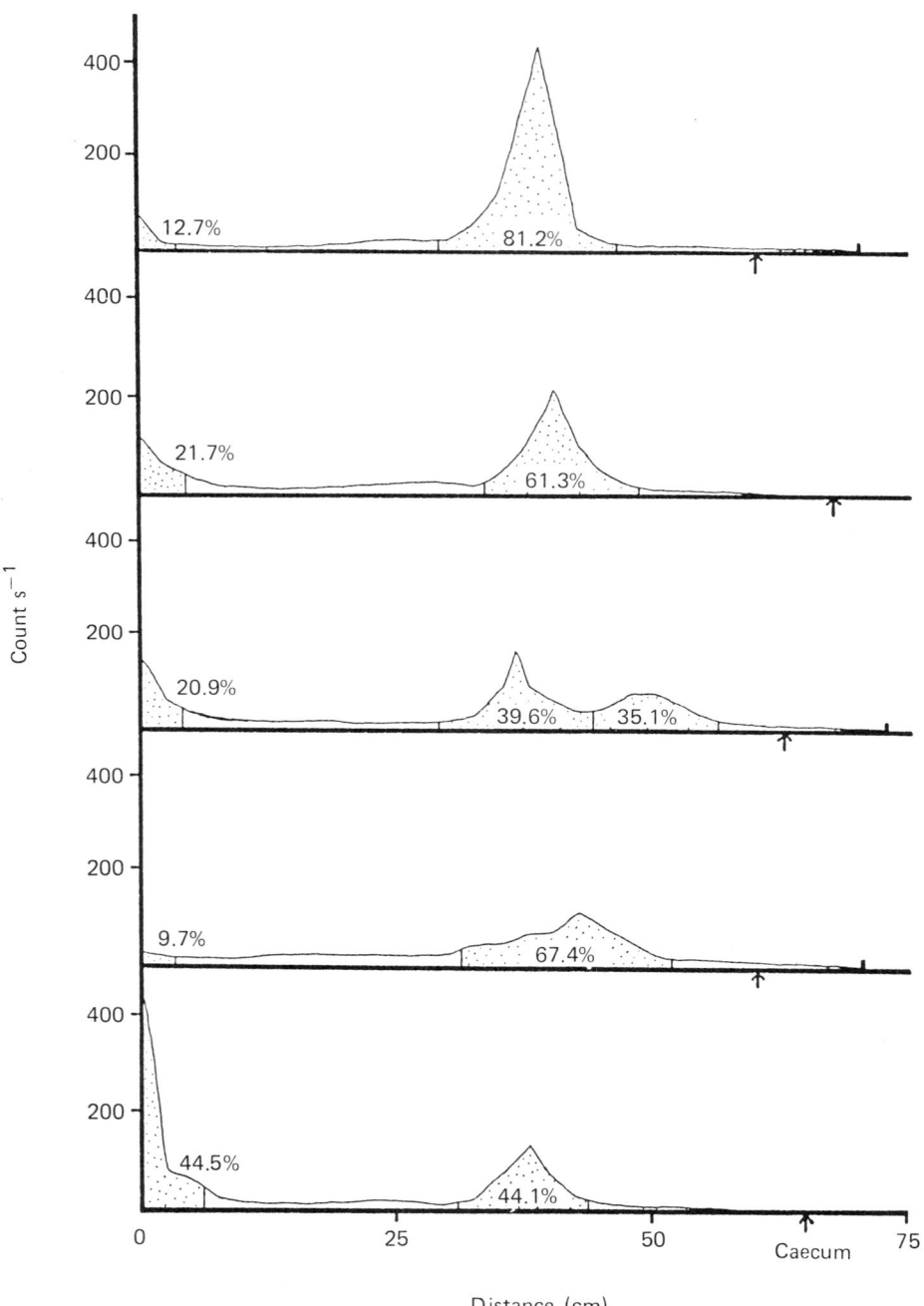

Fig. 3 — The 1-h transit profiles for 9 μm resin particles. The percentage total
activity associated with the peaks is for five mice.

associated with particles removed from the stomach, which appears as a peak (occasionally two) between the stomach and the caecum.

The presence of P75 SCMC-adsorbed film did not significantly affect GI transit, whilst a Carbopol 934P film almost completely arrested gastric emptying of the test particles (Table 2). Such effects may be due to mucosa-adhesion or to gastric

Table 2 — The effect of adsorbed films on gastrointestinal transit of 9 μm particles, 1 h after administration

Adsorbed film	No. of mice in group	% retained in stomach
None	15	29.7±18.4
P75 SCMC	4	38.7±48.4
Carbopol 934	5	97.7±5.2

obstruction caused by particle aggregates. With a sterically stabilized particle, aggregation would not be expected and, indeed, no evidence was observed *in vitro* at gastric pH.

Further evidence for the gastric retention of polyacrylic acid polymers was obtained by Ch'ng *et al*. [41] using ^{51}Cr-Polycarbophil surgically introduced into the stomachs of fasted rats. ^{51}Cr-Polycarbophil was shown to have a significantly slower GI transit compared with ^{51}Cr-poly(methacrylic acid–divinylbenzene) (Table 3).

Table 3 — Rat stomach half-transit times and emptying rate constants of test materials [41]

Test materials	Stomach half-transit time	Stomach emptying rate constant (h^{-1})
^{51}Cr-Normal saline	12 min	3.47
Amberlite 200 resin beads	2 h 15 min	0.31
^{51}Cr-Poly(metacrylic acid–divinylbenzene)	6 h	0.12
^{51}Cr-Polycarbophil	12 h 15 min	0.06

These authors also claim to have achieved bioadhesion within the small intestine. A bioadhesive formulation of chlorothiazide resulted in plasma levels in the rat which were of longer duration, and greater bioavailability compared with a sustained-release bead formulation and the drug presented as a powder [42].

The gastric emptying of Polycarbophil has also been examined in dogs [33], when only 8% of the dose was shown to empty within 90 min. Further canine studies [44] showed that only 50% of a 90 g Polycarbophil meal emptied in 4 h. The presence of such a large mass of polymer may have elicited motor activity of the stomach with subsequent reduced gastric emptying.

An alternative to using animal models is to employ the oral mucosa of volunteers [37]. Mucoadhesive polymer candidates can be converted to granules by standard processing techniques. Granules (20–25) were placed onto the oral mucosa below the lower lip and counted at regular intervals until dislodged, or for a maximum time of 45 min. Between counts the mouth was closed, the tongue kept behind the teeth and mouth movements, other than swallowing, were kept to a minimum. Photographs were taken on each occasion to permit ease of counting, and to provide an estimate of the rate of swelling of the polymer granules. Table 4 illustrates some results obtained

Table 4 — The duration of mucosa-adhesion and swelling of test granules

Granules	Time for 50% loss (min)	Time for 100% loss (min)	% swelling after 5 min	Max % swelling	Time of max % swelling (min)
Ethylcellulose	2	3	—	—	—
P75 SCMC 50%/ hard paraffin 50%	10	15	33	61	10
P75 SCMC 20%/ pHEMA 80%	7	20	58	98	10
P75 SCMC 50%/ ethylcellulose 50%	6	16	136	159	6
Carbopol 934	—	>45	213	—	—
Carbopol 934 50%/stearic acid 50%	—	>45	35	94	15

for various test formulations. Ethylcellulose, a non-mucoadhesive polymer, was rapidly cleared from the mucosa. Other attempts to prolong the action of P75 SCMC by reducing the water uptake (addition of paraffin and ethyl cellulose) were only partially successful. This was also true for P75 SCMC blends with the hydrogel pHEMA. The clearance rates were of good reproducibility, although considerable variation was found for swelling measurements. In this particular test, Carbopol 934P performed very much better than P75 SCMC.

In a volunteer study employing three subjects, Khosla and S. S. Davis (personal communication) demonstrated that Polycarbophil administered with labelled pellets did not reduce the gastric emptying rate of the pellets compared with pellets without the Polycarbophil.

ACKNOWLEDGEMENTS

G. H. gratefully acknowledges SERC and Merrell Pharmaceuticals Ltd, Egham, Surrey for financial support.

REFERENCES

[1] Mungiu, C., Gogalniceanu, D., Leibovici, M. & Negulescu, I. (1979). On the medical use of cyanoacrylate esters: tonicity of pure *n*-butyl-α-cyanoacrylate. *J. Polym. Sci. Polym. Symp.* **66** 189–193.

[2] Vezin, W. R. & Florence, A. T. (1980). *In vitro* heterogeneous degradation of poly (*n*-alkyl-α-cyanoacrylates). *J. Biomed. Mater. Res.* **14** 93–3106.

[3] Meyer, G., Muster, D., Schmitt, D., Jung P. & Jaeger, J. H. (1979). Bone bonding through bioadhesives: present status. *Biomat. Med. Dev. Art. Org.* **7** 55–71.

[4] Park, J. B. (1983). Acrylic bone cement: *in vitro* and *in vivo* property–structural relationship:— a selective review. *Ann. Biomed. Eng.* **11**, 297–312.

[5] Davis, S. S., Hardy, J. G., Taylor, M. J., Whalley, D. R. & Wilson, C. G. (1984). The effect of food on the gastrointestinal transit of pellets and an osmotic device (Osmet). *Int. J. Pharm.* **21** 331–340.

[6] Read, N. W., Cammack, J., Edwards, C., Holgate, A. M., Cann, P. A. & Brown, C. (1982). Is the transit time of a meal through the small intestine related to the rate at which it leaves the stomach? *Gut* **23** 824–828.

[7] Bechgaard, H. & Ladefoged, K. (1978). Distribution of pellets in the gastrointestinal tract. The influence on transit time exerted by the density or diameter of pellets. *J. Pharm. Pharmacol.* **30** 690–692.

[8] Florey, H. (1955). Mucin and the protectin of the body. *Proc. R. Soc. B.* **143** 147–155.

[9] Davenport, H. W. (1977). *Physiology of the Digestive Tract*, Year Book Publishers Incorporated.

[10] Allen, A., Bell, A., Mantle, M. & Pearson, J. P. (1982). The structure and physiology of gastrointestinal mucus. In: Chantler, E. N., Elder, J. B. & Elstein, M. (eds) *Mucus in Health and Disease II*, Plenum Press, New York, pp. 115–133.

[11] Parke, D. V. (1978). Pharmacology of mucus. *Brit. Med. Bull.* **34** 89–94.

[12] Kulenkampff, H. (1975). The structural basis of intestinal absorption. In: Forth, W. & Rummel, W. (eds) *Pharmacology of Intestinal Absorption: Gastrointestinal Absorption of Drugs,* Pergamon Press, London, pp. 1–70.

[13] Neutra, M. R., Grand, R. J. & Trier, J. S. (1977). Glycoprotein synthesis, transport and secretion by epithelial cells of human rectal mucosa: normal and cystic fibrosis. *Lab. Invest.* **36** 535–536.

[14] Silberberg, A. & Meyer, F. A. (1982). Structure and function of mucus. In:

Chantler, E. N., Elder, J. B. & Elstein, M. (eds) *Mucus in Health and Disease II*, Plenum Press, New York, pp. 35–74.

[15] Bickel, M. & Kauffman, G. L. (1981). Gastric gel mucus thickness: effect of distension, 16, 16-dimethyl prostaglandin E2 and carbenoxolone. *Gastroenterol.* **80**, 770–775.

[16] Allen, A. (1978). The structure of gastrointestinal mucous glycoproteins and the viscous and gel-forming properties of mucus. *Brit. Med. Bull.* **34** 28–33.

[17] Slomiany, B. L. & Meyer, K. (1972). Isolation and structural studies of sulfated glycoproteins of hog gastric mucosa. *J. Biol. Chem.* **247** 5062–5070.

[18] Pearson, J. P., Allen, A. & Parry, S. (1981). A 70,000 molecular weight protein isolated from purified pig gastric mucus glycoprotein by reduction of disulphide bridges and its implication in the polymeric structure. *Biochem. J.* **197** 155–162.

[19] Carlstedt, I. & Sheehan, J. K. (1984). Macromolecular architecture and hydrodynamic properties of human cervical mucins. *Biorheology* **21** 225–233

[20] Starkey, B. J., Snary, A. & Allen, A. (1974). Characterisation of gastric mucoproteins isolated by equilibrium density-gradient centrifugation in caesium chloride. *Biochem. J.* **141** 633–639.

[21] Allen, A., Pain, R. H. & Roberts, T. R. (1976). Model for the structure of gastric mucus gel. *Nature* **264** 88–89.

[22] Bell, A. E., Allen, A., Morris, E. & Rees, D. A. (1982). Rheological studies on native pig gastric mucus gels. In: Chantler, E. N., Elder, J. B. & Elstein, M. (eds) *Mucus in Health and Disease II*, Plenum Press, New York, pp. 97–99.

[23] Meyer, F. A., King, M. & Gelman, R. A. (1975). On the role of sialic acid in the rheological properties of mucus. *Biochim. Biophys. Acta* **392** 223–232.

[24] Williams, S. E. & Turnberg, L. A. (1980). Retardation of acid diffusion by pig gastric mucus: a potential role in mucosal protection. *Gastroenterol.* **79** 299–304.

[25] Kearney, P., Kellaway, I. W., Evans, J. C. & Rowlands, C. (1984). Probing the mucus barrier with spin labels. *J. Pharm. Pharmacol.* **36** 26p.

[26] Allen, A., Foster, S. N. E. & Pearson, J. P. (1986). Interaction of a polyacrylate, Carbomer, with gastric mucus and pepsin. *Brit. J. Pharmacol.* **87** 126P.

[27] Peppas, N. A. & Buri, P. A. (1985). Surface, interfacial and molecular aspects of polymer bioadhesion on soft tissues. *J. Cont. Rel.* **2** 257–275.

[28] Smart, J. D., Kellaway, I. W. & Worthington, H. E. C. (1984). An *in vitro* investigation of mucosa-adhesive materials for use in controlled drug delivery. *J. Pharm. Pharmacol.* **36** 295–299.

[29] Slomiany, A., Slomiany, B. L., Witas, H., Aono, M. & Newman, L. J. (1983). Isolation of fatty acids covalently bound to the gastric mucus glycoprotein of normal and cystic fibrosis patients. *Biochim. Biophys. Res. Commun.* **113** 286–293.

[30] Levine, R. R. (1971). Intestinal absorption. In: Rabinowitz, J. L. & Myerson, R. M. (eds) *Absorption Phenomena,* Wiley-Interscience, New York, pp. 27–95.

[31] Freter, R. (1981). Mechanism of association of bacteria with mucosal surfaces. In: *Adhesion and Microorganism Pathogenicity,* Ciba Foundation Symposium 80, Pitman Medical, pp. 36–47.

[32] Scrivener, C. A. & Schantz, C. W. (1947). Penicillin: new methods for its use in dentistry. *J. Am. Dental Assoc.* **35**, 644–647.

[33] Rothner, J. T., Cobe, H. M., Rosenthal, S. L. & Bailin, J. (1949). Adhesive penicillin ointment for topical application. *J. Dent. Res.* **28**, 544–548.

[34] Kutscher, A. H., Zegarelli, E. V., Beube, F. E., Chiton, N. W., Berman, C., Mercadante, J. L., Stern, I. B. & Roland, N. (1959). A new vehicle (Orabase) for the application of drugs to the oral mucous membranes. *Oral Surg., Oral Med., Oral Pathol.* **12** 1080–1089.

[35] Chen, J. L. & Cyr, G. N. (1970). Compositions producing adhesion through hydration. In: Manly, R. S. (ed.) *Adhesion in Biological Systems*, Academic Press, New York, pp. 163–167.

[36] Park, K. & Robinson, J. R. (1984). Bioadhesives as platforms for oral-controlled drug delivery. *Int. J. Pharm.* **19** 107–127.

[37] Smart, J. D. (1984). The evaluation of mucosa-adhesives for the control of gastrointestinal transit. PhD Thesis, The University of Wales.

[38] Gurny, R., Meyer, J. M. & Peppas, N. A. (1984). Bioadhesive intraoral release systems: design, testing and analysis. Biomaterials **5** 336–340.

[39] Park, H. & Robinson, J. R. (1985). Physico-chemical properties of water insoluble polymers important to mucin/epithelial adhesion. *J. Cont. Rel.* **2** 47–57.

[40] Mikos, A. G. & Pappas, N. A. (1986). Comparison of experimental techniques for the measurement of the bioadhesive forces of polymeric materials with soft tissues. In: Chaudry, I. A. & Phies, C. (eds) *Proc. 13th Int. Symp. Cont. Rel. Bioact. Materials*, Norfolk, USA, p. 97.

[41] Ch'ng, H. S., Park, H., Kelly, P. & Robinson, J. R. (1985). Bioadhesive polymers as platforms for oral controlled drug delivery II: synthesis and evaluation of some swelling, water insoluble bioadhesive polymers. *J. Pharm. Sci.* **74** 399–405.

[42] Longer, M. A., Ch'ng, H. S. & Robinson, J. R. (1985). Bioadhesive polymers as platforms for oral controlled drug delivery III: oral delivery of chlorothiazide using a bioadhesive polymer. *J. Pharm. Sci.* **74** 406–411.

[43] Russell, J. & Bass, P. (1984). Method for the quantitation of gastric emptying time of gel test meals. *Am. J. Clin. Nutr.* **40**, 647–653.

[44] Russell, J. & Bass, P. (1985). Canine gastric emptying of Polycarbophil: an indigestible, particulate substance. *Gastroenterol.* **89**, 307–312.

12

Transdermal drug delivery

B. W. Barry, Postgraduate School of Studies in Pharmacy, University of Bradford, Bradford, West Yorkshire BD7 1DP, UK

1. INTRODUCTION

In this chapter I will deal with the concept of delivering drugs both *into* the skin for their local effects in dermatology, and *through* the integument for the systemic treatment of disease states. This latter process has been brought into sharp focus in recent years by the efforts of pharmaceutical firms to develop transdermal delivery devices to treat motion sickness, angina, hormone deficiency and hypertension. We consider the structure of human skin, skin transport and the difficulties associated with the transdermal route, the theoretical advantages of this mode of treatment and how to optimize percutaneous absorption. We can then move on to develop a theory for penetration-enhancer activity, deal with the hairless mouse as a model for human skin, mention some aspects of transdermal delivery devices and close with a few remarks about the future.

2. STRUCTURE OF HUMAN SKIN

Human skin consists of two distinct layers, the stratified avascular cellular epidermis and an underlying dermis of connective tissue. A fatty subcutaneous layer resides beneath the dermis. Hairy skin develops hair follicles and sebaceous glands and the highly vascularized dermis supports the apocrine and eccrine sweat glands which pass through pores in the epidermis to reach the skin surface. In respect of drug permeation, the most important tissue in this complex membrane is the stratum corneum or horny layer, which usually provides the rate-limiting or slowest step in the penetration process.

3. TRANSPORT THROUGH HUMAN SKIN

The transport mechanisms by which drugs cross the intact skin are still not elucidated despite many years of investigation (comprehensive reviews include refs [1–15]). The possible macro routes comprise the transepidermal pathway (across the horny layer either intracellularly or intercellularly) or via the hair follicles and sweat glands (the appendageal way) — see Fig. 1.

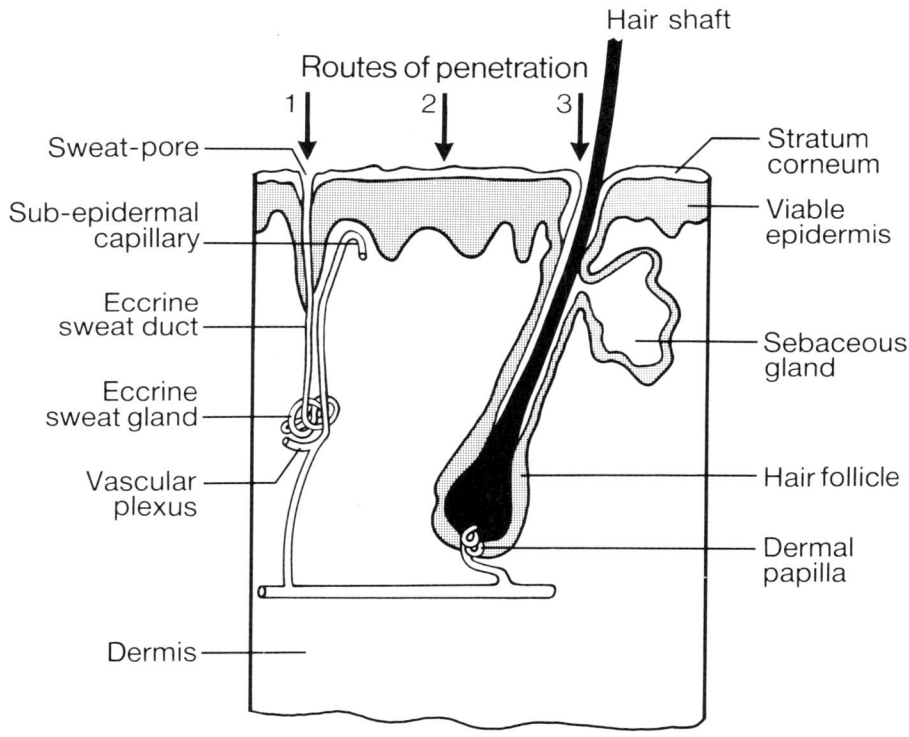

Fig. 1 — The possible macro routes for drug entry through the skin — across the intact stratum corneum or via the hair follicles and sweat glands.

The appendages may be important at short diffusional times and for large polar molecules. For drugs penetrating directly across the intact stratum corneum, entry may be transcellular or intercellular. For many years it was considered that for polar molecules the probable way was through the hydrated keratin of the corneocyte [9]. However, it now seems more likely that the dominant path is the polar region of the intercellular lipid, with the lipid chains providing the non-polar route [16]. Fig. 2 illustrates these possible routes.

The relative importance of these alternatives depends on many factors which include the time-scale of permeation (steady-state versus transient diffusion), the physicochemical properties of the penetrant (for example, its pK_a, molecular size,

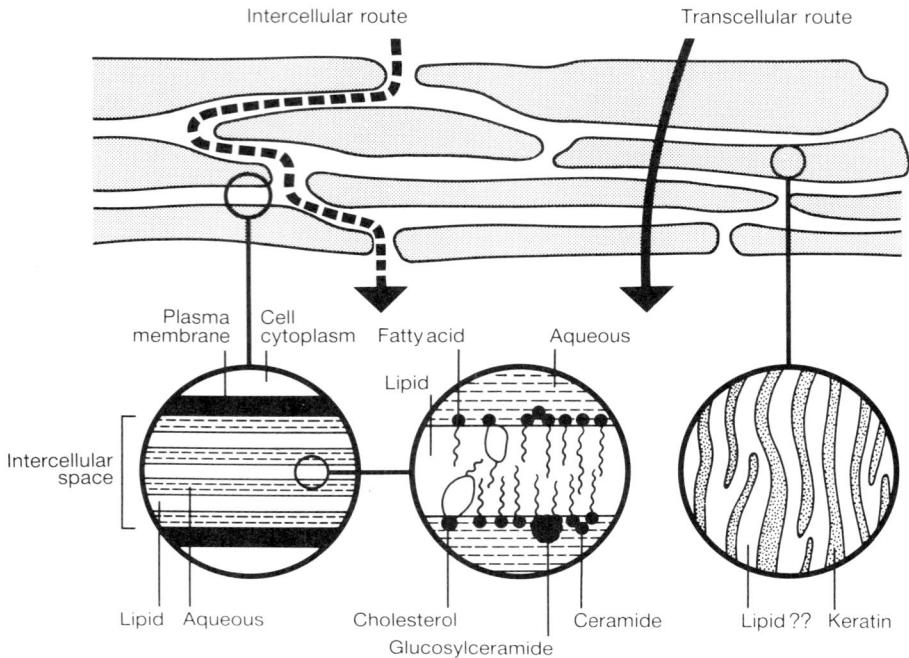

Fig. 2 — The possible micro routes for drug entry through the stratum corneum — transcellular or intercellular. Details are shown of the suggested structure of the intercellular lipid [16] and the intracellular protein fibrils with minimal lipid.

stability and binding affinity, and its solubility and partition coefficient), integrity and thickness of the stratum corneum, density of sweat glands and follicles, skin hydration, metabolism and vehicle effects. We might expect that for most penetrants of intermediate polarity, the molecule will use a variety of routes depending on time of diffusion and skin condition but for simplicity we usually deal with only the predominant route for any particular chemical.

4.   DIFFICULTIES WITH THE TRANSDERMAL ROUTE

One way of considering the problems associated with drug delivery through the skin is for us to accompany in our imagination a stream of drug as it diffuses from a topical vehicle or device on the surface of the skin through the cutis to reach the blood capillaries (Fig. 3). This permeation process is complex and best dealt with in subdivisions.

4.1   Drug in device

In developing a topical system we need a stable preparation of controlled chemical potential with the correct partition coefficient relative to the drug reservoir and any device membrane and the skin layers. In particular, for the type of transdermal

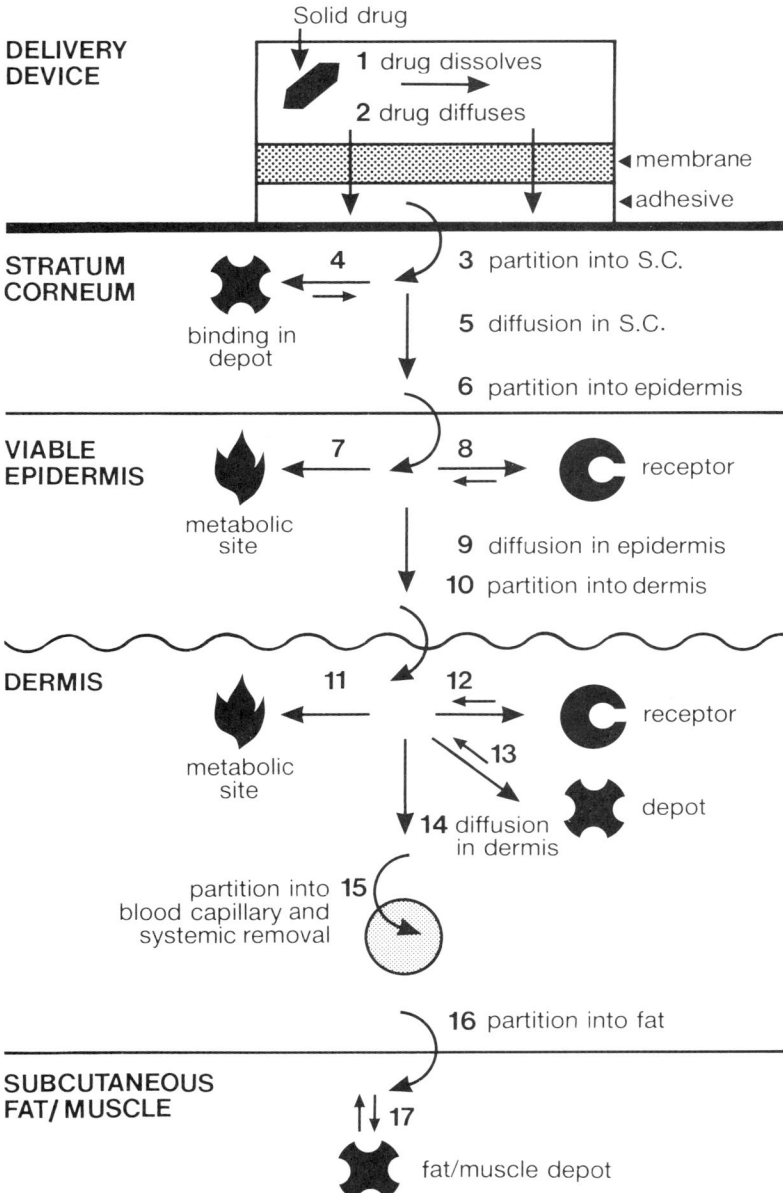

DELIVERY
DEVICE

Solid drug

1 drug dissolves

2 drug diffuses

◀ membrane
◀ adhesive

STRATUM
CORNEUM

4

binding in
depot

3 partition into S.C.

5 diffusion in S.C.

6 partition into epidermis

VIABLE
EPIDERMIS

7   **8**   receptor

metabolic
site

9 diffusion in epidermis

10 partition into dermis

DERMIS

11   **12**   receptor

13

metabolic
site

depot

14 diffusion
in dermis

partition into **15**
blood capillary and
systemic removal

16 partition into fat

SUBCUTANEOUS
FAT/ MUSCLE

↑↓ **17**

fat/muscle depot

Fig. 3 — Percutaneous absorption of drug from a topical device — some factors which influence
the process.

delivery device which incorpoates a rate-controlling membrane, the flux across this
barrier should be low enough that the underlying skin acts as a sink. This is a severe
restriction because of the general impermeability of the stratum corneum. If we do

not make the horny layer act as a sink, then the individual patient's skin will control drug input with the consequences which follow from the significant biological variability existing between people and from skin site to skin site. In the future we will have to design and manufacture new penetration enhancers and dove-tail their delivery with that of the drug so that they precede medicament entry. In this way we may be able to so reduce the resistance of the horny layer that the tissue does in fact perform as a sink. Many pharmacologically active drugs have the incorrect physio-chemical properties to partition into the skin and an important effort in the future will be devoted to synthesizing suitable prodrugs so as to optimize the partition coefficient, stratum corneum : vehicle. In developing new drug entities, more attention should be paid to producing chemicals with low melting points (preferably liquids at biological temperatures) and to including penetration-enhancer groups in the active molecule (E.R. Cooper, personal communication).

4.2   Drug at the skin surface
Light, oxygen and bacteria degrade the microenvironment of the skin surface. To take just two examples, skin microflora can degrade nitroglycerin and steroid esters [17–19]. We may predict that occlusive systems such as the transdermal delivery devices, when applied for several days, will cause problems with changes in skin flora, with maceration and irritation of the skin and because prolonged application can shut down the sweat glands.

4.3   Drug in the stratum corneum
The drug must partition into the stratum corneum and diffuse through this very impermeable barrier. The molecules will interact with many potential binding sites, possibly forming a reservoir operating for days or even weeks. Free drug eventually reaches the interface between the stratum corneum and the viable epidermis, where the medicament must partition into this water-rich tissue. There is a potential problem in that a drug or prodrug designed to partition from a vehicle into the horny layer may then have difficulty leaving the stratum corneum to enter the epidermis. For very lipid-soluble drugs, clearance from the viable tissue may replace diffusion through the stratum corneum as the rate-limiting step.

4.4   Viable epidermis
Living skin is a storehouse of enzymes which may have real activities of 80–90% of those in the liver. Hydrolytic, oxidative, reductive and conjugative reactions all take place [13,14,20,21]. One reason why the activities approach those in the liver is the extreme dilution at which molecules cross the viable epidermis. The process lays them open to attack, although this is counter-balanced by the much greater permeation rates compared with those operating within the stratum corneum. Metabolism may alter permeation pharmacokinetics, activating prodrugs and des-troying active drug while generating active and inactive metabolites [22]. We may speculate that a future possibility would be to incorporate enzyme inhibitors into our devices to protect the drugs. In epidermis the drug meets pharmacological receptors as it permeates to the epidermal/dermal boundary where it partitions into the dermis. As both viable tissues consist mainly of water, we would expect the partition

coefficient to be approximately one, provided that there are no different binding sites in close proximity either side of the interface.

It is probable that sensitization reactions will always occur in time to a fraction of the patient population when any chemical is delivered via an unusual route, i.e. one to which the body is not accustomed. This phenomenon has happened with clonidine and we can predict that it may apply to drugs, enhancers, enzyme inhibitors, adhesives and vehicle components in general.

4.5 Drug in the dermis
After the penetrant partitions into the dermis, additional receptor, metabolic and depot sites may intervene as the drug moves to a blood capillary, partitions into the wall, then out into the blood, finally to be removed by the circulation while undergoing further chemical attack. The lymph system may also aid in drug elimination. We understand little about equilibrium in the dermal environment and the pharmacokinetics which operate there.

4.6 Drug in the subcutaneous fat and muscle
A portion of the penetrant may even partition into the subcutaneous fat and the underlying muscle to form further depots, despite how unlikely this would appear from theoretical considerations [23].

The above scheme is complex even though we have simplified it by representing the process as one of simple unidirectional transport; in practice, the sequence would be more complicated. Factors playing their part include the inhomogeneity of the stratified tissues, the interruption of the stratum corneum by hair follicles and sweat glands, and the division of basal cells, their transport through the horny layer and their loss from the surface. Additionally, drugs penetrate the skin under dynamic conditions. Thus, the medicament, vehicle components, and occlusive hydration effects may progressively change the skin barrier. Sweat, sebum and cellular debris may enter the product, changing its physicochemical characteristics. Volatile solvents may evaporate and emulsions can crack or invert when rubbed into the skin. Such processes will alter the chemical potential of the drug and may even develop super-saturated solutions.

5.   THEORETICAL ADVANTAGES OF THE TRANSDERMAL ROUTE

We can turn now to examine the possible advantages of formulating a satisfactory transdermal device for delivering drugs into the systemic circulation. It is usual to contrast the percutaneous route with oral delivery as the latter regime provides the most popular way for delivering medicaments in general.

Transdermal input of a drug would eliminate several variables which make gastrointestinal absorption a problem. These factors include the dramatic changes in pH as the molecule moves from stomach acid as low as pH 1 to an intestinal pH of up to 8, stomach emptying, intestinal motilities and transit times, the operation of human and bacterial enzymes and the influence of food on drug absorption.

Via skin, the drug enters the systemic circulation without first passing into the portal system and traversing the liver. The route therefore avoids the 'first-pass' phenomenon by which the liver can significantly reduce the amount of intact agent passing into the systemic circulation. Additionally, the medicament avoids the enzymes present in the gut wall. However, as emphasized in the previous section, skin itself is a highly active metabolic organ.

For a correctly formulated product, the percutaneous input of a drug can control administration and so display only one pharmacological action from a medicament that, orally or by injection, may well show several effects, including toxic reactions. Patient compliance may be helped by the continuity of input of drugs with short half-lives.

Transdermal administration under suitable rate control could minimize pulse entry into the bloodstream; undesirable side-effects are particularly associated with peak plasma levels. However, a more difficult matter is deliberately to provide a controlled on/off action because intact skin membranes are intrinsically slow-response systems with prolonged lag times, at least when shunt diffusion via the appendages is negligible.

Percutaneous administration can be valuable for drugs with low therapeutic indices, i.e. those for which the toxic concentration in the plasma is near to the clinical level.

Some investigators claim that it would be easy to terminate therapy by simple removal of a topical device so as to interrupt medicament delivery. However, the stratum corneum would continue to deliver molecules to the viable tissues for some time after device removal, at a declining rate as governed by the properties of the drug reservoir. This is another consequence of the long response times of horny layer membranes.

6.   OPTIMIZATION OF PERCUTANEOUS ABSORPTION

When formulators develop dermatological preparations for optimum bioavailability, they employ two main methods of approach either singly or combined [24]. The first scheme formulates the vehicle or device so that the drug has the maximum tendency to leave the base and to partition into the skin. The scientist does not intend that the vehicle components should affect the physicochemical properties of the stratum corneum. Thus the vehicle design promotes drug release by simply optimizing the chemical potential of the medicament. However, even the most innocuous of vehicles tends to change the nature of the stratum corneum if only by hydrating it. The alternative strategy incorporates into the formulation materials known as penetration enhancers [14,25]. These are chemicals which enter the skin, dynamically and reversibly altering it to promote the penetration of drug. The desirable attributes of such enhancers include the following:

(1)   They should be pharmacologically inert, interacting with no receptors in the skin or in the body generally
(2)   The enhancer should be neither toxic, irritating nor allergenic
(3)   The onset of enhancer activity and the duration of effect should be predictable, controllable and suitable
(4)   The skin should immediately and fully recover its normal barrier property when the enhancer leaves the tissue
(5)   The accelerant should promote penetration into the skin without developing

significant problems of loss of body fluids, electrolytes or other endogenous
materials

(6) The chemical should be compatible with a wide range of drugs and pharmaceutical adjuvants

(7) Where appropriate, the substance should be a suitable solvent for the drugs

(8) For traditional formulations, the material should spread well on the skin and it
should have a suitable skin 'feel'

(9) The chemical should formulate into creams, ointments, gels, lotions, suspensions, aerosols, skin adhesives and delivery devices

(10) It should be odourless, tasteless, colourless and relatively inexpensive.

To illustrate these methods of approach I would like to discuss examples from our
work using the *in vivo* vasoconstrictor assay in human volunteers. This bioassay
provides an excellent procedure for assessing factors which modify the bioavailability of topical steroids by simply scoring with time the pallor induced on the forearms
of volunteers [14,26,27].

6.1   Thermodynamic control

We used the occluded vasoconstrictor assay to test the bioavailability of mechlorisone dibutyrate at 0.1% and 0.2% concentration in six experimental solutions [28].
Various polar solvents (hexylene glycol, propylene glycol, propylene carbonate,
polyethylene glycol 400 and water) were blended so that the steroid was at 90%
saturation in each solvent mixture and thus ideally at the same chemical potential,
even though the overall concentration with a particular solvent system was either
0.1% or 0.2%. From the results of our vasoconstrictor test we constructed blanching
curves of response versus time and determined the area-under-the-curve (AUC)
values as measures of bioavailability. Fig. 4 illustrates a histogram of such AUC
values. We see that within any solvent system there was no significant difference
between preparations containing different *concentrations* of the steroid. This result
accords with our thermodynamic predictions.

6.2   Penetration enhancers

We extended our work on the bioavailability optimization of steroids from the
thermodynamic approach to the alternative strategy of incorporating penetration
enhancers in the formulation. We assessed the bioavailability of betamethasone 17-
benzoate in a number of penetration-enhancer systems, using the *non-occluded*
vasoconstrictor assay, with the steroid at approximate constant thermodynamic
activity (10% saturation). The experimental design used aqueous solutions of 2-
pyrrolidone, N-methylpyrrolidone, dimethylformamide, propylene glycol and
dimethylisosorbide. We also incorporated 2% Azone, 1.5% oleic acid or 5% oleic
acid in some systems; these concentrations produced saturated solutions, i.e.
maximum thermodynamic activities for these enhancers. We took as a standard
solution, the steroid dissolved in dimethylisosorbide (which is not a penetration
enhancer) and expressed the bioavailability as the AUC of the steroid in the test
solvent divided by the AUC in dimethylisosorbide. Fig. 5 illustrates that 2-pyrrolido-
ne,N-methylpyrrolidone, propylene glycol plus oleic acid, propylene glycol plus
Azone, and dimethylformamide increased the bioavailability of the steroid com-

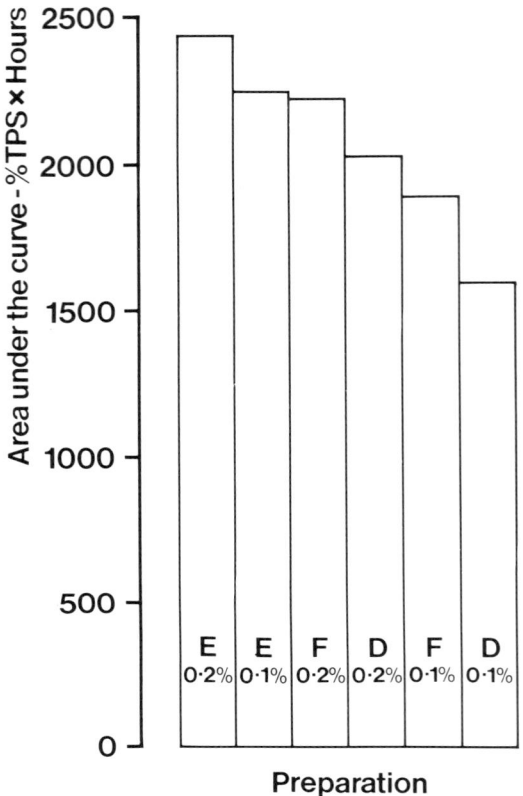

Fig. 4 — Histogram of area-under-the-curve values from vasoconstrictor testing of 0.1% and 0.2% mechlorisone dibutyrate in various solvent systems, which are represented by letters (see Woodford and Barry [28]).

pared with the standard. When oleic acid or Azone were incorporated into dimethy-lisosorbide they did not significantly alter the bioavailability. For optimal effects such enhancers need to be presented to the skin dissolved in suitable specific polar solvents such as propylene glycol.

7.   A THEORY FOR PENETRATION-ENHANCER ACTIVITY

After this brief mention of some of our work with penetration enhancers, I would like to draw on these and other unpublished results together with literature data to develop an overall theory as to how most penetration enhancers act to modify the permeation process through the horny layer barrier. Some of what follows is speculative and requires further experimental proof.

It seems to me that in most situations the crucial events occur in the intercellular

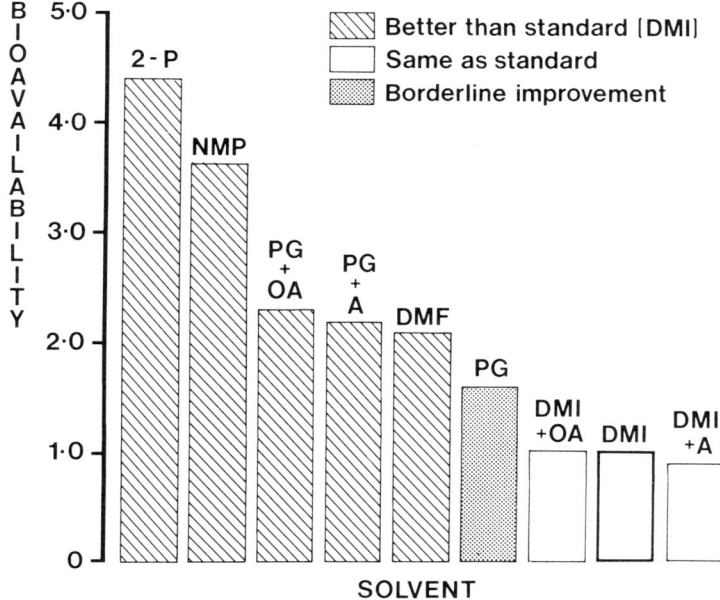

Fig. 5 — Bioavailabilities of enhancer solutions of betamethasone 17-benzoate assessed by the non-occluded vasoconstrictor test; 2-P=2-pyrrolidone, NMP=*N*-methylpyrrolidone, PG=propylene glycol, OA=oleic acid, A=Azone, DMF=dimethylformamide, DMI=dimethylisosorbide.

spaces within the stratum corneum and at three main sites associated with the bilayer lipid structure (Fig. 6).

7.1   Action at site A
Many penetration enhancers will interact with the polar head groups of the lipid via hydrogen bonding and ionic interactions. The consequent disturbance of the hydration spheres of the lipids and alterations in head group interactions will upset the packing at the head region. This disturbance may decrease the retarding action which this domain imposes on the diffusion of polar penetrants. A second response may be to increase the volume of the aqueous layer so that more water enters the tissue. This swelling provides a greater cross-sectional area for polar diffusion (site B) and a larger fractional volume of 'free' water as distinct from the structured water at the lipid interface. This modification may also happen with simple hydration — water itself is a good penetration enhancer! The disturbance of the interfacial structure will tend to alter the packing of the lipid tails such that the lipid hydrophobic route becomes more disordered and more easily traversed by a lipid-like penetrant (site C).

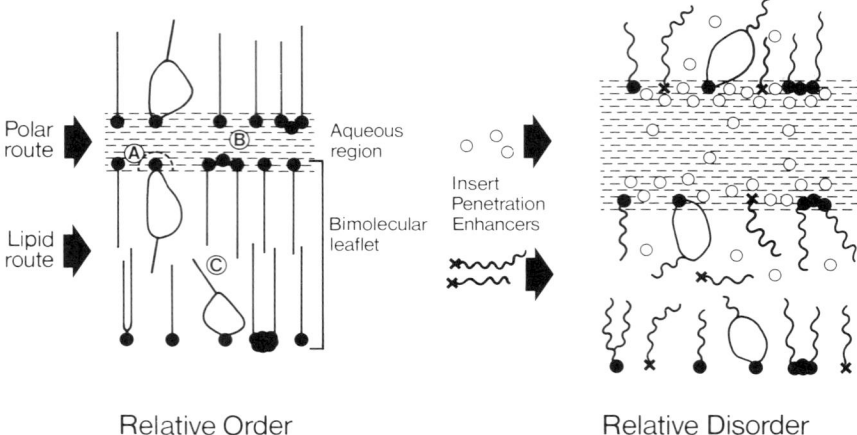

Fig. 6 — Postulated sites for penetration-enhancer activity in the intercellular space, with a change from relative order to disorder on insertion of enhancers (small circles represent polar enhancers such s 2-pyrrolidone and propylene glycol; linear chain represents Azone and bent chain corresponds to *cis*-unsaturated oleic acid).

7.2 Direct influence at site B

Additional to any effect a penetration enhancer has on the aqueous region by increasing its water content, there can be a direct action whereby the domain temporarily changes its bulk chemical constitution. Thus, with high concentration of solvents such as dimethylsulphoxide, propylene glycol or ethanol in a vehicle or device, so much may penetrate into the aqueous region of the tissue that it becomes a better solvent for molecules such as hydrocortisone and oestradiol. In other words, the operational partition coefficient now favour an elevated drug concentration in the skin. The solvent then diffuses out into the dermis followed by the drug diffusing down its concentration gradient.

7.3 Action at the lipid domain (site C)

Penetration enhancers can insert between the hydrophobic tails of the bilayer, upsetting their packing and allowing easier diffusion for lipid penetrants. This alteration in lipid packing can reflect back to provide an element of disorder at the polar head group region of the intercellular domain, promoting polar route permeation.

An important feature of the activity of certain penetration enhancers is the correct choice of a cosolvent for materials such as Azone and *cis*-unsaturated oleic acid. For these enhancers to reach the polar surface of the lipid bilayer (position A) in relatively large amounts, they may need a material such as propylene glycol. This alters the polarity of the aqueous region and so increases its solubilizing ability for lipid-like materials; the cosolvent may also change head group packing. Then the polar heads of the oleic acid and Azone insert between the head groups of the lipid and the enhancer tails flip over to insert between the hydrophobic groups of the membrane lipids, so increasing the fluidity of the lipid domain. Azone is so water insoluble that it may under extreme conditions then move fully into the internal region of the lipid (site C) providing maximum disordering. This cooperation between the elements of cosolvent systems operates particularly with Azone/ propylene glycol mixtures [29]. Not only does propylene glycol aid the penetration of Azone into the stratum corneum, but Azone increases the flux of propylene glycol through the skin which then further increases the amount of Azone in the tissue (R. Evens, personal communication; [30]).

When very dramatic effects occur such that the resistance of the horny layer reduces to that of an equivalent thickness of viable tissue, we may suspect even more drastic disorder in the intercellular domain. It may be that the bimolecular structure completely breaks down and the components form globular micelles dispersed in a relatively extensive continuous phase rich in polar or aprotic solvent. This situation would permit drug permeation at rates which are orders of magnitude greater than those operating in the unaffected horny layer (Fig. 7).

The final stage in this process would be the dissolution of the lipid to form a homogeneous phase with little resistance to molecular diffusion. This extreme disruption would occur only in the presence of high concentrations of molecules with good solvent properties for lipid components.

If, for a particular penetrant, the *intra*cellular route provided a significant permeation pathway, the enhancer could interact with whatever lipid remains within the corneocyte; modern concepts are that the amount is small [16]. As regards the keratin fibrils, we would need to consider the typical spread of interactions which materials such as the aprotic solvents (for example dimethylsulphoxide) and surfactants undergo with proteins. These mechanisms include interactions with polar groups, relaxation of binding forces and alterations in helix conformation. Pore routes may form through this tissue. Most investigators no longer consider that the transcellular route presents a significant pathway for molecular diffusion through the stratum corneum, though presumably the corneocyte may sequester and retain certain molecules within its structure. However, we should guard against a too hasty dismissal of the transcellular route of penetration.

The above theory is not exclusive and has concentrated on agents delivered in amounts which alter the permeability of the stratum corneum without producing frank damage. However, aprotic solvents such as dimethylsulphoxide at high concentrations may damage the skin or produce gross structural changes in it, while the high osmotic activity of the sulphoxide may induce channels in the stratum corneum and so form a continuous network throughout the tissue. Please note also that Fig. 6 is a composite diagram illustrating many effects — a particular enhancer would not produce all the alterations shown.

Incidentally, human skin shows great variation in permeability [31] and in respect of its modification by enhancers. I have a suspicion that mankind is divided into two subgroups — one is susceptible to enhancer activity and the other much less so. Within each subset there is then the usual biological variability. It would be informative to perform a large-scale investigation to look for such a bimodal distribution of permeabilities.

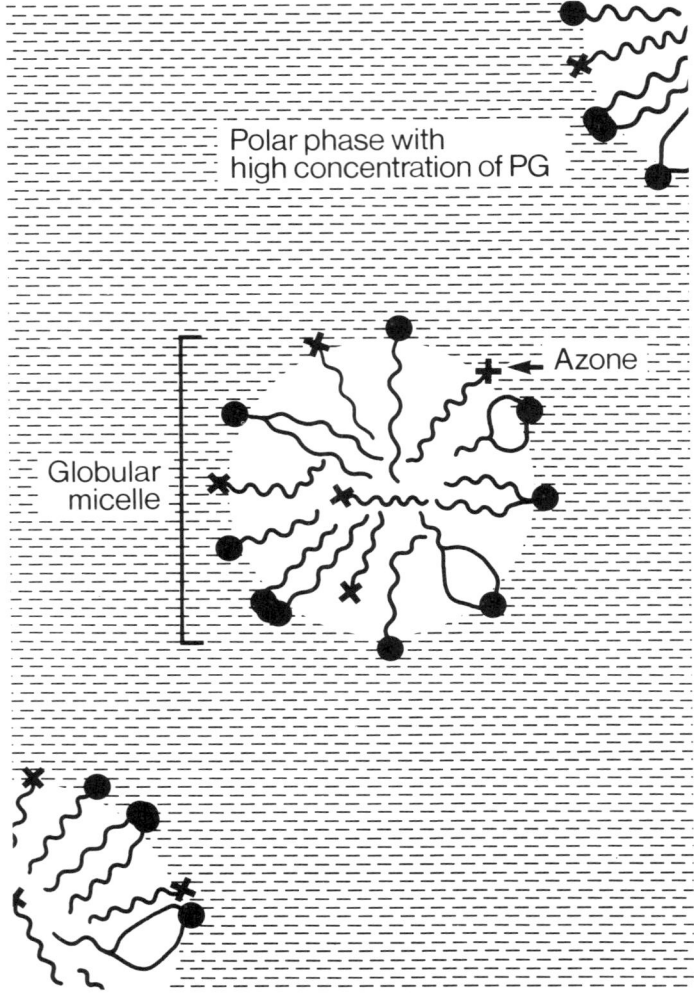

Fig. 7 — Postulated micelle formation in the intercellular domain caused by mixtures such as
Azone in propylene glycol (PG).

8.   HAIRLESS MOUSE SKIN — A CAUTIONARY TALE

In recent years hairless mouse skin has gained a reputation as a good model for
human skin in permeation studies. In certain circumstances this is justified but we
need to be cautious. In our laboratories in several test situations we have found that
the tissue is particularly susceptible to perturbation compared with human cadaver
skin. In particular, we have found that extensive hydration, acetone treatment and
penetration enhancers dramatically increase the permeability of the horny layer
barrier.

8.1 Hydration

Extensive hydration over time destroys the barrier resistance of the tissue. Thus Fig. 8 shows plots of the permeability coefficient for tritiated water as a function of time of hydration for human cadaver skin and hairless mouse skin. The values for human tissue change little over 10 days, emphasizing the remarkable stability of this biological membrane. However, the coefficents for hairless mouse skin, although initially similar to those for human skin, increase dramatically after 2 days of hydration as the tissue disintegrates [32]. This dissimilar behaviour has obvious implications for testing transdermal delivery systems designed to remain on the skin for several days when they will extensively hydrate the stratum corneum.

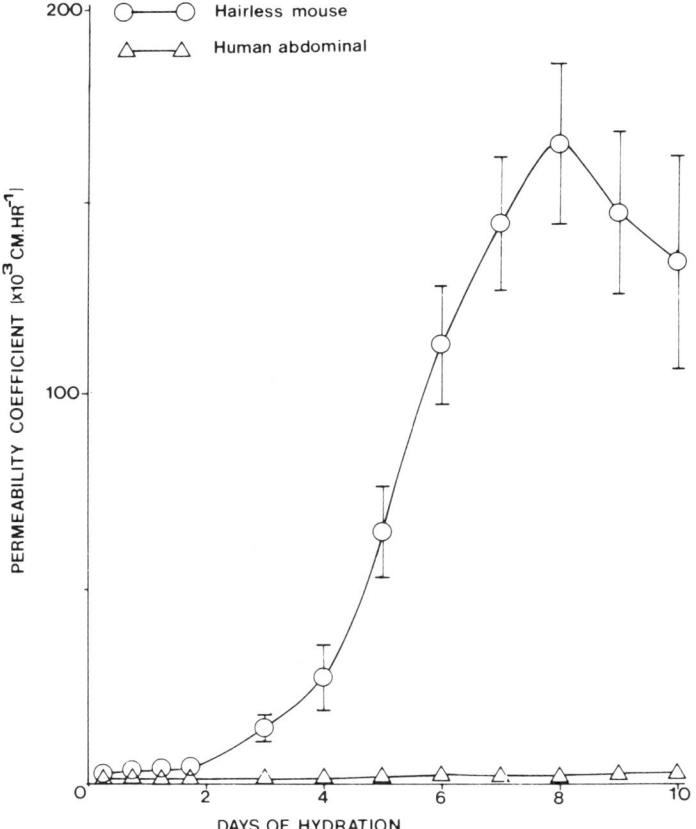

Fig. 8 — Permeability coefficients for tritiated water as a function of hydration time; human cadaver skin and hairless mouse skin.

8.2   Acetone treatment

Depositing drugs onto human skin from acetone either *in vivo* or *in vitro* is a common protocol in skin permeation studies and the solvent seems to produce negligible damage. However, in hairless mouse skin there can be a dramatic response. Thus, in one experiment we treated batches of human skin and hairless mouse skin with acetone for 2 min only, removed the acetone and then determined the permeability coefficients for radiolabelled 5-fluorouracil penetrating from saturated aqueous solution (Fig. 9). Treatment of hairless mouse skin with acetone yielded a 15-fold increase in permeability compared with the control, a much greater effect than for human skin [33].

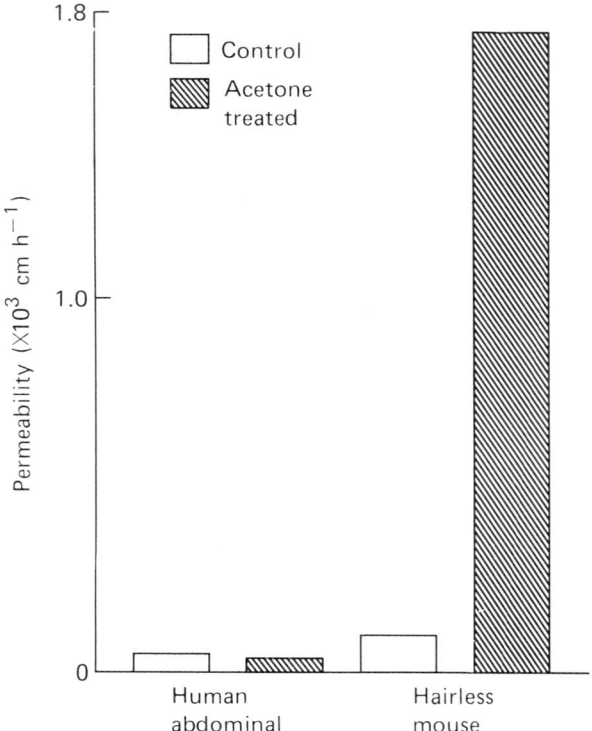

Fig. 9 — Permeability coefficients for 5-fluorouracil penetrating from saturated aqueous solution; prior treatment of hairless mouse skin and human skin with acetone.

8.3   Enhancer activity

When we used hairless mouse skin to investigate the action of penetration enhancers, it always overemphasized the accelerant activity compared with treating human tissue — sometimes markedly so. Thus, in one experiment, we compared the effects of Azone, decylmethylsulphoxide, propylene glycol and oleic acid on the penetration of 5-fluorouracil through both skin types. The technique was a steady-state design with 12-h pretreatment of the skins with the test enhancers; normal saline was the control. We defined an enhancement ratio as the permeability coefficient for treatment/permeability coefficient for control. Fig. 10 illustrates histograms of this ratio. Mixtures of Azone in propylene glycol and oleic acid in propylene glycol increased the permeability coefficient of the drug through both skins, but the effects in hairless mouse were seven-fold greater than for cadaver membranes [34].

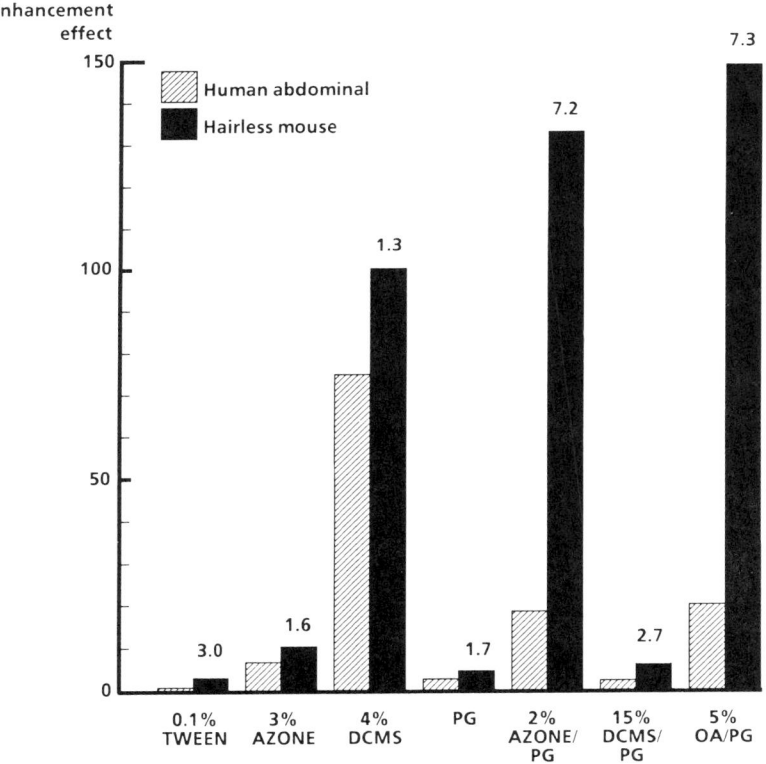

Fig. 10 — Effects of penetration enhancers on the steady-state penetration of 5-fluorouracil through hairless mouse skin and human skin. The numbers above the histogram pairs represent the ratios of effects, hairless mouse to man. DCMS=decylmethylsulphoxide; PG=propylene glycol; OA=oleic acid.

The results of these three experiments caution us against directly applying hairless mouse data to man without confirming the results in humans. Only a few workers appear to have tested the membrane for its suitability as a mimic of human skin [35–37]. The particular danger with hairless mouse experiments is that they often appear to correlate well with cadaver skin, particularly for straightforward experiments, and they may lull the investigator into a false sense of security. I believe that we should always undertake at least some pilot experiments in any research programme to confirm the validity of the mouse data with reference to those of man.

9.   TRANSDERMAL DELIVERY SYSTEMS

Transdermal drug delivery systems are topical devices designed originally to deliver drug to the surface of the skin at a controlled rate. This flux was intended to be well below the maximum that the skin can accept. In this sense the device, not the stratum corneum, controls the rate at which drug diffuses through the epidermis and dermis and passes into the general circulation via the capillaries. On the world market today, there are patches which deliver hyoscine (scopolamine), nitroglycerin, clonidine and oestradiol (some representative references include [12,38–50]). Unfortunately, none of these patches achieves full flux control, mainly because of the relative impermeability of human skin complicated by its biological variability, patient to patient, site to site and even centimetre by centimetre [9, 10, 13–15]. Many other drugs are under investigation for patch use — including testosterone, fentanyl and timolol — and it remains to be seen if these perform more ideally.

Starting our examination of devices by *assuming* that the skin acts as a perfect sink for permeating molecules, we can look at the two main designs for transdermal systems, the monolithic or matrix system and the device which incorporates a rate-limiting membrane.

In the monolith system, no rate-controlling membrane separates the sink from the drug reservoir and the concentration of drug in the device decreases with time. Fig. 11 illustrates the general shape of the cumulative release curve as a function of time where 'sheet' represents the plot for patch geometry. Such devices follow the well-known 'square root of time' law. The inset represents a releasing system with large circles corresponding to solid particles and the dots representing dissolved molecules.

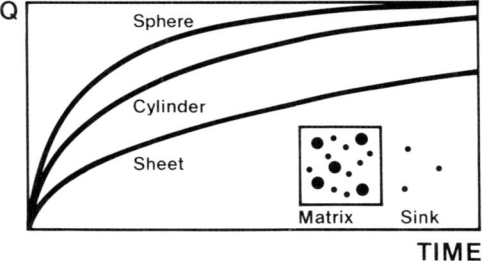

Fig. 11 — Cumulative release curves for monolith systems of different geometries. The inset shows a releasing system with solid particles represented by large circles and dissolved molecules by dots.

Fig. 12 depicts the theoretical delivery profile for a membrane-controlled device (such as that typified by the Alza Transderm system) when the membrane is initially free of drug. The intercept indicates the time required for the membrane drug concentration to equilibrate with the reservoir during the release process. However, on storage of such a device, the membrane and adhesive equilibrate with the reservoir and this readily available amount of drug produces a 'burst' effect. This effect is greater the higher the concentration of drug in the membrane and adhesive (Figs. 13 and 14).

9.1 Hyoscine

The first device used clinically delivered hyoscine from behind the ear, a relatively permeable skin site in humans. In the usual dosage form of injections or tablets, hyoscine can induce confusion, excitement and even hallucinations; the controlled input from the Transderm tries to eliminate these effects. The hyoscine patch went into space with the American astronauts, it can also control radiation sickness and the side-effects of anticancer drugs, but its main users are the travelling public. Prominent display of the patch provides a status symbol for those about to leave on their world cruises. Two-thirds of its users still experience a dry mouth, but even this has been turned to advantage by a recorder-playing doctor who suppressed his salivation by applying the patch.

9.2 Nitroglycerin

A second major use of patch technology is to deliver nitroglycerin and other nitrates (isosorbide dinitrate and mononitrate) to treat angina, congestive heart failure and acute myocardial infarction. There is much dispute about the relative merits of the various nitroglycerin transdermal devices, ointments and tablets. However, the patches have such an attraction for certain patients that their wide use in the USA has been termed discomania.

Several questions relating to the use of nitroglycerin devices are under active discussion. One is whether or not these systems deliver suboptimal drug plasma levels and presumably we will have to await wider clinical trials to answer this query. A second question relates to whether or not tolerance develops within 24 h of use, as claimed by some investigators — again we await further evidence to settle this matter.

A fundamental enquiry asks — exactly where is the rate-limiting step in the overall process of percutaneous absorption from a nitroglycerin patch? Is it in the product or in the skin? In brief, *no* currently marketed transdermal nitroglycerin device fully controls the input of the drug through the skin. As an example of the problem that arises in relation to flux control, we can follow the treatment of Good [40] and compare predicted plasma profiles of glyceryl trinitrate arising from a monolith patch with no control and a membrane device with some control (Fig. 15). For low permeable skin, steady-state level and duration are nearly the same for both systems. However, it is clear that highly permeable skin restricts the duration of steady state to a short time and generates quite high plasma levels for a device which does not limit drug release (Fig. 16). Ciba argues that for the patient with highly permeable skin some system rate control is desirable to extend duration of control and to avoid excessive blood levels of drug.

It is interesting that the variability of plasma levels in volunteer trials is similar for a nitroglycerin ointment and a Transderm-Nitro patch [40]. This suggests that the

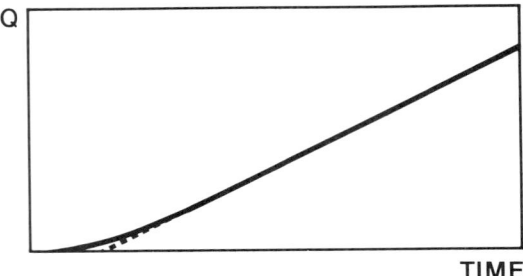

Fig. 12 — Cumulative release curve for membrane-controlled device with membrane and adhesive initially free of drug.

DELIVERY DEVICE - 'PATCH'

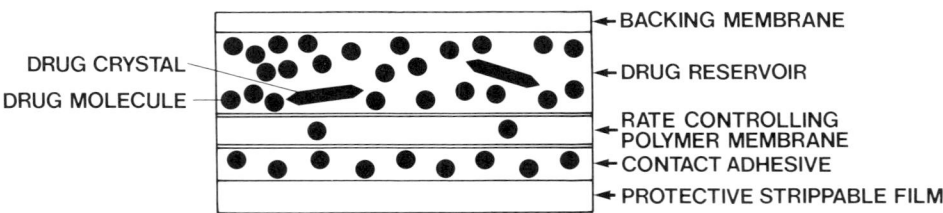

Fig. 13 — Typical membrane-controlled device at equilibrium illustrating crystals of undissolved drug in reservoir and dissolved molecules throughout system.

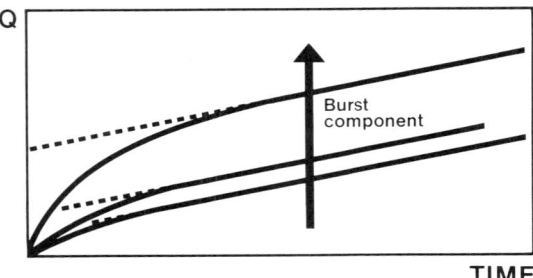

Fig. 14 — Release plots for membrane-controlled device stored to equilibrium; the higher the concentration of drug in the membrane and adhesive, the greater the 'burst' effect.

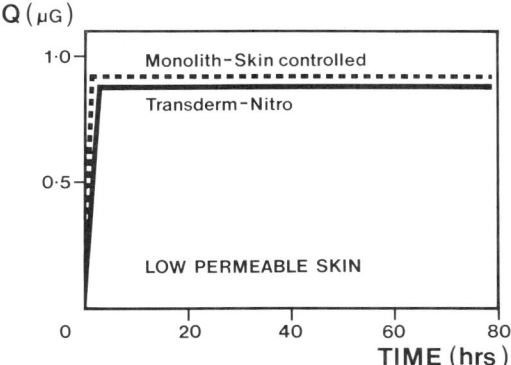

Fig. 15 — Predicted plasma profiles of glyceryl trinitrate from a monolith patch with no control and a membrane device with some control — low permeable skin (after Good [40]).

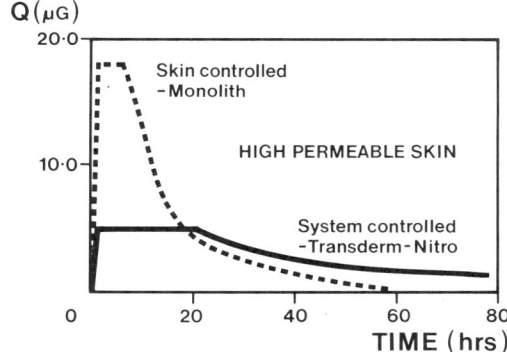

Fig. 16 — Predicted plasma profiles of glyceryl trinitrate from a monolith patch with no control and a membrane device with some control — high permeable skin (Good [40]).

high-technology device is not such an advance on the traditional dosage form. Presumably a major factor here is that the skin essentially controls the drug input from both types of formulation.

9.3 Clonidine
There are supposed to be some 20 transdermal devices in development, but a problem which arose with a recently marketed preparation, Catapres-TTS, is instructive. The patch produced sensitivity reactions which Alza first thought arose from a sensitizing component in the patch adhesive, possibly polyisobutylene. However, recently published work has shown a high incidence of local allergic skin

reactions to topical clonidine itself [42]. A fraction of the patient population always reacts, with time, to any chemical delivered to the body via an unusual route for that molecule.

10.   THE FUTURE

Transdermal therapy appears to be on the brink of a rapid expansion for the rate-controlled administration of potent, non-allergenic agents, with suitable physicochemical properties, where current methods of administration cause problems. One unreasonably optimistic estimate is that, by the mid-1990s, 70% or more of all drugs will be delivered by the transdermal patch system. However, because of the constraints arising from drug potency, skin permeability, or topical reactions, I do not think that transdermal administration will become the preferred dosage route for a high percentage of drugs. There are additional problems with, for example, cutaneous metabolism and the fact that a small volume of the skin has to suffer the entire body load of a drug. Possibilities for the future include making more use of prodrugs, penetration enhancers and specific non-toxic enzyme inhibitors to diminish drug degradation. We need a significant expansion in research work on the fundamentals of skin metabolism as it effects drug destruction and prodrug activation.

A challenge for drug therapy in the future is to deliver efficiently the peptide drugs arising from the biotechnology revolution. At present it seems highly unlikely that simple application to the skin of a peptide in a vehicle would produce suitable clinical effects. One possible approach would be to develop delivery devices which would synchronize the insertion of a suitable penetration enhancer into the stratum corneum together with the peptide. Another possibility would be to employ iontophoresis, a technique which has been used for a number of ionic drugs, and possibly combine it with the use of suitable penetration enhancers. Whatever the technology used, I think that the efficient delivery through the skin of the new peptide drugs will prove to be the most challenging project in skin permeation science to date.

REFERENCES

[1] Idson, B. (1971). Percutaneous absorption. In: Rabinowitz, J. L. & Myerson, R. M. (eds) *Adsorption Phenomena,* Wiley (Interscience), New York, p. 181.
[2] Idson, B. (1975). Percutaneous absorption. *J. Pharm. Sci.* **64** 901.
[3] Katz, M. (1973). Design of topical drug products: pharmaceutics. In: Ariens, E. J. (ed.) *Drug Design,* Academic Press, New York, p. 93.
[4] Katz, M. & Poulsen, B. J. (1971). Absorption of drugs through the skin. In: Brodie, B. B. & Gillette, J. (eds) *Handbook of Experimental Pharmacology,* vol. 28, pt. 1, Springer-Verlag, New York, p. 103.
[5] Katz, M. & Poulsen, B. J. (1972). Corticoid, vehicle, and skin interaction in percutaneous absorption. *J. Soc. Cosmetic Chem.* **23** 565.
[6] Poulsen, B. J. (1973). Design of topical drug products: biopharmaceutics. In: Ariens, E. J. (ed.) *Drug Design,* Academic Press, New York.
[7] Higuchi, T. (1977). Pro-drug, molecular structure and percutaneous delivery.

In: Roche, B. (ed.) *Design of Biopharmaceutical Properties Through Prodrugs and Analogs,* American Pharmaceutical Association, Washington, p. 409.

[8] Dugard, P. H. (1977). Skin permeability theory in relation to percutaneous absorption in toxicology. *Adv. Mod. Toxicol.* **4** 525.

[9] Scheuplein, R. J. (1972). Properties of the skin as a membrane. *Adv. Biol. Skin* **12** 125.

[10] Scheuplein, R. J. (1978). The skin as a barrier, skin permeation, site variation in diffusion and permeability. In: Jarrett, A. (ed.) *The Physiology and Pathophysiology of the Skin,* Academic Press, New York and London, pp. 1669, 1693 and 1731.

[11] Flynn, G. L. (1979). Topical drug absorption and topical pharmaceutical systems. In: Banker, G. S. & Rhodes, C. T. (eds) *Modern Pharmaceutics,* Dekker, New York and Basel, p. 263.

[12] Chien, Y. W. (1982). *Novel Drug Systems,* Dekker, New York and Basel, p. 149.

[13] Schaefer, H., Zesch, A. & Stuttgen, G. (1982). *Skin Permeability,* Springer-Verlag, New York.

[14] Barry, B. W. (1983). *Dermatological Formulations: Percutaneous Absorption,* Dekker, New York and Basel.

[15] Bronaugh, R. L. & Maibach, H. I. (eds) (1985). *Percutaneous Absorption,* Dekker, New York and Basel.

[16] Elias, P. M. (1981). Epidermal lipids, membranes, and keratinization. *Int. J. Dermatol.* **20** 1.

[17] Denyer, S. P., Hugo, W. B. & O'Brien, M. (1984). Metabolism of glyceryl trinitrate by skin staphylococci. *J. Pharm. Pharmacol.* **36,** 61P.

[18] Denyer, S. P., Guy, R. H., Hadgraft, J. & Hugo, W. B. (1985). The microbial degradation of topically applied drugs. *J. Pharm. Pharmacol.* **37** 89.

[19] Brooks, F. L., Hugo, W. B. & Denyer, S. P. (1982). Transformation of betamethasone-17-valerate by skin microflora. *J. Pharm. Pharmacol.* **34** 61P.

[20] Wester, R. C. & Noonan, P. K. (1980). Relevance of animal models for percutaneous absorption. *Int. J. Pharm.* **7** 99.

[21] Noonan, P. K. & Wester, R. K. (1985). Cutaneous metabolism of xenobiotics. In: Bronaugh, R. L. & Maibach, H. I. (eds) *Percutaneous Absorption,* Dekker, New York and Basel, p. 65.

[22] Guy, R. H. & Hadgraft, J. (1984). Pharmacokinetics of percutaneous absorption and concurrent metabolism. *Int. J. Pharm.* **20** 43.

[23] Marty, J.-P., Guy, R. H. & Maibach, H. I. (1985). Percutaneous penetration as a method of delivery to muscle and other tissues. In: Bronaugh, R. L. & Maibach, H. I. (eds) *Percutaneous Absorption,* Dekker, New York and Basel.

[24] Barry, B. W. (1985). Optimisation of percutaneous absorption. In: Bronaugh, R. L. & Maibach, H. I. (eds) *Percutaneous Absorption,* Dekker, New York and Basel, p. 489.

[25] Woodford, R. & Barry, B. W. (1986). Penetration enhancers and the percutaneous absorption of drugs: an update. *J. Toxicol.-Cut. & Ocular Toxicol.* **5** 165.

[26] Barry, B. W. (1976). Bioavailability of topical steroids. *Dermatologica* **152** (Suppl. 1) 47.

[27] Barry, B. W. & Woodford, R. (1978). Activity and bioavailability of topical

steroids. *In vivo/in vitro* correlations for the vasoconstrictor test. *J. Clin. Pharam.* **3** 43.

[28] Woodford, R. & Barry, B. W. (1982). Optimization and bioavailability of topical steroids: thermodynamic control. *J. Invest. Dermatol.* **79** 388.

[29] Barry, B. W. & Bennett, S. L. (1987). To be published.

[30] Hoelgaard, A. & Møllgaard, B. (1986). Dermal drug delivery — improvement by choice of vehicle or drug derivative. In: Anderson, J. M. & Kim, S. W. (eds) *Advances in Drug Delivery Systems,* Elsevier, Amsterdam, p. 111.

[31] Southwell, D., Barry, B. W. & Woodford, R. (1984). Variations in permeability in human skin within and between specimens. *Int. J. Pharm.* **18** 19.

[32] Bond, J. R. & Barry, B. W. (1985). Long-term hydration effects on permeability of hairless mouse skin. *J. Pharm. Pharmac.* **37** Suppl. 77P.

[33] Bond, J. R. & Barry, B. W. (1987). To be published.

[34] Bond, J. R. & Barry, B. W. (1987). To be published.

[35] Stoughton, R. B. (1975). Animal models for *in vitro* percutaneous absorption. In: Maibach, H. I. (ed.) *Animal Models in Dermatology,* Churchill Livingston, New York, p. 121.

[36] Durrheim, H., Flynn, G. L., Higuchi, W. & Behl, C. R. (1980). Permeation of hairless mouse skin I: experimental methods and comparison with human epidermal permeation by alkanols. *J. Pharm. Sci.* **69** 781.

[37] Reifenrath, W. G., Chellquist, E. M., Shipwash, E. A., Jederberg, W. W. & Krueger, G. G. (1984). Evaluation of animal models for predicting skin penetration in man. *Br. J. Dermatol.* **111** Suppl. 27, 123.

[38] Chien, Y. W. (1984). Pharmaceutical considerations of transdermal nitroglycerin delivery: the various approaches. *Am. Heart J.* **108** 207.

[39] Chien, Y. W., Keshary, P. R., Huang, Y. C. & Sarpotdar, P. P. (1983). Comparative controlled skin permeation of nitroglycerin from marketed transdermal delivery systems. *J. Pharm. Sci.* **72** 968.

[40] Good, W. R. (1983). Transderm®-Nitro; controlled delivery of nitroglycerin via the transdermal route. *Drug Development and Industrial Pharmacy* **9** 647.

[41] Shaw, J. E. & Mitchell, C. (1983–84). Dermal drug delivery systems: a review. *J. Toxicol.-Cut. & Ocular Toxicol.* **2** 249.

[42] Groth, H., Vetter, H., Knüsel, J., Foerster, E., Siegenthaler, W. & Vetter, W. (1984). Transdermal clonidine application: long-term results in essential hypertension. *Klin. Wochenschr.* **62** 925.

[43] Breimer, D. D. (1984). Rationale for rate-controlled drug delivery of cardiovascular drugs by the transdermal route. *Am. Heart J.* **108** 196.

[44] Shaw, J. E. (1984). Pharmacokinetics of nitroglycerin and clonidine delivered by the transdermal route. *Am. Heart J.* **108** 217.

[45] Hollenberg, M. & Go, M. (1984). Clinical studies with transdermal nitroglycerin. *Am. Heart J.* **108** 223.

[46] Weber, M. A. & Dreyer, J. I. M. (1984). Clinical experience with rate-controlled delivery of antihypertensive therapy by a transdermal system. *Am. Heart J.* **108** 231.

[47] Whitehead, M. I., Padwick, M. L., Endacott, J. & Pryse-Davies, J. (1985). Endometrial responses to transdermal estradiol in postmenopausal women. *Am. J. Obstet. Gynecol.* **152** 1079.

[48] Padwick, M. L., Endacott, J. & Whitehead, M. I. (1985). Efficacy, acceptability, and metabolic effects of transdermal estradiol in the management of postmenopausal women. *Am. J. Obstet. Gynecol.* **152** 1085.

[49] Place, V. A., Powers, M., Darley, P. E., Schenkel, L. & Good, W. R. (1985). A double-blind comparative study of Estraderm and premarin in the amelioration of postmenopausal symptoms. *Am. J. Obstet. Gynecol.* **152** 1092.

[50] Powers, M. S., Schenkel, L., Darley, P. E., Good, W. R., Balestra, J. C. & Place, V. A. (1985). Pharmacokinetics and pharmacodynamics of transdermal dosage forms of 17-beta-estradiol: comparison with conventional oral estrogens for hormone replacement. *Am. J. Obstet. Gynecol.* **152** 1099.

13

Recent advances in intranasal drug delivery systems

Kenneth S. E. Su, Harve C. Wilson and **Kristina M. Campanale**, Pharmaceutical Research Department and Cardiovascular Research Division, Lilly Research Laboratories, Eli Lilly and Company, Indianapolis, IN 46285, USA

1. ABSTRACT

Research efforts have been directed toward assessing the feasibility of administering drugs intranasally for some time in our laboratories. Like any other drug delivery system, the success of an intranasal delivery system also requires the selection of logical drug candidates. Several examples — a polar quaternary ammonium compound, proteins and peptides, and a catecholamine — will be reviewed and illustrated. In this chapter, nasal absorption of these various types of molecules in animals under a variety of conditions will be described. In addition, utilizing the intranasal administration route and applying sustained-release formulation techniques, some insights into the relationship between deposition, *in vivo* absorption, and the resulting pharmacological response will be discussed.

2. INTRODUCTION

Over the last 5–6 years, the possibility that intranasal administration might be useful for many compounds which are not absorbed orally has received a great deal of attention. In particular, with the availability of proteins and peptides from advanced biotechnology, the research and development of intranasal drug delivery systems has become even more vital. In a review of the literature, it has been demonstrated that systemically active drugs can be administered nasally. For instance, the nasal absorption of salicyclic acid and aminoprine was comparable to that by injection [1]. It was also reported that sulbenicillin, cefazolin, and other orally non-absorbable antibiotics had nasal absorption that was about 50% of the intramuscular dose [1]. The excellent bioavailability of propranolol after intranasal administration in rats, dogs, and humans was reported [2,3]. A good nasal absorption of progesterone [4,5], hydralazine [6], sodium guiazulene-3-sulfonate [7], 17 beta-estradiol [8], and clofilium tosylate [9] was also demonstrated by several investigators. Rapid pharmacological action of nitroglycerin after nasal administration to patients has been observed [10]. The nasal absorption of proteins and peptides, such as oxytocin [11] and synthetic lysine vasopressin [12] was reported nearly 20 years ago. More recently, the nasal absorption of synthetic luteinizing hormone-releasing hormone [13,14], pork and beef insulin [15,16], human insulin [17], enkephalin analogues [18], growth hormone-releasing factor [19], and interferon [20] was also demonstrated. This chapter primarily aims to review the nasal absorption data of various types of compounds under different conditions. Furthermore studies on the relationship of nasal absorption, deposition, and pharmacological responses after nasal administration of different formulations will be discussed.

3.   ANIMAL MODELS FOR INTRANASAL ADMINISTRATION

In view of the literature, generally, there are two types of animal models which could be used for intranasal absorption studies.

3.1   *In vivo* model — rat and dog

The rat model is, in essence, adapted from the literature with some minor modifcation [2]. The surgical preparation for *in vivo* nasal absorption is outlined as follows: the rats are anaesthetized by intraperitoneal injection of sodium pentobarbital. After an incision is made in the neck, the trachea is cannulated with a polyethylene tube. Another tube is inserted through the oesophagus toward the posterior part of the nasal cavity, as shown in Fig. 1. The passage of the nasopalatine tract is sealed to prevent the drainage of the drug solution from the nasal cavity into the mouth. The drug solution is delivered to the nasal cavity through the oesophagus cannulation tubing instead of from the nostril as described in the literature. The blood samples are then collected periodically from the femoral vein.

As described, since all the outlets in this rat model are blocked after surgical preparation, the only possible passage for the drug to be absorbed and transported into the systemic circulation is penetration and/or diffusion through the nasal membrane.

The *in vivo* dog model for nasal absorption studies is briefly described as follows: male beagle dogs are anaesthetized or maintained in the conscious state depending upon the characteristics of the drug and the purpose of the study. In the anaesthetized dog model, the dogs are anaesthetized by IV. injection of sodium thiopental and maintained with sodium phenobarbital. A positive pressure pump provides ventilation through a cuffed endotracheal tube and a heating pad keeps the body temperature at 37–38°C. The blood samples are collected periodically from the jugular vein. Cardiac contractility, when measured, was obtained with a Walton--Brodie strain gauge arch attached to the right ventricle.

Rat Model

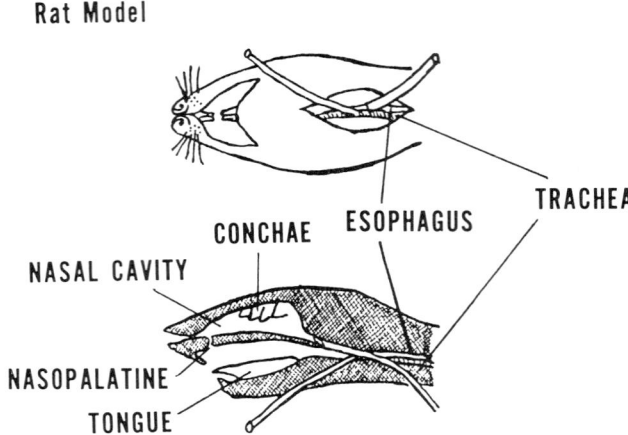

Fig. 1 — The top and side views of the cannulation arrangement in the rat model. From Hussain *et al.* [2], reproduced with permission of the copyright owner, *J. Pharm. Sci.*

3.2 *In situ* **nasal perfusion technique**
Fig. 2 shows the experimental set-up for the *in situ* nasal perfusion studies [2]. The surgical procedure is that described previously in the *in vivo* rat model. As shown in Fig. 2, a funnel is provided between the nose and the reservoir. The testing sample is placed in the reservoir and maintained at 37°C. The drug solution is circulated through the nasal cavity of the rat by means of a peristaltic pump. The perfusion solution passes out from the nostrils, through the funnel, and back into the reservoir. The drug solution in the reservoir is stirred constantly. The amount of drug absorbed is then determined by measuring the drug concentration remaining in the perfusion solution.

4   EXAMPLES AND ILLUSTRATIONS

4.1   Nasal absorption of a quaternary ammonium compound
The influence of the administration route on the absorption of clofilium tosylate has been investigated. Clofilium tosylate is a newly synthesized quaternary ammonium compound (Fig. 3), shown to selectively increase refractoriness of cardiac tissue [21]. It is known that the oral absorption of quaternary ammonium compounds is generally low and irregular [22]. Predictability of oral absorption of clofilium tosylate in rats was poor [23]. A total of 79% of the dose was unchanged and excreted in the faeces within 72 h after oral administration.
     Comparison of the disappearance of radioactivity in the blood of rats following various routes of administration of [14C]clofilium tosylate is shown in Fig. 4. The poor absoption as well as the variations in blood levels following oral administration are clearly demonstrated. Nasal administration of the drug resulted in much higher

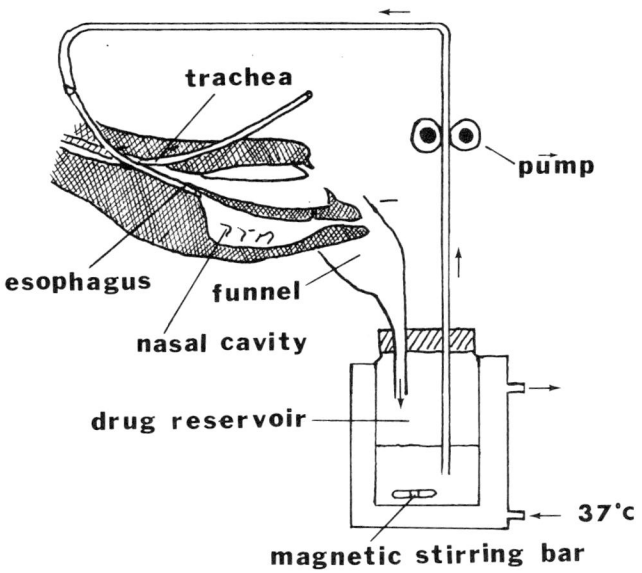

Fig. 2 — The experimental set-up for in situ nasal perfusion studies is the rat model. From Hirai
et al. [1[, reproduced with permission of the copyright owner, *Int. J. Pharm.*

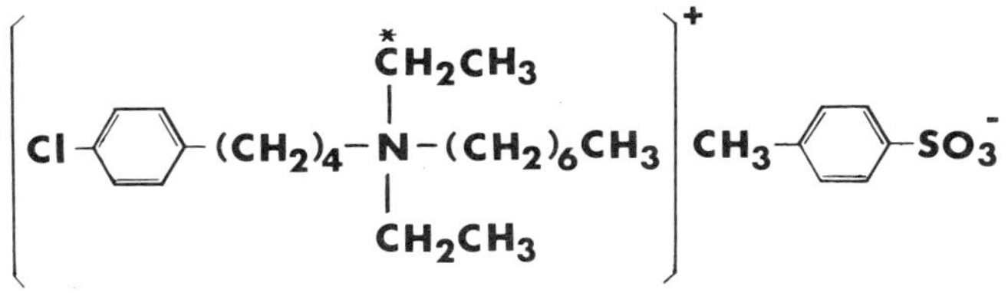

$$\left[Cl-\bigcirc-(CH_2)_4-\overset{\overset{\overset{*}{C}H_2CH_3}{|}}{\underset{\underset{CH_2CH_3}{|}}{N}}-(CH_2)_6CH_3\right]^{+} CH_3-\bigcirc-SO_3^{-}$$

Fig. 3 — Structure of clofilium tosylate. The position of [^{14}C] is shown at the asterisk.

levels of radioactivity than levels after oral adminstration. As shown in Fig. 4, the
blood radioactivity levels of the clofilium ion after oral administration of the tosylate
were about 1% of the levels obtained from the IV dose, whereas the radioactivity
levels after nasal administration were about 70% of the levels obtained from the IV
dose. Furthermore, the difference in levels following intravenous and intranasal
administrations were statistically insignificant ($p > 0.05$).

The effect of dose on nasal absorption indicates that the area under the blood
radioactivity levels versus time curve (AUC) increased with dose in a non-linear

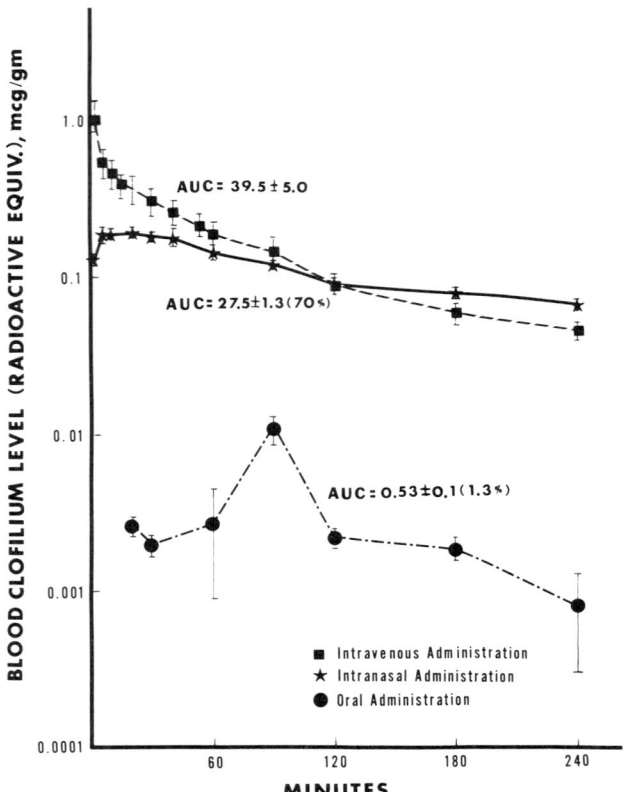

Fig. 4 — [^{14}C]Clofilium ion in blood of rats after various routes of administration of 1.2 mg/kg dose ($n = 3$). From Su *et al.* [9], reproduced with permission from the copyright owner, *J. Pharm. Sci.*

manner (Table 1). However, a linear dose–response relationship appeared in the lower concentration ranges. The non-linear portion of the curve and good absorption at the higher concentration of 1.2 mg/kg were attributed to damage of the nasal mucosa with exposure of the membrane to the quaternary ammonium compound.

The observation is illustrated in Figs 5–7, where at the highest concentration of clofilium tosylate, large portions of mucosa became necrotic. At the lower concentrations, only occasional epithelial cell damage was seen with the majority of mucosa remaining unaffected. Furthermore, histological examination showed no difference between nasal mucosa exposed to the dose of 0.3 or 0.6 mg/kg.

In summary, the intranasal delivery of clofilium tosylate in rats is as follows:

(a) Absorption after nasal administration is rapid and superior to oral delivery.
(b) Histopathological studies suggest that higher doses damage the nasal mucosa

Table 1 — Comparison of $[^{14}C]$clofilium ion blood concentrations[a] in rats — effect of dose

Route of administration	Dose (mg/kg)[b]	AUC (μg/min per g)[c]	Mean specific AUC[d]	Absortion (%)
Intravenous	1.2	39.5 ± 4.98	32.9	—
Nasal	1.2	27.5 ± 1.30	22.9	69.6
Nasal	0.6	5.70 ± 1.06	9.50	28.9
Nasal	0.3	2.81[e] ± 0.28	9.37	28.5

[a] Expressed as microgram equivalents of carbon-14 per gram of blood.
[b] Formulated in solution form.
[c] Mean ± SEM of three rats.
[d] mean specific AUC: (μg/min per g)/(mg/kg) =mean AUC/administration dose.
[e] $p > 0.05$, compared with an an AUC of 0.6 mg/kg.
From Su et al. [9], reproduced with permission of the copyright owner, *J. Pharm. Sci.*

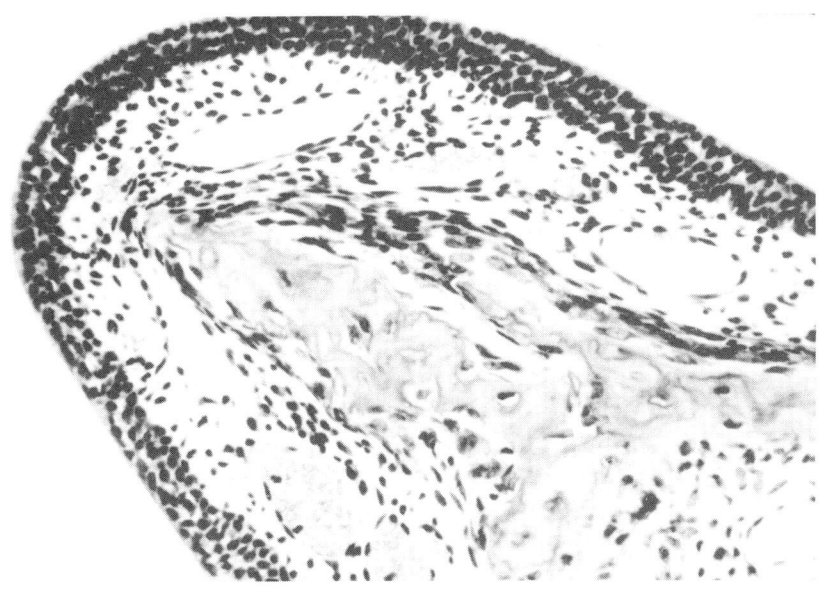

Fig. 5 — Nasal mucosa of rats: the control group. From Su *et al.* [9], reproduced with permission from the copyright owner, *J. Pharm. Sci.*

and the necrosis may facilitate nasal absorption. Whether the therapeutic dose damages the nasal mucosa in man needs to be determined.
(c) Nasal administration may be a possible route for delivery of quaternary ammonium drugs.

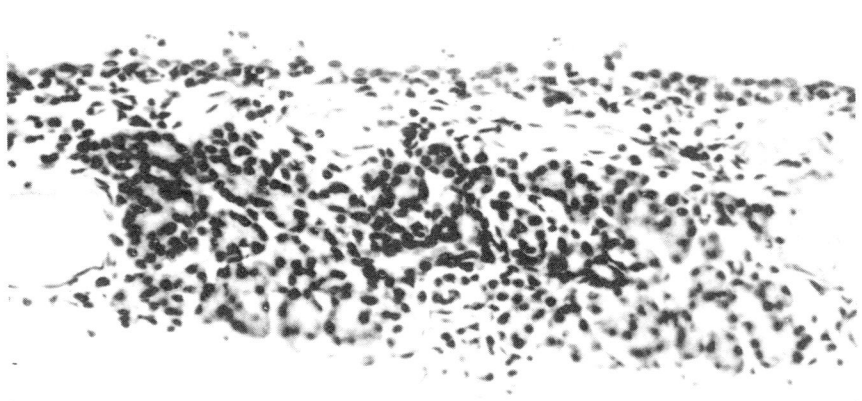

Fig. 6 — Nasal mucosa of rats administered clofilium at a dose of 0.6 mg/kg. From Su *et al.* [9], reproduced with permission from the copyright owner, *J. Pharm. Sci.*

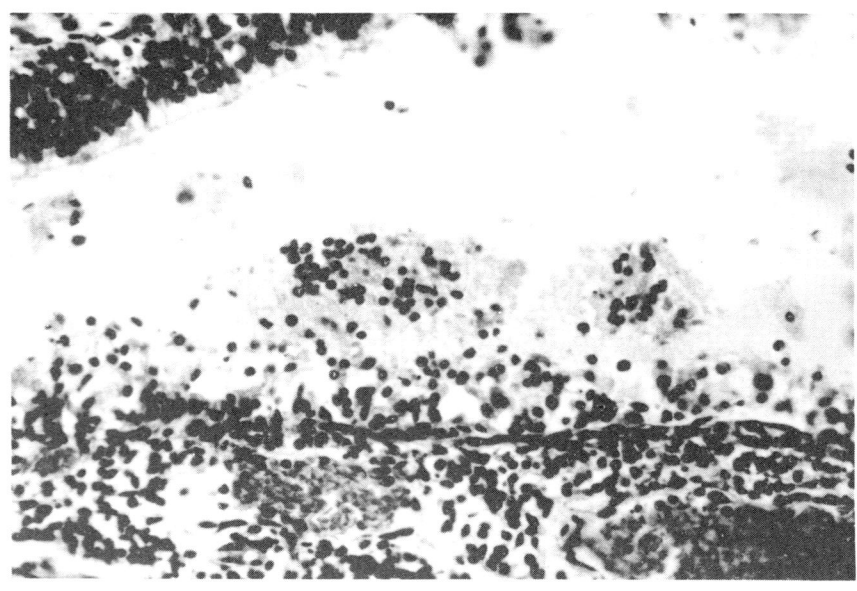

Fig. 7 — Nasal mucosa of rats administered clofilium at a dose of 1.2 mg/kg. From Su *et al.* [9], reproduced with permission from the copyright owner, *J. Pharm. Sci.*

4.2   Nasal absorption of proteins and peptides

In the past 10–15 years, analogues of the naturally occurring enkephalins have been evaluated for their analgesic activity [24–27]. These peptides have to be administered parenterally to have measurable activity. Two enkephalin analogues were chosen for nasal absorption studies. They are: [³H]Tyr*-D-Ala-Gly-L-Phe-D-Leu-OH ([³H]DADLE, mol.wt. = 569.7), and Tyr-D-Ala-Gly-Phe-N-Me-Met-NH_2CH_2COOH (metkephamid, mol. wt. = 660.8). Both are pentapeptides with short plasma half-lives. Although low-molecular-weight peptides, their oral absorption is extremely poor.

The effect of surfactant on nasal absorption of drugs is well known. Surfactants can influence drug absorption and membrane transport, and may also reduce proteolytic activity. A number of publications reported that conjugated bile salts, such as sodium glycocholate and sodium deoxycholate, enhanced the nasal absorption of peptides [15,16]. The nasal absorption data, for [³H]DADLE, in the presence and absence of sodium glychlolate as a promoter, is summarized in Table 2.

Table 2 — Comparison of blood concentrations[a] of total radioactivity equivalents of [³H]DADLE in rats after various routes of administration of 2 mg/kg dose[b]

Route of administration	n	AUC[c] (μg/min per g)	Relative absorption (%)
Subcutaneous			
[³H]DADLE in saline	3	590.4 ± 41.4	—
Nasal			
[³H]DADLE in saline	3	348.1 ± 48.3	59.0
[³H]DADLE in saline plus 1% sodium glycocholate	4	555.9 ± 85.1	94.1

[a] Expressed as microgram equivalents of tritium in blood.
[b] The dose volume was maintained at 0.1 ml.
[c] AUC: mean ± SEM.
From Su et al. [18], reproduced with permission of the copyright owner, *J. Pharm. Sci.*

In the absence of sodium glycocholate, a nasal absorption of about 59% of the subcutaneous dose was found based on the total amount of labelled compound appearing in the blood. However, in the presence of 1% sodium glycocholate, the nasal absorption was enhanced to 94% of the subcutaneous dose. Obviously, the total radioactivity detected in the blood included both the parent molecule and its metabolites. A typical quantitative analysis of radioactivity of [³H]DADLE in rat serum following intransal administration is shown in Fig. 8. The disappearance of parent peptide and the appearance of its metabolites can be followed kinetically.

Fig. 9 shows the comparison of radioactivity of intact DADLE serum concen-

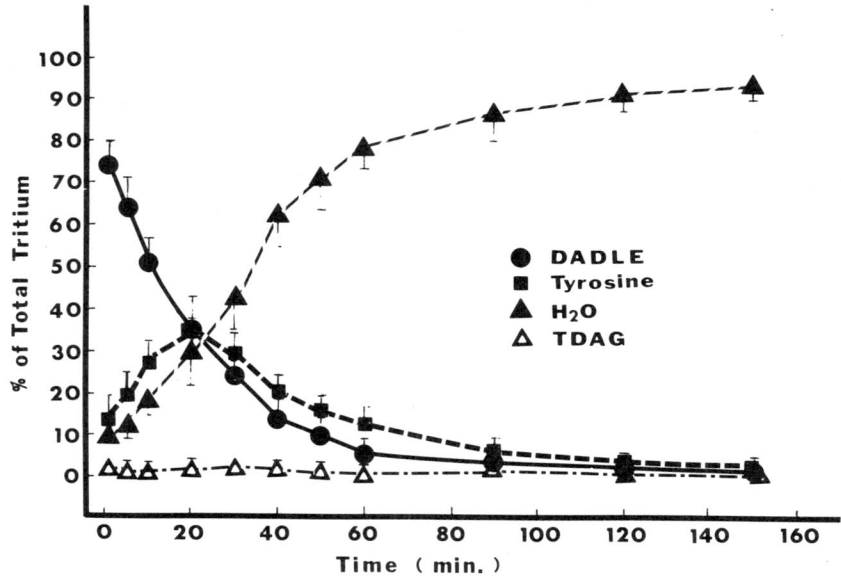

Fig. 8 — Absorption and distribution of [^{3}H]DADLE in rat serum following intranasal administration of 2 mg/kg dose ($n = 3$). From Su *et al.* [18], reproduced with permission from the copyright owner, *J. Pharm. Sci.*

tration in rats after intravenous and intranasal administrations. The peak concentration at 1 min was about 3.4 μg/ml and 0.6 μg/ml for IV and nasal administration, respectively. Therefore, there was a 5.4-fold higher serum DADLE concentration in the intravenously dosed animals as compared to animals administered nasal solution. However, the difference in the extent of absorption (AUC) between intravenous and nasal administration was statically insignificant ($p > 0.1$), with the bioavailability of DADLE after intranasal administration being about 93% of the intravenous dose.

The nasal absorption of metkephamid in rats was different from that of DADLE. As shown in Table 3, there was no influence of surfactant on the nasal absorption of metkephamid. The difference in serum concentrations after nasal administration of metkephamid, in the presence or absence of promoter in the formulation, was statistically insignificant ($p > 0.1$). The data suggested that there is no need to incorporate a surfactant in the formulation to enhance the absorption, as compared to the other pentapeptide described previously (Table 2).

This observation is consistent with the reported data that metkephamid is a more stable enkephalin analogue and less susceptible to enzymatic degradation [28].

Comparison of serum concentrations of metkephamid following various routes of administration in rats is shown in Fig. 10. No metkephamid could be detected in the serum after oral administration. The difference in the extent of absorption after intravenous, subcutaneous, and intranasal administrations was statistically insignificant ($p > 0.1$).

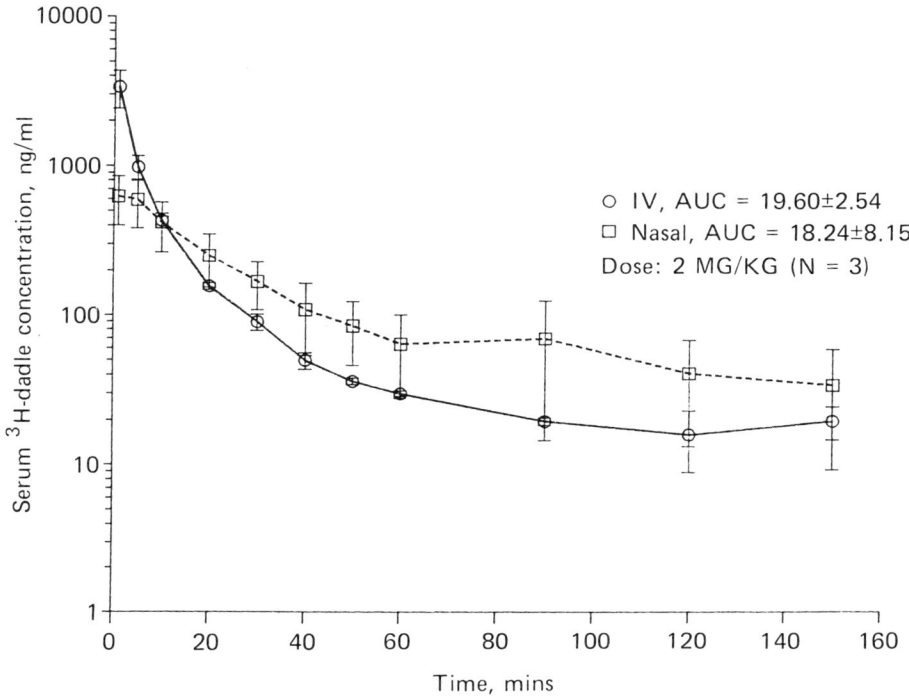

Fig. 9 — Comparison of radioactivity of intact [³H]DADLE serum concentration in rats after intravenous and intranasal administration.

Table 3 — Effect of promoter on nasal absorption of metkephamid in rats after administered of 25 mg/mg dose

Route of administration	n	AUC[a] (μg/min per g)	Relative absorption (%)
Intravenous			
Metkephamid in saline	3	186.71 ± 34.74	—
Nasal			
Metkephamid in saline plus 1% sodium glycocholate	3	144.24 ± 4.77	77.2
Metkephamid in saline	4	$190.38^{b} \pm 65.33$	101.9

[a] AUC: mean $\pm$ SEM.
[b] $p > 0.1$, comparison between two nasal formulations.

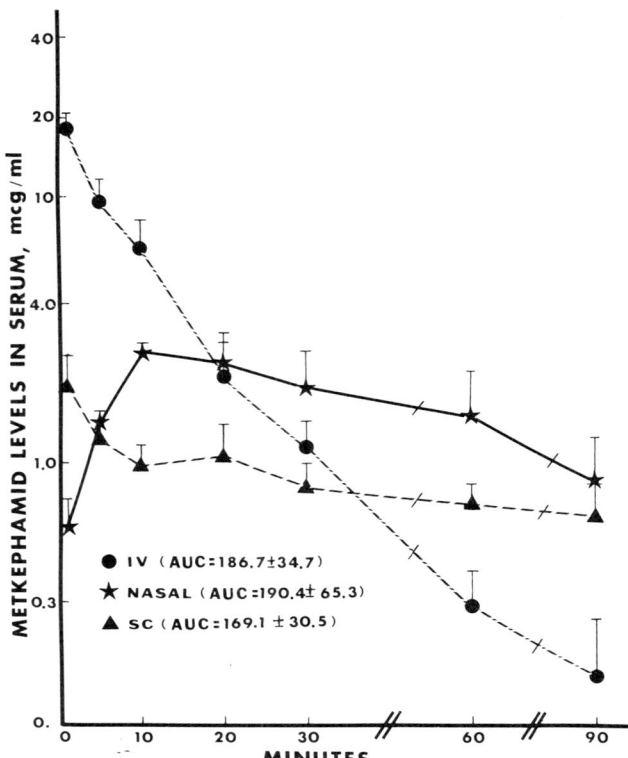

Fig. 10 — Comparison of serum concentrations of metkephamid after various routes of administration in rats. From Su *et al* [18], reproduced with permission from the copyright owner, *J. Pharm. Sci.*

The effect of dose on the nasal absorption is shown in Table 4. The area under the curve of serum metkephamid concentrations versus time increased with increasing dose.

The extent of absorption expressed as AUC per unit dose remained relatively constant. Thus, the amount of metkephamid absorbed nasally was directly proportional to the dose administered according to the law of diffusion. Therefore, a linear relationship between the dose and the AUC was observed in the range of concentration studied with a correlation coefficient of 0.950.

In summary, the intranasal delivery of enkephalins in rats is as follows:

(a) Promoters may be necessary for effective nasal absorption of some small peptides
(b) Future studies need to address mucosal integrity following long-term administration
(c) Nasal delivery of proteins and peptides, once again as shown in the literature, may offer a useful route for systemic medication.

Table 4 — Effect of dose on the nasal absorption of metkephamid[a] in rats

Route of administration	n	AUC[b]	Mean specific AUC[c]	Bioavail- ability (%)
Intravenous				
25 mg/kg	3	186.71 ± 34.74	7.47	—
Intranasal				
50 mg/kg	3	273.40 ± 35.57	5.47[d]	73.2
25 mg/kg	4	190.38 ± 65.33	7.61[d]	101.9
12.5 mg/kg	3	60.51 ± 15.57	4.84[d]	64.8

[a] Metkephamid was dissolved in saline.
[b] AUC: μg/min per ml, mean ± SEM.
[c] Mean specific AUC: (μg/min per ml)/(mg/kg) = mean AUC/administered dose.
[d] $p > 0.1$, comparison between various doses of nasal administration.
From Su et al. [18], reproduced with permission of the copyright owner, *J. Pharm. Sci.*

4.3 Nasal absorption of a catecholamine

Dobutamine hydrochloride (Fig. 11) is a synthetic catecholamine with strong stimulation of the beta-1 adrenergic receptor and mild stimulation of the beta-2 and alpha-1 receptors [29]. It is a relatively selective positive inotropic drug that increases ventricular contractility and cardiac output without substantially increasing heart rate and systemic blood pressure [30]. Because of the extremely short half-life, the clinical utility is currently limited to intravenous infusion only.

The influence of administration route on absorption in anaesthetized rats given a 2.5 mg/kg dose is shown in Fig. 12. The intravenous infusion was performed at the infusion rate of 8.3 μg/kg per min over 5 h. The average dobutamine plasma concentrations produced by each dose after intravenous bolus, intravenous infusion, and intranasal route are shown for the duration of the study.

The intravenous bolus administration route produced a very high dobutamine plasma concentration, which was greater than 1000 ng/ml within 0.5 min after dosing, and a duration of only 30 min. However, an equivalent dose following intranasal administration produced a moderate dobutamine plasma concentration of about 100 ng/ml by 20 min and remained elevated after 2 h. For intravenous infusion, the plasma concentration of dobutamine reached 10 ng/ml by 30 min after infusion and remained at that level for the 5-h infusion period. The comparison of the extent of absorption (AUC) following these three administration routes revealed dramatic differences. It would appear that nasal absorption is about 500% of that by intravenous bolus and 300% of that by intravenous infusion. The interpretation of these data requires further investigation.

The effect of method of nasal administration on absorption was also studied. As shown in Fig. 13, the extent of absorption when giving dobutamine at the dose of 2.5 mg/kg from the oesophagus is larger than that from the nostril. In a review of the anatomy and physiology, of the nose, the posterior part of the nasal cavity is populated by pseudo-stratified columnar epithelium, which is a highly vascularized

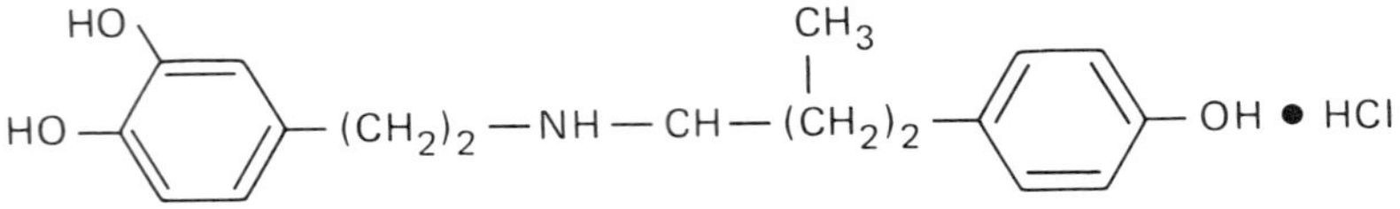

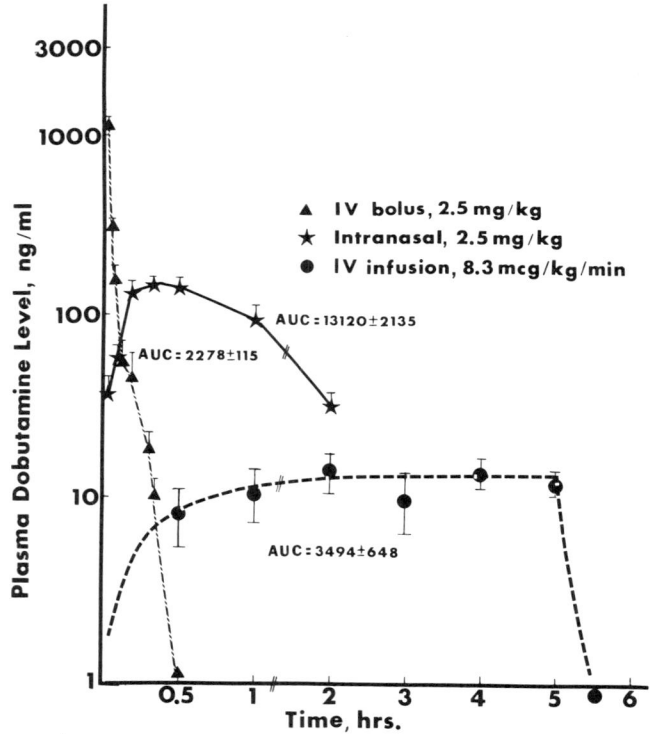

Fig. 11 — Structure of dobutamine hydrochloride.

Fig. 12 — Plasma concentrations of dobutamine after various routes of administration of 2.5 mg/kg dose in rats (n = 3–4).

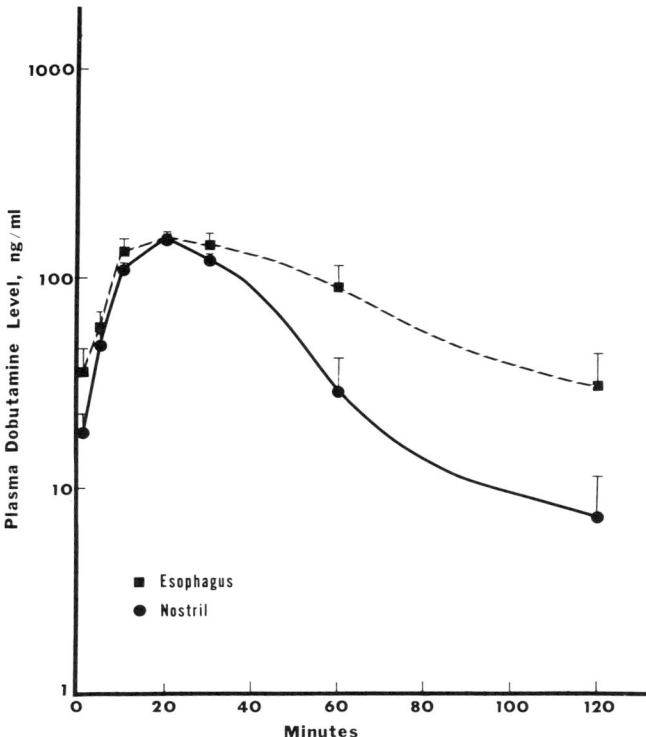

Fig. 13 — Comparison of nasal administration method on nasal absorption of dobutamine in rats.

surface for absorption, likely to provide good nasal absorption. The difference in AUC of the two nasal administration methods is statistically significant ($p < 0.05$). On the basis of this, it is proposed that the optimal sites of absorption appear to be in the posterior part of the cavity.

In the earlier studies on the pharmacological activity after intranasal administration of dobutamine, the duration of response lasted only 1 h. It is conceivable that this duration would not be sufficient for chronic dobutamine therapy. A sustained-release formulation is essential to prolong the inotropic effect of dobutamine.

As shown in Fig. 14, the duration of pharmacological response was observed for only 1 h with the regular aerosol formulation. It was surprising to observe that a 4-h duration was achieved with the sustained-release aerosol formulation. Furthermore, the cardiac contractility produced by dobutamine after intranasal administration was comparable to that by intravenous infusion at the rate of 2 μg/kg/per min for 4 h.

Results fom the studies of various sustained-release agents are summarized in Table 5. None of the agents tested so far, with the exception of oleic acid and to a

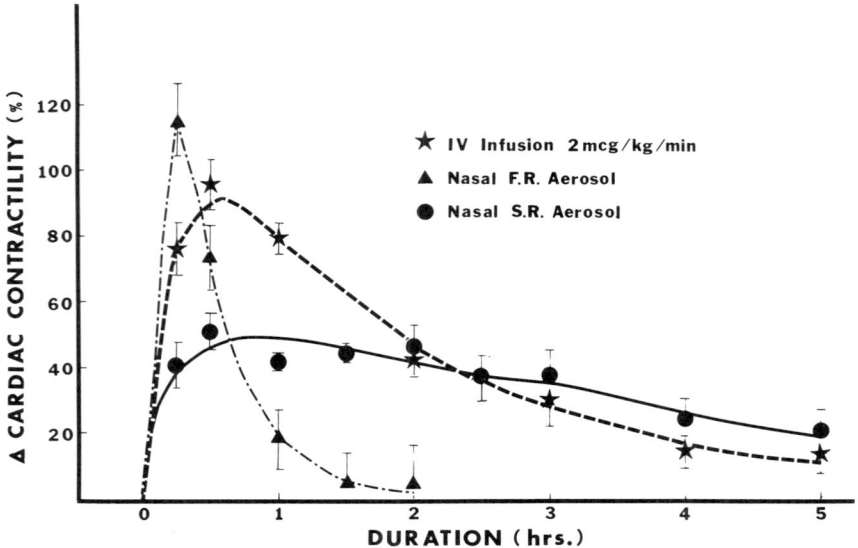

Fig. 14 — Duration of cardiac contractility of dobutamine in dogs after intravenous infusion and administration of various nasal formulations at the dose of 733 $\mu g/kg$ ($n = 4$).

Table 5 — Effect of sustained-release agents on the cardiac contractility parameters of dobutamine in dogs ($n = 3$–5)

Sustained-release agents	Cardiac contractility activity		
	Onset time[a] (min)	Peak time [b] (min)	Duration (min)
None in formulation	5	10–30	60
Triacetin	5	10–30	60
Span 85	5	10–30	60
Coconut oil	5	10–30	60
Ethyl oleate	5	10–30	60
Olive oil	5	10–30	60
Oleic acid	5	15–60	240+
Linoleic acid	5	13–30	210+

[a] The time contractility activity was first observed.
[b] The peak time of contractility activity.

lesser extent linoleic acid, affected the duration of the dobutamine response. The incorporation of oleic acid into the formulation produced an onset of inotropic response within 5 min, which reached a peak within 15–60 min and produced a duration of action of 4–5 h.

The effect of oleic acid on the duration of cardiac contractility in anaesthetized dogs after nasal administration is shown in Table 6. Two to three per cent oleic acid

Table 6 — Effect of oleic acid in dobutamine nasal formulation on inotropic activity in dogs[a] ($n = 4$)

Oleic acid %	Peak of contractility ($\Delta\%$)[b]	Half-life of duration (min)
0	160	30
2	80	45
3	66	75
7	42	180

[a] The data were corrected for variations in cardiac sensitivity in dogs.
[b] The percentage changed from the control.

increased the half-life of duration from 1.5- to 2.5-fold. A much more favourable response was observed with oleic acid concentrations from 3 to 10% (the response with 10% oleic acid, although not shown, was the same as that shown for 7% oleic acid). The 3–10% oleic acid produced a moderate inotropic response, peaking at 30 min, and having a duration 3–5 h above control. The mechanism of prolonging the duration of cardiac contractility of dobutamine in the presence of oleic acid needs further study.

The bioavailability of dobutamine after adminstration of an intranasal sustained-release formulation in dogs is shown in Fig. 15.

After intranasal administration, a dobutamine plasma concentration of 29 ng/ml at 15 min and a peak concentration of 112 ng/ml at 1 h following dosing were obtained. This dobutamine plasma concentration then decreased to 18 ng/ml by 6 h. The average dobutamine plasma levels from the dobutamine intravenous infusion studies at an infusion rate of 5 μg/kg per min for 6 h in dogs results in a constant plasma dobutamine concentration throughout most of the study. The comparison of the intranasal and intravenous routes of administering dobutamine shows the similarities of these two routes. However, the extent of absorption as measured by AUC per unit dose revealed that the bioavailability of nasal absorption is about two-fold that of intravenous infusion. However, when the metabolite is taken into account, then the total amount of dobutamine absorbed following intranasal administration is essentially equivalent to intravenous infusion.

In the summary, the intranasal delivery of dobutamine in rats and dogs is as follows:

(a) It is readily absorbed from the nasal mucosa with rapid onset of absorption

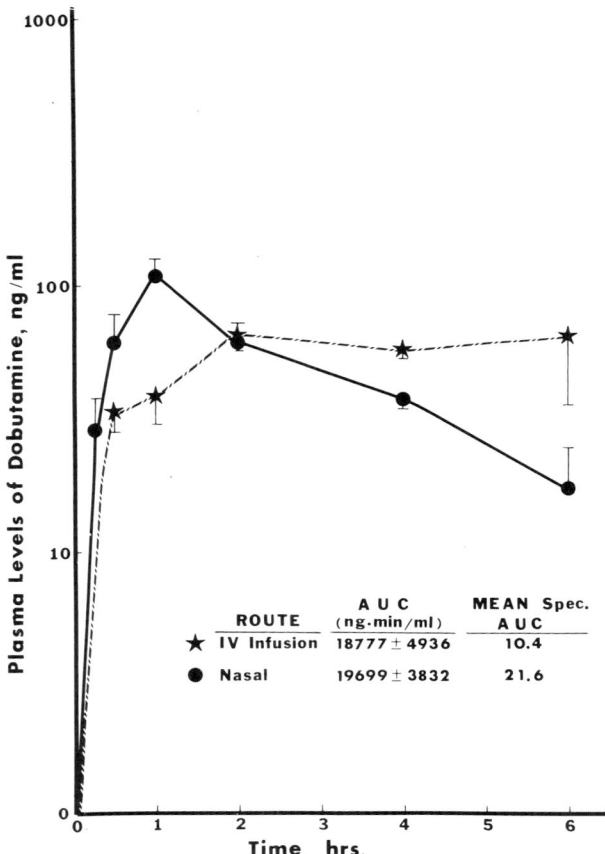

Fig. 15 — Plasma concentrations of dobutamine after intravenous infusion and nasal administration of dogs (*n* = 4–12).

(b) Bioavailability after nasal administration is theoretically equivalent to the IV infusion route
(c) These data, along with other studies on dobutamine, suggested that catecholamines may be intranasally delivered.

5 CONCLUSION

It is evident that the intranasal route of administration could be considered as potentially useful for delivering drugs to the systemic circulation. The highly vascularized surface of nasal mucosa for absorption, the bypass of hepatic first-pass metabolism, the rapid onset of action after nasal administration, and the avoidance of injection therapy show that the intranasal drug delivery system offers several advantages. In particular, we have demonstrated that a short biological half-life compound can be designed for mimicking intravenous infusion by applying an intranasal sustained-release formulation approach. Our observations along with those of other researchers, suggest that a growing potential for the intranasal delivery of systemic medication is foreseeable.

ACKNOWLEDGEMENTS

The authors would like to acknowledge the collaboration and contributions of Dr C. L. Gries, Dr. L. G. Mendelsohn, Ms G. A. Kerchner, Ms K. Brune, Mr W. C. Coffman, Mr W. C. Raper, and the discussion and suggestion of Dr A. Bingham and the assistance of Mrs A. Simpson in the preparation of this manuscript.

REFERENCES

[1] Hirai, S., Yashiki, T., Matsuzawa, T. & Mima, H. (1981). Absorption of drugs from the nasal mucosa of rat. *Int. J. Pharm.* **7**, 315–325.

[2] Hussain, A., Hirai, S. & Bawarshi, R. (1980). Nasal absorption of propranolol from different dosage forms by rats and dogs. *J. Pharm. Sci.* **69** 1411–1413.

[3] Hussain, A., Foster, T., Hirai, S., Kashahara, T., Batenhorst, R. & Jones, M. (1980). Nasal absorption of propranolol in humans. *J. Pharm. Sci.* **69** 1240.

[4] David, G. F. X., Puri, & Anand Kumar, T. C. (1981). Bioavailability of progesterone enhanced by intranasal spraying. *Experientia* **37** 533–534.

[5] Hussain, A., Hirai, S. & Bawarshi, R. (1981). Nasal absorption of natural contraceptive steroids in rats — progesterone absorption. *J. Pharm. Sci.* **79** 466–567.

[6] Kaneo, Y. (1983). Absorption from the nasal mucous membrane, I. Nasal absorption of hydralazine in rats. *Acta Pharm. Suec.* **20** 379–388.

[7] Mukai, H., Sugihara, K. & Sugiyama, M. (1985). Studies on the absorption of sodium guiazulene-3-sulfonate. I. *J. Pharmacobio.-Dyn.* **8** 329–336.

[8] Rigg, L. A., Milanes, B., Villanueva, B. M. & Yen, S. C. C. (1977). Efficacy of intravaginal and intranasal administration of micronized estradiol-17. *J. Clin. Endocr. Metab.* **45** 1261–1264.

[9] Su, K. S. E., Campanale, K. M. & Gries, C. L. (1984). Nasal drug delivery system of a quaternary ammonium compound: clofilium tosylate. *J. Pharm. Sci.* **73**, 1251–1254.

[10] Hill, A. B. (1979). Intranasal administration of nitroglycerin. *Anesth.* **51** 67.

[11] Talledo, E., Adams, S. F. & Zuspan, F. P. (1964). Response of pregnant human uterus to oxytocin given intranasally. *J. Am. Med. Assoc.* **189** 348–350.

[12] Moses, A. M. (1964). Synthetic lysine vasopressin nasal spray in the treatment of diabetes insipidus. *Clin. Pharmacol. Ther.* **5** 422–427.

[13] Flink, G., Ginnser, G., Liedholm, P., Thorell, J. & Mulder, J. (1974). Comparison of plasma levels of luteinizing hormone-releasing hormone in men after intravenous or intranasal administration. *J. Endocr.* **63** 351–360.

[14] Berquist, C., Nillius, S. J. & Wide, L. (1979). Intranasal gonadotropin-releasing hormone agonist as a contraceptive agent *Lancet* **II**, 215–216.

[15] Hirai, S., Yashiki, T. & Mima, H. (1981). Effect of surfactants on the nasal absorption of insulin in rats. *Int. J. Pharm.* **9** 164–172.

[16] Moses, A. C., Gordon, G. S., Carey, M. C. & Flier, J. S. (1983). Insulin administered intransally as an insulin-bile salt aerosol: effectiveness and repro-ducibility in normal and diabetic subjects. *Diabetes* **32** 1040–1047.

[17] Su, K. S. E., Howey, D. C., Campanale, K. M. & Oeswein, J. Q. (1986). Intranasal administration of human sodium insulin (HSI) in rats, dogs, and humans: absorption and possible mechanism. *Diabetes* **35** 64A.

[18] Su, K. S. E., Campanale, K. M., Mendelsohn, L. G., Kerchner, G. A. & Gries, C. L. (1985). Nasal delivery of polypeptides, I: nasal absorption of enkephalins in rats. *J. Pharm. Sci.* **74**, 394–398.

[19] Evans, W. S., Borges, J. L. C., Kaiser, L., Vance, M. L., Sellers, R. P., MacLeod, R. M., Vale, W. & Throner, M. O. (1983). Intranasal administration of human pancreatic tumor GH-releasing factor-40 stimulates GH release in normal men. *J. Clin. Endocr. Metab.* **57** 1081–1083.

[20] Greenberg, S. B., Harmon, M. W., Johnson, P. E. & Couch, R. B. (1978). Antiviral activity of intranasally applied human leukocyte interferon. *Antimic-rob. Agents and Chemoth.* **14** 596–600.

[21] Steinberg, M. I. & Molloy, B. B. (1979). A new antifibrillatory agent that selectively increases cellular refractoriness. *Life Sci.* **25** 1397–1406.

[22] Garrett, E. R., Green, J. R. & Bailer, M. (1982). Bretylium pharmacokinetics and bioavailabilities in man with various doses and modes of administration. *Biopharm. Drug Dispos.* **3** 129–164.

[23] Steinberg, M. I. (1984). In *New Drug Annual*, Raven Press, New York, NY, p. 103.

[24] Frederickson, R. C. A., Smithwick, E. L., Shuman, R. & Bemis, K. G. (1981). Metkephamid, a systemically active analogue of methionine enkephalin with potent opioid delta-receptor activity. *Science* **211** 603–605.

[25] Leander, J. D. & Wood, C. R. (1982). Metkephamid effects on operant behavior. *Peptides* **3** 771–773.

[26] Gesellchen, P. D., Tafur, S. & Shields, J. E. (1979). In: Gross, E. & Meienhofer, J. (eds) *Peptides: Structure and Biological Function*, Proc. of the Sixth Am. Peptide Symp., Pierce Chemical Company, Rockford, IL, pp. 117–120.

[27] Frederickson, R. C. A. (1979). Enkephalin pentapeptides — a review of current evidence for a physicological role in vertebrate neurotransmission. *Life Sci.* **21** 23–42.

[28] Gesellchen, P. D., Parli, C. J. & Frederickson, R. C. A. (1980). In: Rich, D. H. & Gross, Ed. (eds) *Peptides: Synthesis-Structure-Function*, Proc. of the Seventh Am. Peptide Symp., Pierce Chemical Company, Rockford, IL, pp. 637–640.

[29] Ruffalo, R. R., Spradlin, T. A., Pollock, G. D., Waddell, J. E. & Murphy, P. J. (1981). Alpha and beta adrenergic effects of the stereoisomers of dobutamine. *J. Pharmacol. Exp. Ther.* **219** 447–452.

[30] Tuttle, R. R. & Mills, J. (1975). Dobutamine: development of a new catechola-mine to selectivity increase cardiac contractility. *Cir. Res.* **36** 185–196.

14

New systems for the ocular delivery of drugs

John W. Shell, Iolab Pharmaceuticals, 861 South Village, Oaks Drive, Covina, CA 91724, USA

1. INTRODUCTION

Most ophthalmic drugs are applied topically in the form of eyedrops. The typical administration pattern is one of pulse entry of the drug, followed by a rapid decline of drug concentration in the tears, the kinetics of which approximate first order (Fig. 1).

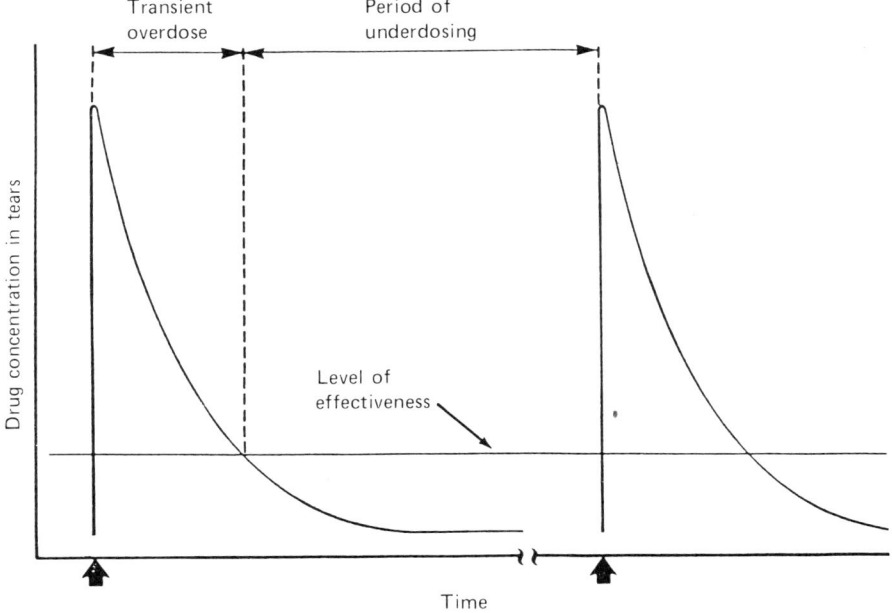

Fig. 1 — Typical drug concentration–time profile from eyedrop administration.

Adequate therapy from eyedrops may be achieved either by providing a sufficient magnitude of the pulse, so that its effect is extended for a useful period of time, or by giving more frequent applications of a less concentrated pulse.

Some of the new ophthalmic drug delivery systems that have recently been reported provide for an enhanced pulse entry, with enhanced initial corneal absorption of the drug. While these systems prolong the desired effect with less frequent applications than eyedrops require, the side-effects are also enhanced; thus the systems are limited to use with drugs whose dose-related side-effects are not serious, or can be tolerated by the patient. Representative examples of these delivery systems are described below.

Other ophthalmic systems that have been developed aim at avoiding the pulse entry with which side-effects are associated, and at providing only the optimum amount of drug, as indicated by the 'level of effectiveness' shown in Fig. 1, for an extended time period. These are 'controlled-delivery' systems, and are reveiwed as a separate group.

2. SYSTEMS THAT EXTEND DURATION OF DRUG ACTION BY ENHANCING INITIAL CORNEAL ABSORPTION

Many delivery systems, some recently developed, incorporate a drug homogeneously distributed within a hydrophilic matrix. Tears can enter the matrix of such systems when they are placed in the cul-de-sac of the eye and, through a leaching action, rapidly remove a soluble drug. Thus, upon exposure of the system to the tears, the release rate of the drug is initially high but quickly declines (the pulse entry).

A number of approaches have been employed that provide an enhanced drug pulse, either by increasing corneal penetration, or by temporarily prolonging the absorption phase. Some of these approaches are old, and some are new. They include the addition of soluble polymers to eyedrop solutions; the use of presoaked matrices and soluble gels; ointments, emulsions and suspensions; and systems that facilitate drug transport, such as ion pairs, some liposome systems, prodrugs, and chemical derivatives other than prodrugs. All of these systems have similar drug release patterns, an example of which is illustrated in Fig. 2. This figure shows the release of pilocarpine from soft contact lenses previously soaked in 4% pilocarpine solution, and provides a comparison of experimentally determined values (encircled points) and the theoretical release pattern, as calculated by the following predictive equations [1].

$$\frac{M_t}{M_\infty} = 4\left(\frac{D_t}{l^2\pi}\right)^{\frac{1}{2}} \tag{1}$$

$$\frac{M_t}{M_\infty} = 1 - \frac{8}{\pi^2}\exp\left(-\frac{\pi^2 D_t}{l^2}\right) \tag{2}$$

Equation 1 is valid for the first 60% of the drug released and equation 2 is valid for the final 60%, with both equations giving almost identical results over the middle

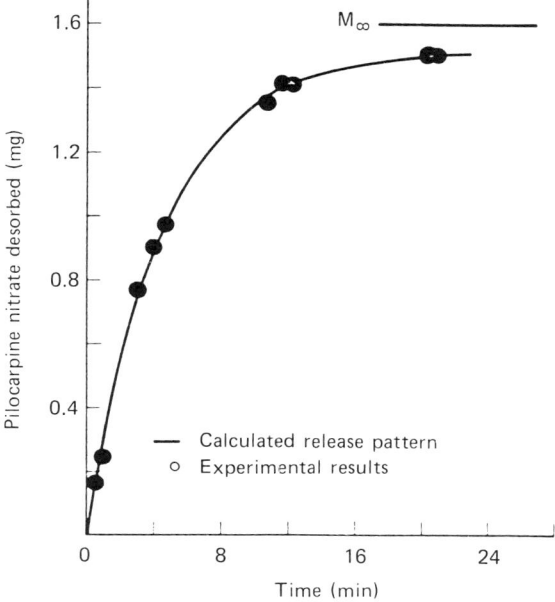

Fig. 2 — Drug release from hydrophilic matrix.

20% of the drug release. In these equations M_t represents the mass of drug released after time t in the release medium, and M_∞ represents the mass of drug released after an infinite time. l is the thickness of the device and D is the diffusion coefficient of the drug in the matrix. More than 90% of the drug is desorbed within the first 20–30 min.

The pattern is similar for all hydrophilic matrices. Their use extends the time that the dissolved drug will continue to be effective, as compared with an eyedrop; for instance, soft contact lenses presoaked in a 2% pilocarpine solution and placed on the cornea can maintain a significant reduction in intraocular pressure for almost 24 h. As noted above, however, 90% of the drug is desorbed within a half-hour, and the modification of the pulse necessary to achieve a full day's hypotensive therapy produces significant pilocarpine side-effects, such as increased miosis and myopia.

2.1   The addition of soluble polymers to eyedrop solutions

There have been numerous claims of prolongation of drug–corneal contact time of an eyedrop formulation by the addition of soluble polymers, such as methylcellulose, polyvinyl alcohol, hydroxypropyl cellulose, and polyvinylpyrrolidone. Most of these agents presumably increase the tear viscosity, which decreases the otherwise rapid initial drainage rate, and thus sustain to some extent the initial tear concentration of the drug [2,3]. Polyvinyl alcohol, is apparently an exception, as its favourable influence on pilocarpine bioavailability has recently been shown not to be due to viscosity effects [4]. Whereas the claims for enhanced drug bioavailability by addition of these agents to eyedrop formulations are valid as measured in animals [5], the effects are minimal in humans [6], and their clinical significance in humans is at best modest [2].

2.2 Soluble gels

The development of two soluble gels for the delivery of pilocarpine has been reported. One of these systems, containing 4% pilocarpine in a high viscosity acrylic vehicle, has recently become available commercially, and delivers a 24-h pilocarpine dose from a single, night-time placement in the cul-de-sac [7–9]. As is usual with hydrophilic matrices, the effect is greatest immediately after instillation, and diminishes with time [7]. The approach does allow for only a single administration per day, as opposed to a four-times-daily eyedrop application, and a choice of night-time administration diminishes patient-perceived pilocarpine side-effects, such as initial miosis and induced myopia. To date, neither the drug release mechanism nor the kinetics of drug release from this system have been reported; thus information is not yet available as to whether the prolonged drug action described results from an increased (but short-term) surge in corneal absorption, or prolongation at a lower level of the drug absorption phase, a question upon which the usefulness of the system for the delivery of more potent drugs will depend. In requiring only once-daily application, this system does offer a significant advantage in patient conve-nience, which is believed to improve patient compliance favourably [9].

A second ophthalmic gel, also recently reported for the delivery of pilocarpine, is poloxamer 407 [10]. This vehicle was reportedly chosen because of its low viscosity, optical clarity, and mucomimetic properties, and for its previous acceptability in ophthalmic preparations. This formulation enhanced pilocarpine activity, as indi-cated by miosis measurements in rabbits, compared to an aqueous pilocarpine solution of equal drug concentration.

2.3 Ointments

Ophthalmic ointments represent a common topical dosage form. Their obvious disadvantages include interference with vision, and aesthetic considerations. Nevertheless, ointments offer the clinical advantage of prolonged medication from each instillation. Thus, with drugs whose maximum efficacy depends upon constant presence, such as antiviral agents, night-time ointment use combined with daytime eyedrop use is a common regimen. Drug bioavailablility usually peaks later [11] with ointment vehicles than with solutions or suspensions, and total bioavailability (i.e., area under the curve) is significantly greater than that from aqueous solutions or suspensions. The fundamental relationship governing the diffusion of finely dis-persed drugs from ointment bases has been described [12].

The superior bioavailability of drugs from ointment bases is due to several factors: higher effective concentration; increased tissue contact time; inhibition of dilution by the tears [13]; and resistance to nasolacrimal drainage [14]. Whereas the physiological turnover rate of tears is about 16% per min, the turnover rate in the cul-de-sac for drugs administered in ointment form is as low as 0.5% per min [15]. The shearing action from blinking significantly enhanced drug release from ointments [16].

2.4   Emulsions and suspensions

A pilocarpine emulsion in eyedrop form (Piloplex) has been reported to prolong therapeutic effect compared to pilocarpine hydrochloride eyedrops, such that it may be administered only twice, rather than four times daily [17–20]. In this formulation, pilocarpine is bound to a polymeric material and this complex makes up the internal, dispersed phase of the emulsion system. *In vitro* studies have indicated that the release time of 80% of the pilocarpine from this system is 6 h, compared to 80% released in only 1 h from pilocarpine hydrochloride solution [18]; thus the prolonged therapeutic effect is apparently due both to an enhanced pulse entry of drug, and to a prolongation of drug release from the vehicle.

Again using pilocarpine as a model drug, an eyedrop formulation has been described that consists of an aqueous suspension of particles (average diameter 0.3 microns) of a cellulose acetate hydrogen phthalate latex, onto the surface of which pilocarpine HCl was previously adsorbed [21]. The suspension had a low viscosity (180 cP), and was readily delivered as an eyedrop. The latex particles reportedly coagulate upon instillation due to a pH change, and therefore resist drainage from the eye. This system, containing 2% pilocarpine HCl, reportedly caused significant enhancement of the miotic response in rabbit eyes, with the leaching-out process extending past 4 h.

2.5   Facilitated transport: ion pairs, prodrugs, liposomes, and chemical derivative formation

Facilitated transport, in general, refers either to chemical modifications, or to the use of additional agents (in some instances, carrier vehicles) that, when reacted with or coadministered with an otherwise poorly absorbed drug, enhance its absorption. One example is the formation of an *ion pair*, a coulombic association between large organic ions of opposite charge. In such an association the charges are, for practical purposes, no longer manifested and the ion pair can behave as if it were a lipophilic substance. Thus together the ions are both transported well, but neither is transported well without the other. In animals, the method has been used successfully to enhance the transport of the anti-inflammatory agent sodium chromoglycate (the dianion) across the cornea by first associating it with dodecylbenzyldimethylammonium chloride, a quaternary ammonium compound (the cation) [22,23]; of penicillin, using cetylpyridinium chloride [24]; and of chloramphenicol, using phosphonium salts [25].

A useful approach to improve a number of characteristics of a given drug is by latentiation through formation of a *prodrug*: a chemical derivative of the drug, usually an ester, that is synthesized to improve some specific physical property (solubility and thus bioavailability, chemical stability, taste, volatility). The drug in its original form is regenerated *in vivo* after its administration, sometimes during the course of its absorption, sometimes afterwards.

The use of prodrugs in medicine is not new. However, the first ophthalmic prodrug, dipivalylepinephrine, was only recently introduced (dipivefrin, Propine). By diesterification, the compound was made more lipophilic, resulting in a ten-fold increase in its corneal absorption. Thus, a 0.1% solution of this prodrug is equivalent to a 1% solution of the parent compound. Moreover, enhanced absorption allows for less frequent administration. Upon absorption, esterases within both the cornea and the aqueous humor act rapidly to regenerate the epinephrine, freeing it to elicit the desired response. Pivalic acid, also regenerated, has been shown to be non-toxic.

Epinephrine is a known sensitizer, and many patients experience significant adverse reactions from its topical use. Yet it is a naturally occurring hormone. The apparent paradox of an endogenous agent eliciting widespread allergic reactions may possibly have its explanation in the chemical instability of exogenous epinephrine preparations, with the adverse effects apparently caused by the degradation products always present in at least trace quantities in multidose epinephrine eyedrop solutions. Thus, reports of fewer side-effects with the more stable ester of this agent appear well founded.

Another means of facilitating the transport of drugs is by incorporating them into *liposomes*, which then serve as carrier vehicles [26]. Liposomes are highly ordered assemblages that form when water-insoluble polar lipids, such as phospholipids, are combined with water under favourable conditions. In structure, they may consist of one or a number of concentric lipid bilayers, separated by aqueous layers. The carrying capacity of unilamellar structures is greater than that of multilamellar structures, however, the procedures such as sonication, or more recently, reverse-phase evaporation, have been used to produce the smaller, more efficient unilamellar structures, which then persist in water without further change. Extrusion of the final structures through polycarbonate membranes with defined pore size adds the advantage of size homogeneity. By formation of the liposomes in the presence of a selected drug, the latter becomes incorporated, concentrated in either the aqueous or lipid layer, depending upon its solubility characteristics. Liposomes of defined size, stability, and permeability properties can be prepared by appropriate methodology, as recently reviewed [27]. They have been proposed as drug carriers for a variety of agents, and their uses for this purpose have also been reviewed in detail [28, 29].

Some recent studies on the mechanisms by which topically applied liposomes deliver drugs to the eye disclose that the drug–liposome affinity as well as the affinity between the liposomes and ocular tissues markedly affect the bioavailability of the delivered drug [30]. Inasmuch as both of these separate affinities vary greatly, wide variations in the degree of absorption of liposome-associated drugs occur. It has been found [31] that liposomal incorporation of epinephrine reduces by half the conjunctival and corneal absorption it would otherwise have, while inulin absorption in these tissues is increased ten-fold when topically applied in a liposome carrier. Barza, Baum and Szoka (Szoka, personal communication, 1982) have compared the ocular tissue levels of gentamicin in rabbit eyes following application of either unincorporated drug or drug incorporated in reverse-phase evaporation liposomes. The two forms produced similar drug levels in the cornea, but the liposome form provided only one-fourth as much drug in the aqueous humor. Following subconjunctival injection, however, the liposome form resulted in a drug level a full order of magnitude higher after 24 h in the cornea, sclera, and choroid.

Other investigators [32] found at least a four-fold increase in the passage of penicillin G across rabbit corneas from unilaminar liposome compared to non-incorporated drug, and a ten-fold enhancement of indoxole passage across rat corneas. In the latter instance the lipoidal drug was incorporated directly into the vesicle membranes. These investigators have presented evidence that the liposome–

corneal surface affinity is based on electrostatic attraction, being greater for positively charged liposomes, less for negatively charged, and least for neutral liposomes.

Techniques have recently been investigated to add specificity of lipsomal binding to selected target tissues. For this purpose, concanavalin A has been shown to bind negatively charged large unilamellar liposomes selectively to the lenses of experimental animals, allowing the selective delivery of tetracycline [33] and aldose reductase inhibitors [34] to the lens.

The above reports relate to the influence of liposome carriers on drug absorption and binding to tissues. In one reported study of the therapeutic efficacy from a liposomal system, it was shown that idoxuridine delivered by liposome carrier was more effective than idoxuridine alone in experimentally induced epithelial and stromal herpes simplex keratitis, and also in the prevention of stromal lesions [35]: and liposome incorporation prior to delivery has provided reduced toxicity of amphotericin B [36].

Transport of drugs across the corneal barrier can sometimes be facilitated by *chemical derivative formation* without loss of activity. Distinction is made between temporary derivatives, from which the active parent compound is expected to be regenerated following absorption (prodrugs, above), and derivatives which are made to improve some useful property, such as their bioavailability, but which maintain both their new form and their activity in the new form. A recently reported success with the latter approach involved removing one alkyl group from the quaternary nitrogen of carbachol, and converting this group into a tertiary nitrogen compound. The new derivative, N-demethylated carbachol, possesses an enhanced ability to penetrate the cornea, but with retention of miotic activity [37,38].

2.6 Solid, hydrophilic ocular inserts

A number of soluble, solid-state drug carriers have been utilized for ophthalmic medication. 'Lamellae', described as early as 1948 in the *British Pharmacopoeia,* were atropine-containing gelatin wafers intended for placement beneath the eyelid. A Russian study [39] revised the approach with pilocarpine-impregnated discs of polyvinyl alcohol (PVA), which were reported to provide sustained miosis and reduction of intraocular pressure. Other investigators [40] also used PVA, but apparently in a less soluble form. They achieved antibiotic concentrations in the tear fluid 3 h after removal of the carrier that were 65 times greater than that found 3 h after the instillation of a 1% oily tetracycline solution. Twenty-four hours after removal, the residual concentration from the carrier was 11 times that obtained from the solution alone.

Other water-soluble ocular inserts have been developed using hydroxypropyl cellulose as a matrix material. They have been tested for ocular tolerance, for acceptance based on size and shape [41], and for delivery of pilocarpine from the lower cul-de-sac [42]. In general, smaller devices were better retained in the eye than larger ones, and rod-shaped devices were better retained than those that were oval-shaped. They remained in position in the lower cul-de-sac, but were often extruded from the upper sac. The devices were well tolerated, and generally dissolved within 12 h. Units containing up to 2 mg of pilocarpine base were reported to provide an intraocular pressure reduction for a period that in some cases exceeded 24 h, and investigation of the use of these inserts to deliver anti-inflammatory, anti-infective, and antiglaucoma drugs has also been reported. Ocular inserts consisting of only this polymer matrix alone, without an incorporated drug, have recently become available (Lacrisert) for treatment of the dry eye syndrome.

Delivery of an antibiotic by an ocular insert made of succinylated, enzyme-solubilized collagen has also been described [43], and this approach appears promising for the treatment of ocular infection. One study compared [14C] gentamicin levels in rabbit tear film and in ocular tissue when the drug was administered by eyedrops, ointments, subconjunctival injection, or by the solid wafers of solubilized collagen. The collagen wafers gave superior levels of drug in the tears, sclera, and cornea. Prolongation of the pulse entry as compared to eyedrops and enhancement of the pulse magnitude as compared to ointment delivery or periocular injection, are evident from Fig. 3. Ocular inserts made of this same matrix material have also been

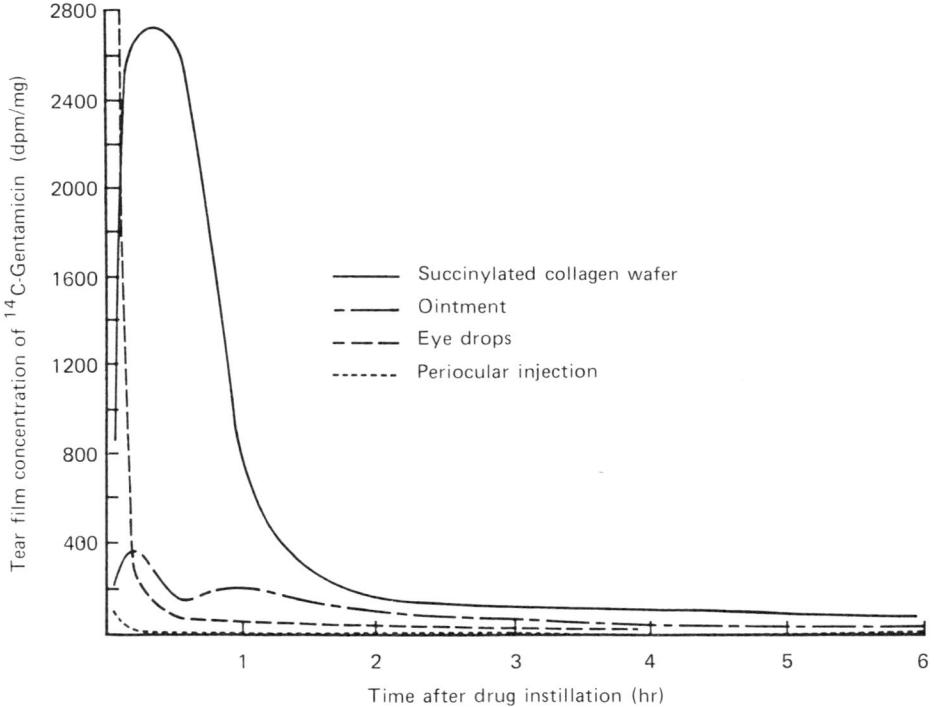

Fig. 3 — [14C]Gentamicin sulfate concentration in tear film versus time.

investigated for treating tear film abnormalities [44].

Fibrin film has also been evaluated as a carrier for prolonging drug action [45], and has been shown to possess good biocompatibility with ocular tissues. Systems containing pilocarpine HCl released some 87–97% of their total drug content within the first hour of use, but the system maintained drug activity several hours longer than pilocarpine eyedrops.

As previously noted, the kinetics of drug release from soluble ocular inserts are essentially those from hydrophilic matrices; the pattern is characterized by a very high initial rate that rapidly declines. Hydrophilic devices, whether they dissolve or not, release soluble drugs at a rapidly declining rate because of the leaching action of the tears. With reference to delivery time, the half-life of most water-soluble drugs in hydrophilic matrices is less than 30 min. In general, the release rate is an inverse function of the square root of the time, unless additional measures are taken to inhibit the leaching action of the tears.

One approach to delaying the release of drug from hydrophilic matrices (i.e., delay the leaching action of the tears) is to use sparingly soluble drugs or less-soluble derivatives of the drugs. In this situation the drug release rate is more closely related to the dissolution rate of the drug. This approach has been used with hydrocortisone acetate, a sparingly soluble drug dispersed in a polypeptide matrix that was cross-linked to provide a slow matrix-dissolution rate. The efficacy of this system was demonstrated in both the prevention of corneal xenograft rejection in rabbits, and in the total suppression of this reaction after it was allowed to reach full severity [46]. The onset and development of corneal and uveal inflammation were inhibited to an equal extent by 0.25–2.5% eyedrops four times daily or by continuous steroid delivery rates of 0.1–7.0 μg/h. When corneal xenograft reaction and uveitis were allowed to reach full severity, ocular inserts that released 2 or 9 μg/h of hydrocortisone acetate had a therapeutic effect equal to 0.25 and 2.5% eyedrops, respectively. The amounts of the drug delivered as eyedrops at these concentrations ranged from approximately 700 to 7000 μg every 24 h, respectively, whereas the ocular insert units delivered 2.5 and 215 μg every 24 h.

Similar results have been obtained in comparisons to steroids in ointment form. In a rabbit model of phlyctenulosis [47], hydrocortisone acetate released continuously from the matrix at 20 μg/h compared well in efficacy with a 2.5% hydrocortisone ointment, where the dose from the ocular inserts was from one-sixth to one-seventh the amount present in the ointment. The lower total dose required from continuously delivered steroids is significant in view of the dose-related side-effects of corticosteroids in the eye.

3.   SYSTEMS THAT PROVIDE FOR A RATE-CONTROLLED RELEASE OF DRUGS

3.1   Rationale for rate-controlled drug release

As previously described, in the absence of any efforts to modify it, the administration pattern of drugs given by conventional eyedrops will be one of pulse entry, as shown in Fig. 1. The pattern is characterized by a transient overdose, followed by a prolonged period of underdosing. The side-effects of ophthalmic drugs, which are for the most part dose-related, are associated with the initial overdose and the high tissue levels it provides. Moreover, any patient-perceived side-effects tend to extend the period of underdosing prior to the next drop administration due to the effect of this perception on patient compliance. An objective of controlled-release delivery systems is to provide the drug continuously, but only at the level of its effectiveness as depicted by the horizontal line in Fig. 1. This objective requires a system that delivers the drug with approximately zero-order kinetics; that is, a system from which the amount of drug delivered per unit time is independent of the amount left undelivered. The rate, therefore, remains constant with time until the supply is depleted. To achieve this goal, two approaches have been successful. One is based on drug diffusion across a barrier membrane (Fick's diffusion), and the other on the osmotic properties of the drug.

3.2   Diffusional systems

Diffusional systems prevent a continuous decline in release rate through utilization of a barrier membrane of fixed thickness. Such a system consists of a central reservoir of drug enclosed between specially tailored membranes that allow the drug to diffuse from the reservoir at a precisely determined rate.

It is convenient to classify membrane-controlled devices into two categories, according to the solubility of the drug. The simplest case is with drugs which are sparingly soluble in water. With these drugs the release rate (J) is given by Fick's law as:

$$J = \frac{DA\Delta C_M}{l}$$

where D is the diffusion coefficient of the drug, A is the surface area of the membrane, C_M is the difference in concentration in the membrane at the two surfaces, and l is the membrane thickness. The concentration just inside the membrane can be related to the solution concentration by the expression:

$$C_M(0) = KC' \text{ at the inner surface and}$$
$$C_M(1) = KC'' \text{ at the outer surface,}$$

where C' and C'' denote the concentration of drug inside and outside the device. K is the distribution coefficient; it is analogous to the more familiar liquid–liquid partition coefficient. Since the concentration outside the device is almost always negligible while the concentration inside is fixed at the drug's solubility $(C' = C_s)$, combining the above gives:

$$J = \frac{ADKC_s}{l}$$

All terms on the right hand side of the equation are constants, and this device delivers a drug at a constant rate as long as the solution inside the device remains saturated, i.e. the device contains excess solid drug, and the membrane serves as a rate-controlling factor.

Fig. 4 illustrates the release patterns obtained with two commonly used sparingly soluble drugs incorporated into membrane-controlled devices. The plot shows accumulated drug release; a plot of release rate would be a straight, essentially

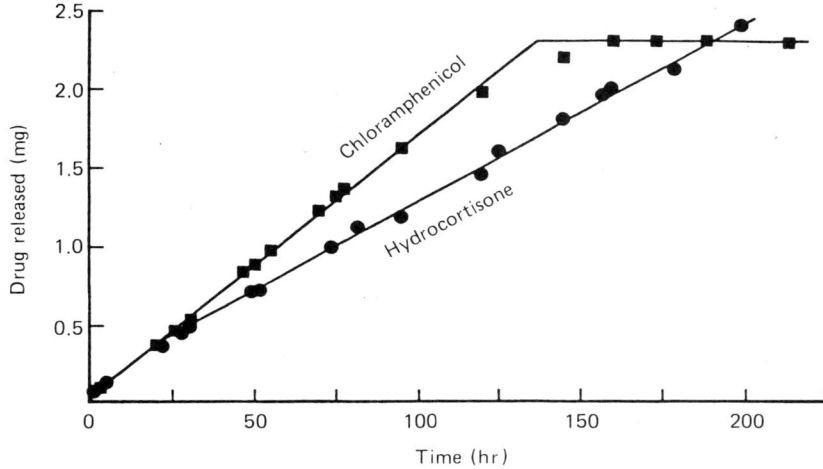

Fig. 4 — Cumulative release of chloramphenicol and hydrocortisone from membrane-controlled devices.

horizontal line. The release rate from these devices is constant over almost the entire lifetime of the device; drug release ends when the reservoir is exhausted (as shown in the figure with chloramphenicol). Thus the lifetime of the device is adjusted by incorporating more or less drug, limited finally by volume constraints related to the size of device which can be comfortably tolerated within the cul-de-sac of the eye. The release can be increased by making the device surface area larger or the membranes thinner.

The situation with soluble drugs is quite different, since a strong driving force to osmotically imbibe water develops with ionic drugs if the membrane is water permeable, resulting in a decline in drug release rate due to the dilution. Accordingly, hydrophobic membranes must be used, but these are permeable only to non-ionized drug molecules. In spite of these constraints, useful systems for soluble drugs are feasible if a non-ionized form of the drug is used. For example, such systems utilizing pilocarpine free base have become available (Ocusert) with release rate values of 20 μg/h and 40 μg/h, for a duration of 1 week. A typical release rate profile for the 20 μg/h dose system is shown in Fig. 5.

Consistent with expectations of systems that deliver drugs at a constant, controlled rate, the pilocarpine diffusional system has been shown to provide effective therapy with significantly less side-effects. Clinical studies have shown the system to induce less miosis and myopia ([48], Figs 6 and 7) and less anterior chamber shallowing [49] when compared to pilocarpine eyedrops.

A comparison of intraocular tissue levels of pilocarpine following administration by eyedrops or by rate-controlled delivery is shown in Fig. 8 [50]. In most tissues the levels of eyedrop-delivered pilocarpine never fell below the level maintained by the continuous delivery systems, with the notable exception of the aqueous humor.

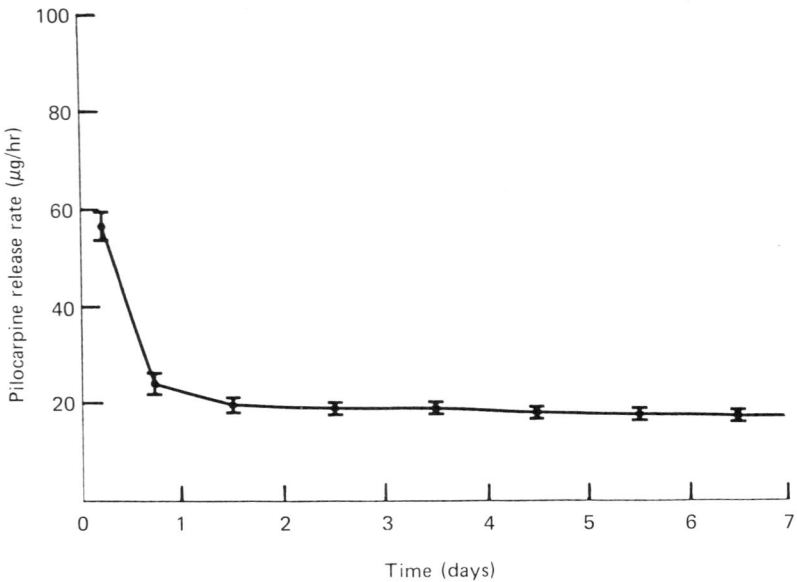

Fig. 5 — Plot of release rate of pilocarpine from a membrane-controlled device, nominal rate (i.e. dose) of 20 μg/h.

Presumably it is the relatively rapid turnover of aqueous humor (and consequent decline in aqueous humor levels of pilocarpine) after eyedrop administration that requires a four-times-daily administration. In most tissues, none having a direct bearing on the hypotensive action of pilocarpine, drug levels from the eyedrop regimen were usually several-fold higher than those maintained by continuous delivery. This is particularly true with the lens, a finding of possible significance in view of the reported cataractogenic activity of pilocarpine [51], and with the vitreous, of possible significance in view of the reported association of retinal detachment with miotic therapy [52,53]. These findings suggest an element of safety favouring a continuous delivery system. Whereas long-term residual hypotensive activity is obtained from pilocarpine delivered in this manner, the reservoir is apparently not in tissues susceptible to unfavourable side-effects.

3.3 Osmotic systems
Experimental continuous delivery systems based upon the osmotic properties of an incorporated drug have been developed, and have undergone early clinical testing [54]. Several sizes and shapes have been developed; they range from a thin, flat layer of different shapes to a contoured, three-dimensional unit designed to conform to the supratarsal space of the upper cul-de-sac. The latter system has been utilized in the delivery of diethylcarbamazine in ocular onchocerciasis [55]. The non-hydrophilic polymer matrix contains the incorporated drug, which is dispersed in the solid state

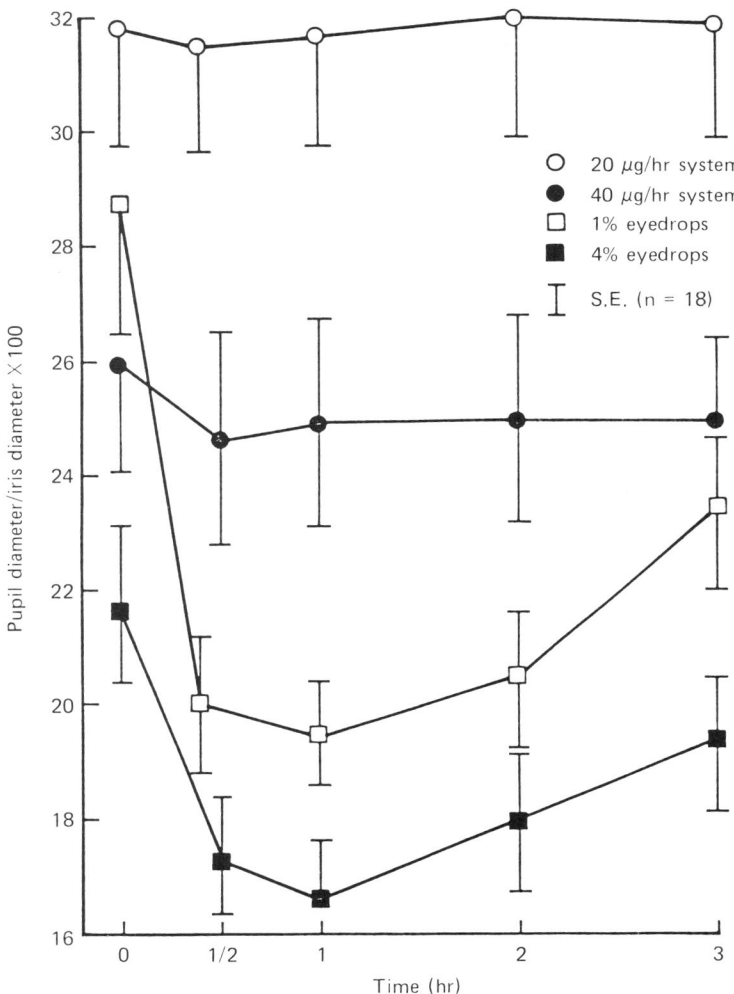

Fig. 6 — Reduced miotic effect from continuously delivered pilocarpine compared to eyedrops.

as numerous, extremely small domains, each as a discrete compartment separated by polymer material. Drug delivery proceeds at a fairly constant rate for the life of the system, at which time the device is removed and replaced. The useful total life of these systems is limited to a large extent by drug volume constraints, there being an upper limit to the size of device the eye will tolerate and retain, but practical systems have been developed that deliver therapeutic levels of drug for 2 weeks.

Ocular therapeutic systems utilizing the osmotic principle offer several advantages over diffusional systems. Many important ophthalmic agents are alkaloids or

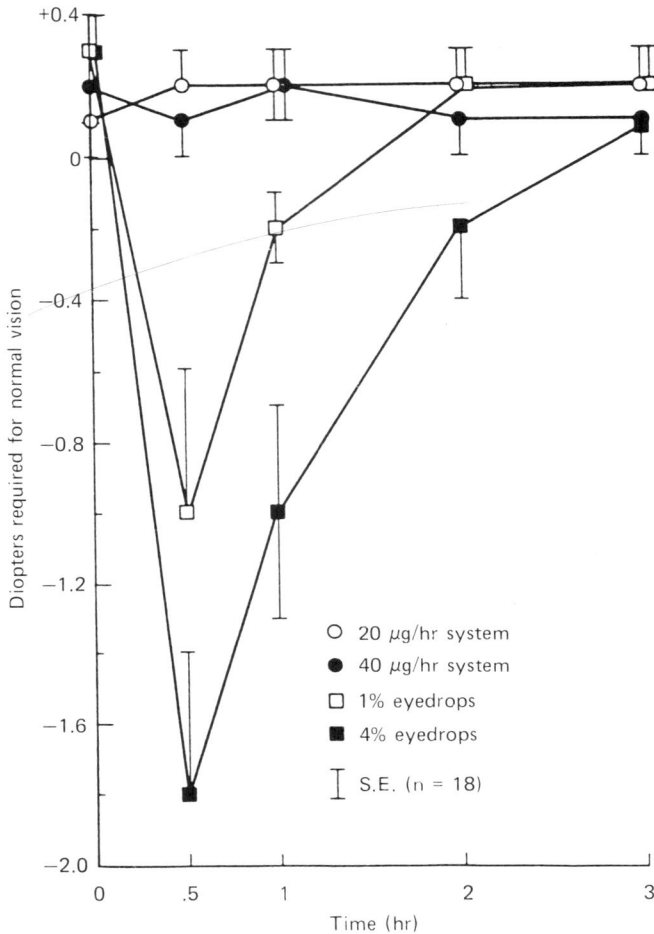

Fig. 7 — Reduced effect of induced myopia from continuously delivered pilocarpine compared to eyedrops.

weak bases, and the free base form is usually needed for diffusion through the required hydrophobic barrier membrane of the diffusional systems. These bases are, however, thermally unstable, and such systems in general require refrigeration. The salt forms used in osmotic systems are thermally much more stable, thus they require no refrigeration. Moreover, imperfections in a system or the leakage infrequently reported from diffusional systems are not factors of concern with osmotic systems, a feature that allows for their use with more potent agents.

3.4 Bioerodible systems
The obvious advantage of soluble, or erodible ocular inserts is that the patient does not have to remove them following use. In contrast to the soluble gels and hydrophilic ocular inserts previously described, which cannot deliver drugs at a

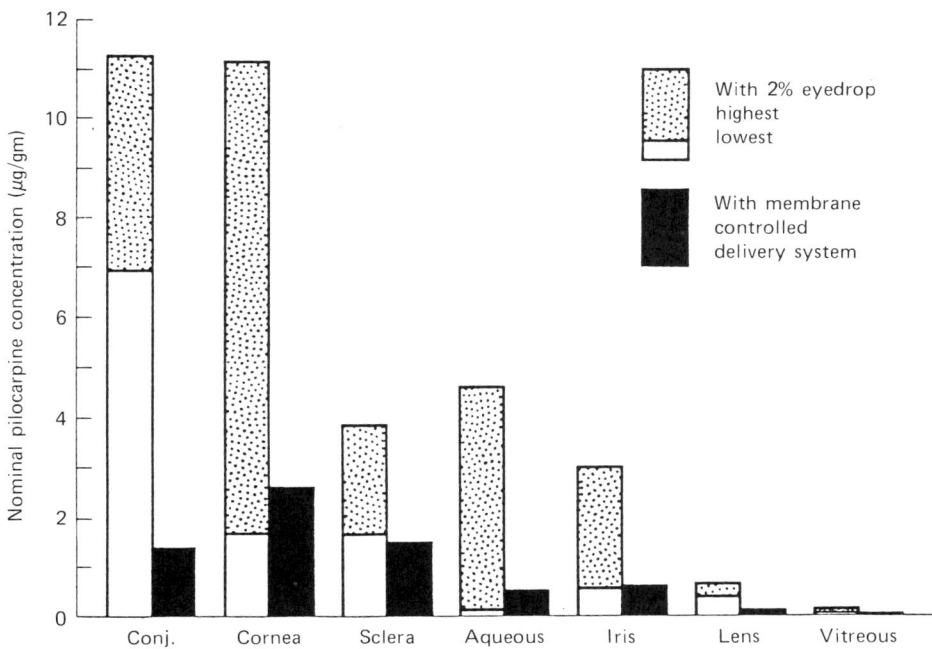

Fig. 8 — Distribution of [^{14}C]pilocarpine in seven ocular tissues of rabbits treated by continuous delivery at 20 μg/h, or by 2% eyedrops given at 6-h intervals.

constant, controlled rate, one method to provide constant-rate drug delivery is by
use of an erodible *hydrophobic* matrix. Such a matrix does not allow leaching of the
drug by the tears of the eye. One such system that has been described undergoes a
surface-only hydrolysis from contact with the tears, resulting in solubilization and
erosion of only the outermost layer, with the release of drug contained therein.
Continuous progress of this process, layer by layer from a reasonably constant
surface, provides a non-pulsed, constant-rate supply of the drug [56].

Another promising approach is based upon a biodegradable polymer to which a
selected drug is attached through a hydrolytically labile linkage [57, 58]. The polymer
matrix ultimately dissolves, but prior to that event the drug is released at a rate
dependent on both the hydrolysis of the drug/polymer linkage and subsequent drug
diffusion through the matrix.

In addition to the use of sparingly soluble drugs to delay their release from
hydrophilic matrices, a separate effect can apparently be utilized involving an ionic
interaction of a drug salt with a soluble polymer matrix [59]. Using a matrix of
hydroxypropyl cellulose, dissociation of an incorporated pilocarpine pamoate salt
has been accomplished with release of only the pilocarpine moiety, a process shown
to proceed with apparent zero-order kinetics. The rate was found to vary inversely
with the molecular weight of the polymer used for the matrix.

Unlike non-soluble, diffusional systems, which can provide reasonably constant drug release up to the time of their replacement in the eye, thus avoiding periodic lapses in the therapy of chronic diseases, erodible systems cannot be expected to deliver a drug at a constant rate during the last period of time before their erosion is complete. Thus while they can be useful for the therapy of chronic conditions, they would seem to offer most promise as systems for the treatment of acute eye conditions.

A totally new application of controlled ocular drug delivery by an erodible matrix may lie in the enhancement of the success rate of one of the surgical procedures currently used for the treatment of refractory cases of glaucoma. A standard filtering procedure consists of introduction of a patency under a limbus-based, triangular conjunctival flap, which subsequently serves as a high-resistance drainage facility for the fluid in the anterior chamber. Unfortunately in many cases, fibroblast prolife-ration eventually diminishes the patency, requiring repeat surgery. It is now known that subconjunctival injections of certain antimetabolites, such as 5-fluorouracil or cytosine arabinoside, inhibit the proliferation of fibroblasts and promote healing without loss of patency. These antimitotic agents are toxic, however, particularly to the cornea; moreover, repeat injections are essential. Thus a reasonable objective is to provide a prolonged delivery of the drug at the surgical site, without transient overdoses, and the implantation of a 5-fluorouracil-containing erodible matrix film under the flap at the close of surgery appears, in the early stages, to have merit (J. W. Shell, unpublished work).

3.5   Summary of rate-controlled drug release features

Continuous, rate-controlled drug delivery devices, whether based on diffusional, osmotic, or bioerodible mechanisns, offer unique therapeutic advantages. In addi-tion to avoiding the pulse entry of the drug with its associated side-effects, and to requiring less-frequent applications, both of which may improve patient compliance, they provide round-the-clock medication, a regimen difficult to achieve by eyedrops due to the improbability of self-medication by patients during the night. Assuming that the accumulated total hours of untreated intraocular pressure over a patient's lifetime can contribute to disc changes and field loss, provision of round-the-clock therapy must be considered an important improvement for the treatment of glaucoma.

The advantage of continuous medication is further exemplified in the treatment of herpes simplex keratitis. The efficacy of most ocular antiviral agents currently in use depends upon isosteric replacement of one or another building block of the viral DNA, which produces a faulty DNA that cannot replicate. This is an intermittent and unpredictable process. Accordingly, constant presence of the agent is highly advantageous.

Some interesting but unanswered questions arise regarding the pharmacodyna-mic aspects of continuous, compared with pulse-entry delivery methods in ocular therapy. For instance, when still-functioning continuous pilocarpine delivery systems are removed, their effect can persist for an additional 2–7 days [60]. When systems are left in place several days in excess of the 7-day life of the system, residual effects are still measurable to a variable degree. In one study that continued for 12 days after therapy was stopped, the hypotensive effect of pilocarpine remained statistically significant up to the 9th day with a 20 μg/h system, and to the 12th day with a 40 μg/h system [61]. Yet the hypotensive effect from pilocarpine eyedrops vanishes within hours. One may postulate greater drug reservoir effects due to ocular tissue binding from continuous delivery systems, and there is some evidence supporting this explanation [50].

4. CONCLUDING OBSERVATIONS AND FUTURE OUTLOOK

The therapeutic advantages offered by the use of ophthalmic drug delivery systems are numerous and significant, as the foregoing review attests. In spite of this, the available systems have not yet gained widespread acceptance, possibly because prescribers have not yet had truly compelling reasons for substituting them for the universally understood and relatively inexpensive eyedrops. This situation may change as improved delivery systems are developed, and as continuous administration systems are mandated by the emergence of important new drugs that have very short biological half-lives. Further, and most particularly, the situation may change as important new ophthalmic drugs emerge that have serious side-effects. The recent introduction into ophthalmic practice of a beta-adrenergic blocking agent exemplifies this issue. The most prevalent use of this class of agents is in oral tablets, prescribed for arterial hypertension. But the amount of drug surviving in active form from *oral* administration of the most frequently used of these agents is only 36% for propranolol [62] and 38% for metoprolol [63], with the remainder accounted for by the 'first-pass effect' — losses caused by intestinal mucosa inactivation and liver metabolism. When such drugs are given in *eyedrop* form, the situation is very different: the 80% or more of the volume of an administered eyedrop, which is known to drain rapidly through the nasolacrimal canal, avoids the first-pass effect, and is totally available for systemic absorption through the highly vascularized mucosa. Thus, an eyedrop is more like an intravenous dose. Fig. 9 shows a comparison of the mean pulse rate of 11 adult volunteers following a standard exercise regimen, after administering one 0.5% timolol eyedrop (commercial size), or a placebo eyedrop. This exercise tachycardia test shows a significant effect of beta-blockade, a systemic parameter that vanishes when the same subjects are treated with a low-level, continuously delivered beta-blocker at a rate which in glaucoma patients is therapeutically equal to 0.5% timolol eyedrops [64]. A concluding observation is that until recently the side-effects of the frequently used and relatively safe ophthalmic drugs have been of little consequence, or at least have not been serious enough to alter prescribing habits in favour of new drug delivery systems. The development and rational use of more potent drugs, however, which may have serious side-effects, may require concomitant development and use of improved methods for their controlled (i.e. non-pulsed) delivery.

Another feature of some ophthalmic delivery systems that may encourage their eventual acceptance is their freedom from the need for preservatives and other vehicle ingredients. The deleterious effects of these agents are not widely appreciated, but they are real. For example, 0.01 and 0.02% concentrations of a common ophthalmic preservative, benzalkonium chloride (in pH 4 buffer), respectively increased the corneal penetration of [^{14}C] inulin in rabbits ten-fold and 18-fold [65], presumably due to corrosive action on the corneal epithelium at this pH value. The

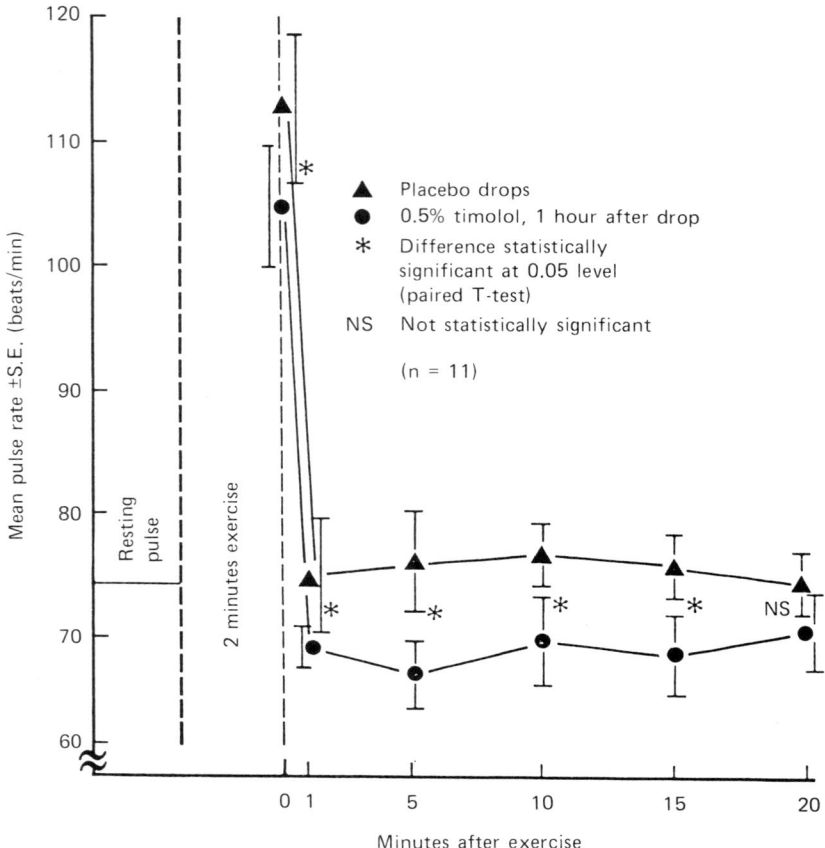

Fig. 9 — Reduction of exercise tachycardia in normal volunteers following administration of 0.5% timolol eyedrops.

finding is significant, as these concentrations and this pH value are frequently used in eyedrop formulations.

Finally, systems that provide continuous, controlled drug release to the eye may in time find important uses in the treatment of ophthalmic diseases which, due to special circumstances, are otherwise difficult to treat effectively. The most important example is trachoma, an infectious ocular disease that is the leading cause of blindness worldwide. This condition, found mostly in arid regions of the world such as North Africa and the Middle East, is caused by an organism for which effective agents are available, but it resists effective treatment due to other factors: an ubiquitous vector; conditions which are often non-hygienic; and a population in which repeated self-medication is not a reasonable expectation. The conditions promote rapid reinfection following otherwise effective therapy. The provision of continuous ocular drug delivery to the eyes of the young children within these populations — for extended periods of time — offers a mechanism to help break the chain of reinfection. Thus advanced ocular drug delivery systems offer some hope for improving the epidemiological picture of this severely debilitating disease, and there is evidence of some success with this approach [66, 67].

ACKNOWLEDGEMENTS

The information in this chapter appears by kind permission of Alan R. Liss Inc., USA.

REFERENCES

[1] Shell, J. W. & Baker, (1974).
[2] Adler, C. A., Maurice, D. M. & Paterson, M. E. (1971). The effect of viscosity of the vehicle on the penetration of fluorescein into the human eye. *Exp. Eye Res.* **11** 34–42.
[3] Benedetto, D. A., Shah, D. O. & Kaufman, H. E. (1975). The instilled fluid dynamics and surface chemistry of polymers in the preocular tear film. *Invest. Ophthalmol. Vis. Sci.* **14** 887–902.
[4] Saetton, M. F., Giannaccini, B., Teneggi, A., Savigni, P. & Tellini, N. (1982). Vehicle effects on ophthalmic bioavailability: the influence of different polymers on the activity of pilocarpine in rabbit and man. *J. Pharm. Pharmacol.* **34** 464–466.
[5] Chrai, S. S. & Robinson, J. R. (1974). Ocular evaluation of methylcellulose vehicle in albino rabbits. *J. Pharm. Sci.* **63** 1218–1223.
[6] Chrai, S. S., Patton, T. F., Mehta, A. & Robinson, J. R. (1973). Lacrimal and instilled fluid dynamics in rabbit eyes. *J. Pharm. Sci.* **62** 1112–1121.
[7] Goldberg, I., Ashburn, F. S., Kass, M. A. & Becker, B. (1979). Efficacy and patient acceptance of pilocarpine gel. *Am. J. Ophthalmol.* **88** 843–846.
[8] Mandell, A. I., Stewart, R. M. & Jass, M. A. (1979). Multiclinic evaluation of pilocarpine gel. *Invest. Ophthalmol. Vis. Sci.* (Suppl.) 165.
[9] March, W. F., Stewart, R. M., Mandell, A. I. & Bruce, L. A. (1982). Duration of effect of pilocarpine gel. *Arch. Ophthalmol.* **100**, 1270–1271.
[10] Miyazaki, S., Ishii, K. & Takada, M. (1982). Use of fibrin film as a carrier for drug delivery: a long-acting delivery system for pilocarpine into the eye. *Chem. Pharm. Bull.* **30** 3405–3407.
[11] Sieg, J. W. & Robinson, J. R. (1975). Vehicle effects on ocular drug bioavailability. I. Evaluation of fluorometholone. *J. Pharm. Sci.* **64** 931–936.
[12] Higuchi, T. (1963). Mechanism of sustained-action medications. Theoretical analysis of rate of release of solid drugs dispersed in solid matrices. *J. Pharm. Sci.* **52** 1145–1149.
[13] Sieg, J. W. & Robinson, J. R. (1977). Vehicle effects on ocular drug bioavailability. II. Evaluation of pilocarpine. *J. Pharm. Sci.* **66** 1222–1228.
[14] Norn, M. S. (1964). Role of the vehicle in local treatment of the eye. *Acta Ophthalmol.* **42** 727–733.
[15] Massey, J. Y., Hanna, C., Goodart, R. & Wallace, T. (1976). Effect of drug

vehicle on human ocular retention of topically applied tetracycline. *Am. J. Ophthalmol.* **81** 151–156.

[16] Sieg, J. W. & Robinson, J. R. (1979). Vehicle effects on ocular drug bioavailability. III. Shear-facilitated pilocarpine release from ointments. *J. Pharm. Sci.* **68** 724–728.

[17] Blumenthal, J., Ticho, U., Zonis, S., Gal, A., Blank, I. & Mazor, Z. (1979). Further clinical trial with piloplex — A new long-acting pilocarpine salt. *Glaucoma* **1** 145–148.

[18] Mazor, A., Ticho, U., Rehany, U. & Rose, L. (1979). Piloplex — A new long-acting pilocarpine salt: B. Comparative study of the visual effects of pilocarpine and piloplex eyedrops. *Br. J. Ophthalmol.* **63** 48–51.

[19] Ticho, U., Blumenthal, M., Zonis, S., Gal, A., Blank, I. & Mazor, Z. (1979). A clinical trial with Piloplex — a new long-acting pilocarpine compound. Preliminary report. *Ann. Ophthalmol.* **11** 555–561.

[20] Ticho, U., Blumenthal, M., Zonis, S., Gal, A., Blank, I. & Mazor, Z. (1979). Piloplex, a new long-acting pilocarpine polymer salt: a long-term study. *Br. J. Ophthalmol.* **63** 45–47.

[21] Gurny, R. (1981). Preliminary study of prolonged acting drug delivery system for the treatment of glaucoma. *Pharm. Acta Helv.* **56** 130–132.

[22] Davis, S. S., Tomlinson, E. & Wilson, C. G. (1978). The effect of ion association on the transcorneal transport of drugs. *Br. J. Pharmacol.* **64** 444–445.

[23] Wilson, C. G., Tomlinson, E., Davis, S. S. & Olejnik, O. (1981). Altered ocular absorption and disposition of sodium cromoglycate upon ion-pair and complex coacervate formation with dodecylbenzyldimethylammonium chloride. *J. Pharm. Pharmacol.* **31** 749–753.

[24] Godby, R. E. W., Green, K. Hull, D. S. (1979). Influence of cetylpyridinium chloride on corneal permeability to penicillin. *J. Pharm. Sci.* **68** 1176–1178.

[25] Davis, S. S., Kinkel, J. F. M., Olejnik, O. & Tomlinson, E. (1981). Enhancement of drug distribution by ion-pair formation. *J. Pharm. Pharmacol.* **33** (Suppl), 104.

[26] Bangham, A. D., Hill, M. W. & Miller, N. G. A. (1974). Preparation and use of liposomes as models of biological membranes. In: Korn, Ed. (ed.) *Methods in Membrane Biology*, Plenum Press, New York, pp. 1–68.

[27] Szoka, F., Jr. & Papahadjopoulos, D. (1980). Comparative properties and methods of preparation of lipid vesicles (liposomes). *Ann. Rev. Biophys. Bioeng.* **9** 467–508.

[28] Kimelberg, H. K. & Mayhew, E. G. (1978). Properties and biological effects of liposomes and their uses in pharmacology and toxicology. *CRC Crit. Rev. Toxicol.* **6**, 25–78.

[29] Knight, G. G. (ed.) (1981). *Liposomes: From Physical Structure to Therapeutic Applications,* Elsevier/North-Holland, Biomedical Press, Amsterdam.

[30] Stratford, R. E., Yang, D. C., Redell, M. A. & Lee, V. H. L. (1982/83). Ocular distribution of liposome-encapsulated epinephrine and inulin in the albino rabbit. *Curr., Eye Res.* **2** 377–386.

[31] Stratford, R. E., Yang, D. C., Redell, M. A. & Lee, V. H. L. (1983). Effects of

topically applied liposomes on disposition of epinephrine and inulin in the albino rabbit eye. *Int. J. Pharmaceutics.* **13** 263–272.

[32] Schaeffer, H. E. & Krohn, D. L. (1982). Liposomes in topical drug delivery. *Invest. Ophthalmol. Vis. Sci.* **22** 220–227.

[33] Megaw, J., Gardner, K. & Lerman, S. (1981). Intraocular liposome drug delivery system. *Invest. Ophthalmol. Vis. Sci.* **20** (Suppl.), 66.

[34] Megaw, J. (1983). Delivery of liposomally encapsulated drugs to the ocular lens. *Lens R.* **1**(3) 221–234.

[35] Smolin, G., Okumoto, M., Feiler, S. & Condon, D. (1981). Idoxuridine/ liposome therapy for herpex simplex keratitis. *Am. J. Ophthalmol.* **91** 220–225.

[36] Barza, M., Baum, J., Tremblay, C., Szoka, F. & D'Amico, D. J. (1985). Ocular toxicity of intravitreally injected liposomal amphotericin B in Rhesus monkeys. *Am. J. Ophthalmol.* **100** 259–263.

[37] Chiou, G. C. Y., Trzeciakowski, J. & Gelatt, K. N. (1980). Reduction of intraocular pressure in glaucomatous dogs by a new cholinergic drug. *Invest. Ophthalmol. Vis. Sci.* **19** 1198–1203.

[38] Trzeciakowski, J. & Chiou, G. C. (1980). Effects of demethylated carbachol on iris and ciliary muscles. *J. Pharm. Sci.* **69** 332–334.

[39] Yakovlev, A. A. & Lenkevich, M. M. (1966). Use of pilocarpine impregnated alcohol films in the treatment of glaucomatous patients. *Vestn. Oftalmol.* **79** 40.

[40] Maichuck, Y. F. & Tishina, I. F. (1971). Polyacrylamide, prolongating vehicle for eyedrops. *Vestn. Oftalmol.* **6** 60–83.

[41] Katz, I. M. & Blackman, W. M. (1977). A soluble sustained-release ophthalmic delivery unit. *Am. J. Ophthalmol.* **83** 728–734.

[42] Bensinger, R., Shin, D. H., Kass, M. A., Podos, S. M. & Becker, B. (1976). Pilocarpine and ocular inserts. *Invest Ophthalmol.* **15** 1008–1010.

[43] Bloomfield, S. E., Miyata, T., Dunn, M. W., Bueser, N., Stenzel, K. H. & Rubin, A. L. (1978). Soluble gentamicin ophthalmic inserts as a drug delivery system. *Arch. Ophthalmol.* **96** 885–887.

[44] Bloomfield, S. E., Miyata, T., Dunn, M. W., Bueser, N., Stenzel, K. H. & Rubin, A. L. (1977). Soluble artificial tear inserts. *Arch. Ophthalmol.* **95** 247–250.

[45] Mindel, J. S., Cohen, G., Barker, L. A., Lewis, D. E., Jacobs, M. & Heaton, R. B., Jr. (1982). Non-enzymatic and enzymatic conversion of dipivefrin. *Invest. Ophthalmol. Vis. Sci*; (Suppl.), 22.

[46] Dohlman, C. H., Pavan-Langston, D. & Rose, A. (1972). A new ocular insert device for continuous-rate delivery to the eye. *Ann. Ophthalmol.* **4** 823–832.

[47] Lerman, S., Davis, P. & Jackson, W. B. (1973). Prolonged release hydrocortisone therapy, *Can. J. Ophthalmol.* **8** 114–118.

[48] Brown, H. S., Meltzer, G., Merrill, R. C., Fisher, M., Ferre, C. & Place, V. A. (1976). Visual effects of pilocarpine in glaucoma. Comparative study of administration by eyedrops or by ocular therapeutic systems. *Arch. Ophthalmol.* **94** 1716–1719.

[49] Drance, S. M., Mitchell, D. W. A. & Schulzer, M. (1977). The effects of Ocusert pilocarpine on anterior chamber depth, visual acuity, and intraocular pressure in man. *Can. J. Ophthalmol.* **12** 24–28.

[50] Sendelbeck, L., Moore, D. & Urquhart, J. (1975). Comparative distribution of pilocarpine in ocular tissues of the rabbit during administration by eyedrop or by membrane controlled delivery systems. *Am. J. Ophthalmol.* **80** 274–283.

[51] Levene, R. Z. (1975). Uniocular miotic therapy. *Trans, Am. Acad. Ophthalmol. Otolaryngol.* **79** OP376–380.

[52] Alpar, J. J. (1979). Miotics and retinal detachment. *Ann. Ophthalmol.* **11** 395–401.

[53] Beasley, H., Fraunfelder, F. T. (1979). Retinal detachments and topical ocular miotics. *Ophthalmology* **86** 95–98.

[54] Gale, R., Chandrasekaran, S. K., Swanson, D. & Wright, J. (1980). Use of osmotically active therapeutic agents in monolithic systems. *J. Membr. Sci.* **7** 319–331.

[55] Jones, B. R., Anderson, J. & Fuglsang, H. (1978). Effects of various concentrations of diethylcarbamazine citrate applied as eyedrops in onchocerciasis, and the possibilities of improved therapy from continuous non-pulsed delivery. *Br. J. Ophthalmol.* **62** 428–439.

[56] Capozza, R. C., Sendelbeck, L. & Balkenhol, W. J. (1978). Preparation and evaluation of a bioerodible naltrexone delivery system. In: *Polymeric Delivery Systems: Midland Macromolecular Monographs*, vol. 5, Gordon and Breach, New York, pp. 59, 57–73.

[57] Kim, S. W., Petersen, R. V. & Feijen, J. (1979). In: Ariens, A. (ed.) *Drug Design*, vol. X. Academic Press, New York, pp. 193–250.

[58] Petersen, R. V., Anderson, C. G., Fang, S. M., Gregonis, D. E., Kim, S. W., Feijen, J., Anderson, J. M. & Mitra, S. (1980). Controlled release of progestins from poly (α-amino acid) carriers. In: Baker, R. (ed.) *Controlled Release of Bioactive Materials*, Academic Press, New York, pp. 45–60.

[59] Harwood, R. J. & Schwartz, J. D. (1982). Drug release from compression molded films: preliminary studies with pilocarpine. *Drug Dvlp.-Indust. Pharm.* **8** 663–682.

[60] Quigley, H. A., Pollack, I. P. & Harbin, T. S., Jr. (1975). Pilocarpine Ocuserts. Long-term clinical trials and selected pharmacodynamics. *Arch. Ophthalmol.* **93** 771–775.

[61] Chen, T. T. & Lee, P. F. (1976). Clinical experience on Ocusert pilocarpine system. A long-term evaluation. *Invest. Ophthalmol. Vis. Sci.* **15** (Suppl.) 48.

[62] Kornhauser, D. M., Wood, A. J. J., Wood, R. E., Vestal, G. R., Wilkinson, R., Branch, A. & Shan, D. G. (1978). Biological determinants of propranolol disposition in man. *Clin. Pharmacol. Ther.* **23** 165–174.

[63] Regardh, C. G., Borg, K. O., Johansson, R., Johansson, G. & Palmer, L. (1974). Pharmacokinetic studies on the selective β-1-receptor antagonist metoprolol in man. *J. Pharmacokin. Biopharm.* **2** 347–364.

[64] Shell, J. W. (1982). Pharmacokinetics of topically applied ophthalmic drugs. *Surv. Ophthalmol.* **26** 207–218.

[65] Keller, N., Moore, D., Carper, D. & Longwell, A. (1980). Increased corneal permeability induced by the dual effects of transient tear film acidification and exposure to benzalkonium chloride. *Exp. Eye Res.* **30** 203–210.

[66] Jones, B. R., Darougar, S., Mohsenine, H. & Poirier, R. H. (1976). Commu-

nicable ophthalmia: the blinding scourge of the middle east. *Br. J. Ophthalmol.* **60** 492–498.

[67] Jones, B. R. (1975). The prevention of blindness from Trachoma (The Bowman Lecture, 1975). *Trans. Ophthalmol. Soc. UK* **95** 16–33.

15

Drug delivery: advances and retreats

A. T. Florence, Department of Pharmacy, University of Strathclyde, Royal College Building, 204 George Street, Glasgow G1 1XW

Periodically there is a need to review progress in a field. There have been many developments in drug delivery in the last decade, a natural consequence perhaps of the 'discovery' of biopharmaceutics in the nineteen-sixties, but stimulated by more recent developments in biotechnology, and driven by hopes of achieving the ultimate, targeted drug therapy.† There have been many conferences and proceedings volumes devoted to individual systems for drug delivery, particularly liposomes [1,2], or to individual routes of administration, in which progress has not always been measured in the context of alternative approaches. Sometimes extravagant claims have been made in describing the future potential of some of these delivery systems; in hindsight one could perhaps claim that some work has been flawed because the goals were too distant and, because of that, ill-defined.

An Icarus complex has been most evident in relation to the possibility of targeting of non-specific drugs to specific sites in the body. It has taken several years for the community to accept that some of the biological impediments to targeting with colloidal carriers [3] are at present insurmountable. However, sometimes too severe a test is applied to the pharmaceutical sciences: the criterion of successful research is sometimes considered to be a marketable product. Other areas of scientific activity do not suffer such constraints. To achieve the ultimate aim of a useful medicine, toxicological, pharmacological and financial factors come into the equation alongside the pharmaceutical factors. Perhaps we should more often consider the work done in drug delivery which has not led to the market place as necessary scientific endeavour. Occasionally, however, the lure of the market attracts the scientist and has led to uncritical claims and to a minimization of problems, to the extent that **Gardner** was moved to make a plea at this conference that 'good science and not entrepreneurial zeal be our guide in determining future directions of drug delivery'.

The conference did not succumb to the lures of drug targeting or to descriptions of commonplace technology. As **Gardner** pointed out, too much work on carrier

---

† This overview by Professor Florence includes references to papers presented at the meeting at Churchill College, Cambridge, in July 1986 that have not appeared as chapters in this published volume.

systems for targeting has been based on naive physical approaches and a failure to take into account the physiological processes employed by the body to deal with particulate matter. He predicted the success of some areas of interdisciplinary research. After some 20 years of work on liposomes as drug carriers, clinical trials are now underway, and companies set up to exploit them. From this we can conclude that completely new technologies require much scientific proving, that original aims are not always achieved and that more modest goals may need to be defined. In the case of liposomes, the extravascular targeting potential, which was always somewhat flawed in concept, has been replaced with the more realistic aims of providing vehicles to modify the release rate or toxicity of drugs: Liposome Technology's research and development programme [4] aims in the immediate future to address delivery to the respiratory tract via aerosols, intravenous and ophthalmic delivery of drugs, and delivery of peptides. Should products with clinical benefit emerge from these programmes, as they undoubtedly will if preliminary results with amphotericin B are anything to go by, then the work, initiated perhaps by false promise, will have proved to have been worthwhile. However, if the concepts of vesicular delivery had been critically assessed at an earlier stage, liposomes might have made an earlier debut in man.

It is vitally important that scientists working in drug delivery accept and publicize the limitations as well as the potential of the systems with which they work. It is possible for the scientific community to be led down false trails; one example of scientific embarrassment in another field involved the study of polywater, which turned out not to be a new form of water but an artefact due to the leaching of silicate impurities from capillary tubes. Research into the targeting of liposomes, microspheres and monoclonal antibody drug carriers could fall into that category unless we find out more about the nature of the systems which we attempt to target, and the physical and anatomical factors that determine the destination and migration of drug carriers. Nevertheless we must continue to probe biological systems with synthetic or natural carriers so that facets of the organism, the opsonization of foreign particles, their adhesion to epithelial surfaces, uptake by cells of the reticuloendothelial system (RES), biodegradation, and translocation, can be explored. Many of these topics were covered in this conference.

In spite of advances in drug delivery by parenteral routes, the mouth will still be the portal of entry of choice for patients who have a choice. The complexities of the oral route are indicated by the fact that it has taken to the present time for an understanding of the nature of the transit of dosage forms down the gastrointestinal (GI) tract to emerge. The advent of gamma-scintigraphy aided this work, as **Davis** and his colleagues have admirably shown. In investigations of carrier systems the oral route has frequently been overlooked, yet several systems which have been extensively studied by the parenteral route, might be used orally. We heard of the oral use of albumin microspheres, for example, at this meeting.

In spite of the progress that has been made in understanding the oral route and its vagaries, more still must be learned about the dynamic system. There is a need to refine predictive powers by determining the optimal release rates of drugs *in vivo* in relation to rates of transit down the GI tract and the variable conditions for absorption in different sectors of the gut. The approach of Merkle and his colleagues will undoubtedly prove valuable in this context.

Much of what has been achieved by the oral route has probably been adventitious. It must be agreed that in the future drug delivery should be approached, like drug design, on a more rational basis than hitherto. It is largely impossible now because the appropriate information relating to the three elements of drug delivery systems (Fig. 1), the carrier, the route and the target, is not always accessible.

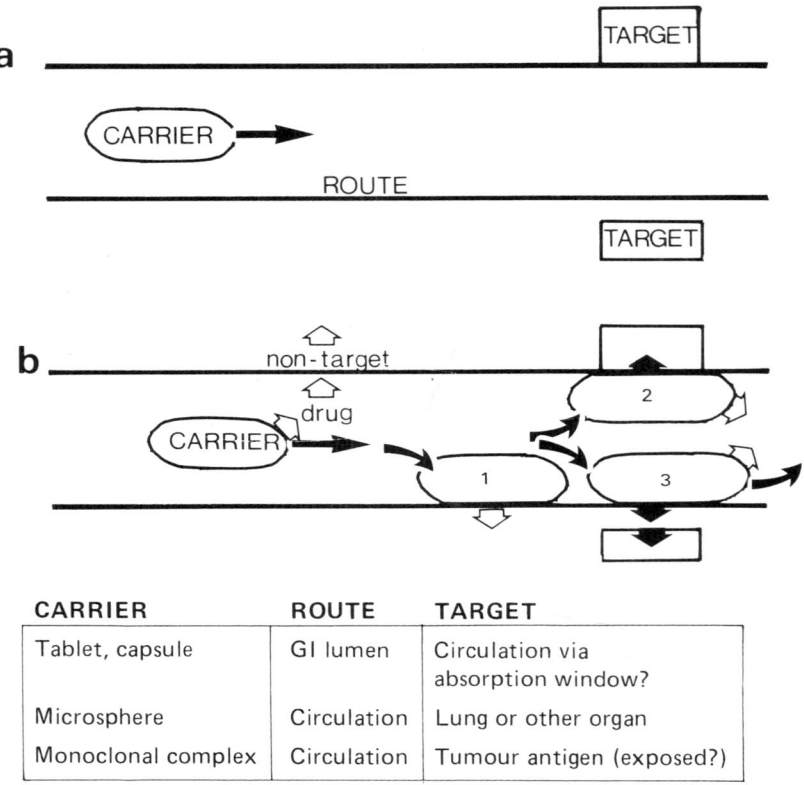

CARRIER	ROUTE	TARGET
Tablet, capsule	GI lumen	Circulation via absorption window?
Microsphere	Circulation	Lung or other organ
Monoclonal complex	Circulation	Tumour antigen (exposed?)

Fig. 15.1 — (a) The elements of drug delivery: the carrier, the route and the target. Two targets are shown, the upper site having direct access to the supply route; the lower target is at a distance from the supply route. (b) Shows the leakage of drug from the carrier as it moves in the systemic circulation or gastrointestinal tract and consequent loss of drug to non-target tissues, and the adhesion of the carrier (1) to the walls of the route and loss of drug to non-target sites. For successful targeting the carrier must locate at the target (2) and (3), but even here loss of drug to tissues other than the target can occur.

These elements must be considered whether one deals with a novel targeting system or a conventional oral tablet. Table 1 shows the main groups of drug carrier. Free drugs and prodrugs are freely diffusible. Other delivery systems may be categorized as mobile or static. Pharmaceutical laboratories have devoted their energies in the past to studying the properties of the carrier *in vitro* and have largely ignored the

Table 15.1 — Categories of drug delivery systems

Free drug	Diffusable
Prodrug	species
Macromolecular complexes	
Vesicles	
Nanoparticles	Mobile carriers
Microspheres	
Slow-release tablets	
Implants	
Mini-pumps	
Pumps	Static pumps
Transdermal patches	
Ocular devices	

nature of the target, which may simply be an absorption window in the case of orally administered drug. Certainly the location and access to target sites have until recently received little critical attention. It has been fortunate that it is of little concern in many cases whether the target and all surrounding tissues are saturated, but even with, for example, antibiotics of low toxicity, more precise delivery would seem to be in order, as most drugs are foreign entities.

In the case of colloidal and super-colloidal carriers, microspheres, vesicles, nanoparticles and other particulate systems, which are generally administered parenterally, the route to the target is the circulation, which, with its traps and sinks, has been underestimated. Escape routes are ill-understood. It is the ability or otherwise of mobile colloidal carriers to leave the systemic circulation and translocate to their target cell or organ which is the greatest problem facing those who quest for extravascular targeting. The problem of access—in sufficient concentration—is not one confined to carrier systems, but is shared by free drug and prodrug molecules. The problem to be addressed with carrier systems is more complex, as the dissociation of the drug has to be achieved at or in the target rather than *en route*, and rate control should optimally be achieved. Table 15.2 summarizes the factors which determine the success for drug delivery to one target, a solid tumour.

If we consider a spherical tumour as a target, even if the tumour can be bathed in drug solution, drug must diffuse in sufficient concentrations to kill aberrant cells. This is a process that needs further study [5,6]. When a carrier system is employed, not only must it approach the target, but drug must be released from it at an appropriate rate to maximize diffusion. Instantaneous release of drug from the carrier is unlikely, unless externally triggered. No microspherical device has yet been fabricated which can achieve this, although progress has been made towards responding systems. Liposomes have been prepared which respond to raised temperature [7] or pH change, and polymers whose permeability is influenced by

Table 15.2 — Factors controlling success of tumour therapy

Vascularization of tumour
Permeability of capillaries in tumour
Blood flow
Rate of drug release from delivery system
Physical homogeneity of tumour
Drug penetration
Cell sensitivity: optimal c–t relationships
Drug metabolism and binding in tumour
Drug escape from tumour

---

ultrasound [8] or magnetic fields [9] have been described. These form the basis of possible future responding systems.

Interactive systems are still something of a curiosity, although a reversible glucose-responsive delivery system was described at this meeting by Fischel-Ghodsian, Jacobs and Langer. It is clear that whatever the system and its aims, the *in vitro* and *in vivo* characteristics of the carrier, soluble or insoluble, disintegrating or non-disintegrating, such as those outlined in Fig. 2, must be determined.

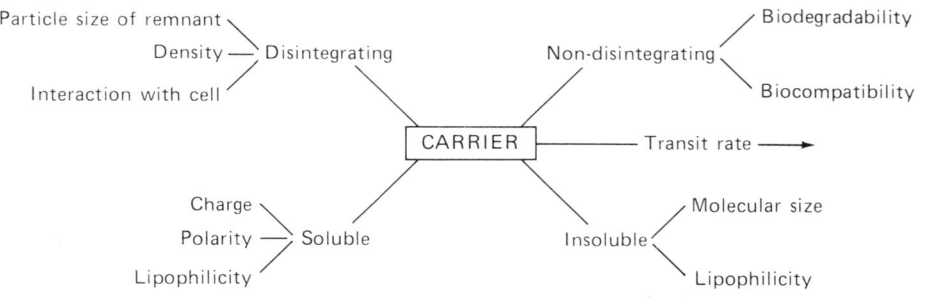

Fig. 15.2 — Properties of importance in evaluating carrier systems for drugs.

Yates [10] disagreed with the concept that we should 'design toward delivery of drugs locally where they act and then use the body as a universal sink'. 'If God had known that principle', he said 'He might not have invented the endocrine system. It uses the blood as a general channel and pours everything into it.' Selectivity is achieved at the target. This of course suggests chemical specificity, and a solution to targeting through medicinal chemistry. Dr Gardner was inclined to this view also, but it is fair to say that medicinal chemists have probably succeeded more often than pharmaceutical scientists only because they have prepared more bullets in the form of chemical compounds. It is rather more difficult to produce the same proliferation of delivery systems.

Although neither medicinal chemistry nor formulation is yet an exact science, it is time for medicinal chemists and formulation scientists to collaborate more closely. Whether one deals with a new chemical entity or a new carrier system, the array of physiological, chemical and physical problems to be overcome is similar. Drugs designed from the standpoint of receptor fit might not be transportable to the receptor. Specific drugs with selectivity for given cell types in optimized delivery systems are surely the aim. This can be argued as a general case even when many drugs can function apparently superbly in the simplest of tablets. Many of the delivery systems that have been the subject of extensive work are carriers waiting for the appropriate drug; the more potent the drug, the more the formulation scientist can do with it. The overall lack of clinical success with cancer chemotherapy suggests the need for continued attack on all fronts even though some avenues will turn out to be cul-de-sacs.

There are several elements to a review of progress. Critical approaches to past achievements is one and the proper comparisons of any system with alternatives another. Yet another is the examination of the range of behaviour of individual systems. Liposomes, for example, cannot be considered in a generic sense, because of the variety of phospholipids and adjuvants that can be used in their construction; a monoclonal antibody may behave differently with different drug molecules. **Rowland** pointed out at this conference that 'each antibody must be individually evaluated for any particular type of drug-coupling procedure requiring chemical manipulation', and **Lloyd** found that the nature of the drug altered the structural requirements for the essential spacer molecules between drug and polymeric carrier.

It seems that there is a need for a re-evaluation of success in drug delivery. A recent report observed the preferential localization of insulin in the ipsilateral lymph node when it was administered in small liposomes by the intramuscular route. But the capture in the lymph node represented only 3–4% of the dose. Is this targeting? Similar results have been noted with imaging and therapeutic radiolabelled carriers [11]. While the results on monoclonal antibody–drug complexes presented by **Rowland** at this meeting were promising, the more general finding is that the amount of specific antibody which locates in tumour tissue is low; one recent report [11] estimates that 0.05–0.2% of administered antibody located in the tumour. One hundred per cent of 25 μm diameter albumin microspheres lodge in the lung minutes after injection, but the drug released from them is free to locate elsewhere [12]. Perhaps we need a better index of targeting, and a better convention for expressing success.

The importance of comparison is all the more evident when a variety of systems is available. Experiments on one cannot produce the necessary comparative data. Direct comparison of perhaps complex systems with simpler systems should be advocated. Kovach *et al.* [13] reported on the regional targeting of bisantrene by directed intravascular precipitation following rapid injection into the internal ileac vein of a solution of the drug at pH 4.5. This resulted in concentrations of the drug in the urinary bladder wall supplied by the artery that were more than 1000 times those in the same tissue supplied by the artery following injection of the same dose of drug intravenously. Could sorption promotors, liposomes, or microspheres or prodrugs have achieved such a result? This simple expedient of causing a drug to precipitate produced an element of targeting which, by any measure of success, was significant. **Ganderton**, in his paper, made a plea for simplicity of approach, and gave as examples slow-release tablets patented by Mead-Johnson and Syntex which comprised in one case virtually 100% drug, achieving an effect without recourse to unnecessary technology.

It is tempting to think, and perhaps true, that the problems of oral, nasal and topical delivery are soluble. The problems of implants and implanted devices are within reach of the technology of this century. The problems of targeting seem so immense that we should be honest about it and define the problems that beset us.

TARGETING

Rowland pointed out in his paper some of the remaining concerns, but also the potential with monoclonal antibodies as carriers: problems remain with (i) antigenic heterogeneity, (ii) antigen expression outwith the target, (iii) cross-reactivity and (iv) the stability of the drug–antibody complex during transit to the site and its lability at the site, and (v) loss of potency of the complex. In spite of being able to administer without toxicity higher doses of conjugated vindesine than when free, this monoclonal conjugate at its highest dose led at best to 85% suppression of tumour growth leading Rowland to the conclusion that 'improving the therapeutic index does not guarantee a cure'. A selectivity of ten-fold was obtained with a vindesine anti-carcino-embryonic antigen antibody complex, and the concentration remained high for several days. Tumour levels of drug were found to be 1000 times greater. The mechanism of this has still to be explained. But whatever it is, other indices are improved: the LD50 increased by a factor of 15 and bone marrow depression and GI mucosal toxicity were absent. Levels in the liver and spleen and systemic toxicity with some systems might prove to be a problem.

Lloyd clearly distinguished between pinocytosis and phagocytosis, mechanisms of uptake of importance to soluble and particulate carriers respectively. Phagocytosis, unlike pinocytosis, is restricted to a few specialized cell types. Pinocytosis, though a more generalized activity, can nevertheless be substrate-specific. The attachment of a targeting moiety to particulate carriers is doomed to have little effect on body distribution, Lloyd avers. Davis and Illum [14] have, however, found that adsorbed macromolecules, such as the poloxamers, can indeed influence distribution of colloids by minimizing interactions with the RES. Similar problems of guaranteeing the destination of soluble carrier systems exist, particularly if non-specific adsorption to cells takes place. Intravascular aggregation of molecules can also occur, as the macromolecules become involved with the complex chemistry of the blood. Polymer interaction with cells requires further investigation as the role of factors such as molecular weight, shape and charge of the polymer has not been elucidated. Lloyd's view is that the major obstacle to targeting is our knowledge of the specific properties of cell types within the body.

Roerdink and coworkers have shown how the properties of liposomes can be engineered. Results with doxorubicin were ascribed to differential rates of drug release when vesicles with different fluidities are entrapped within hepatocytes. The reduction in cardiotoxicity of the drug following liposomal administration is possibly due to the sustained-release properties of the carrier, rather than to any targeting potential. Liposomal doxorubicin is one drug in clinical trial. Our own work [15] has shown that the presentation of the drug in niosomes (non-ionic surfactant vesicles) leads to a reduced level of the cardiotoxic metabolite. The possibility of altering metabolic profiles of drugs such as methotrexate and doxorubicin in niosomes [15–17] through altered kinetics and organ distribution perhaps opens up some additional horizons for carrier systems. It suggests, too, that this type of work must continue because we know so little of what is likely to happen on injection of the various drug complexes. The organism is probed. Drug is presented in new ways, at different rates for different durations to individual organs, sometimes in particles, and then released often from new sites. It would be a brave person who reckoned he could predict the outcome.

Ryman [18] pointed out that, on the one hand, while both RES and circulating monocytes would consume circulating liposomes which if they contained cytotoxic drugs would have serious implications for hopes of cancer chemotherapy with carriers, on the other hand liposomes have been found [19] to be capable of delivering macrophage-activating factor and muramyl dipeptide. As the circulating monocytes penetrate the alveolar space they are able to reduce lung metastases in mice and dogs. The liposome is therefore capable of delivering molecules which activate the natural defence mechanism of the body. Several speakers at this meeting have presented similar unpredictable findings, so there must be some measure of disagreement with any contention that the work with carrier systems is unlikely to lead far. **Tomlinson**, in his comprehensive paper, emphasizes this point, reminding us how knowledge of carrier systems can be applied not only to drug delivery, but to diverse objectives such as cellular delivery of genetic information, sorting of diseased cells from normal cells, and vaccines. His list of accessible biological targets for particulate carriers must be a sufficient challenge for the scientific and medical community.

The scope for the medication of discrete compartments and the treatment of accessible epithelial surfaces is great; even intralesional administration with carrier systems can lead to beneficial results [12].

The area of implantable systems is more dependent on technology than on the physiological responses of the surroundings, although these are not unimportant. In the papers by **Feijen, Hutchinson** and **Furr, Theeuwes,** and **Blackshear** was evident the ingenuity of the polymer scientist and chemical engineer in designing systems whose function depends on control over membrane permeability or matrix release. Semipermeability and osmotic flux determine the performance of osmotic pumps, and vapour pressure may control mechanical elements in an implanted pump. The task in the next decade will be to miniaturize some systems, as has already been achieved with the osmotic pump in the Oros device, so that they can be applied to routes other than the subcutaneous and to produce systems whose permeability can be remotely controlled.

Devices such as the implantable osmotic pump allow us to probe the biological response in more depth and have already shown their worth, as **Ray** and **Theeuwes** point out, in studying the temporal aspects of animal toxicology, an area of drug delivery which is much neglected. Microperfusion can lead to high local concentrations of drug, although it can never be generally true that selective drug delivery, however achieved, avoids the consequences of systemic administration, the problems of penetration, transport, scheduling and metabolism. The design of the delivery catheters of osmotic pumps to allow pulsed delivery of drug indicates what can be achieved. Pulsed-release systems based on controlled-release glasses have been described by Drake and others [20].

It is true that the majority of drugs will continue to be given by the oral route wherever this is possible. Patients will accept other routes where benefits can be shown or where there is no alternative. **Ganderton** reviewed the technological advances of systems for oral use and concluded that there was little place for some of the 'overelaborate' devices described in the patent literature and elsewhere. Systems can only be justified by their 'simplicity and consistency'. He emphasizes the need for pharmaceutical scientists not to lose sight of what some might call conventional technology.

Whenever technology results in non-disintegrating products, techniques are now available for the evaluation of their mode of transit and release characteristics in the GI tract, as **Davis** has shown. The work of his group has elucidated many of the factors that control the descent of dosage form. To modify the transit of oral dosage forms or to achieve retention of dosage forms say in the oral cavity, bioadhesives have been proposed. **Kellaway** has presented data on some potential adhesives and has investigated means of measuring the interaction between the dosage form and mucosal surfaces. However, it is possible that pharmacological control of gastric emptying may be the most likely approach in the future [21].

Drugs that are not absorbed well or at all from the GI tract may be absorbed by other routes, for example the intranasal route, which **Su** and colleagues reviewed. Drugs such as propranolol and progesterone that are absorbed orally may also be administered intranasally with some advantage, but the nature of the nasal formulations must be carefully addressed, particularly in relation to possible long-term toxic effects of administration to an organ not designed for such assault. Nasal bleeding and ulceration after administration of peptides are two side-effects that are obvious practical drawbacks. The potential for using some carrier systems to achieve sustained action and minimize local toxicities intranasally is a possibility.

Barry's review of transdermal drug delivery emphasizes the variability of the skin, not only in its permeability to drug molecules but also in its response to penetration enhancers necessary to achieve a therapeutic flux of some drugs across the skin. This makes the design of transdermal devices with rate-controlling membranes a more complex affair. Indeed it may be the physiological variability in patients that will prevent the purely technological solution to controlled-release medication by whatever route, including the oral route. Barry questions the value of some of the recently marketed patches for nitroglycerin, given the variability in plasma levels that result from their use. The tolerance that has been observed to long-term administration by transdermal patch is another example of the unexpected. Iontophoretic means of assisting transdermal penetration may be applied more widely in the future [22].

There is no suggestion that the cornea is a variable organ, but it is obviously less robust and the eye is not a channel for the systemic administration of drugs, but until recently medication of the eye has been a crude affair. **Shell's** review points out interesting differences in the metabolism of agents such as propranolol to the eye, however. Serious attention must be given to the treatment of serious, sight- and life-threatening diseases of the eye where continuous infusion of drug is required.

CONCLUSIONS

Although in many of our pursuits we have to accept the possibility of ultimate failure, we must accept our inability to predict the outcome of any research programme worth its name. Academic research must not be restricted by funding imperatives to pursue short-term goals and development work; it is necessary for groups to pursue drug delivery research even with experimental carrier systems that might be unacceptable in human medicine so that their performance *in vivo* can be analysed. Even if the results are unwelcome, lessons can be learned and better systems devised; much can be learned about the behaviour of drugs in this way. The tolerance to transdermal nitroglycerin, the rebound 'travel sickness' to transdermal hyoscine, the altered metabolism of doxorubicin delivered in microspheres, and the effect of poloxamers on the uptake by the RES of colloids were not predicted. While drug targeting is pursued it is important that pharmaceutical scientists do not abandon their traditional formulation pursuits. Many of the problems with new delivery systems depend on traditional skills for their solution. Above all there should be honesty in the appraisal of the system we work on, and there must exist the freedom to admit that an approach does not and cannot work or is inappropriately complex. When this is the norm, progress towards controlled and targeted drug delivery will be faster.

REFERENCES

[1] Gregoriadis, G. & Allison, A. C. (eds) (1980). *Liposomes in Biological Systems,* John Wiley, Chichester.
[2] Papahadjopolous, D. & Miller, N. (1978). Liposomes and their uses in biology and medicine. *Ann. N. Y. Acad. Sci.* **308**.
[3] Tomlinson, E. & Davis, S. S. (eds) (1986). *Site Specific Drug Therapy,* John Wiley, Chichester.
[4] Liposome Technology, Inc. Company Profile, March 1986. California.
[5] Florence, A. T. (1985). Rate control in targeted drug delivery. In: Prescott, L. & Nimmo, W. S. (eds) *Rate Control in Drug Therapy,* Churchill Livingstone, Edinburgh, p. 103.
[6] Weinstein, J. N., Black, C. D. V., Barbet, J., *et al.* (1986). In Tomlinson, E. & Davis, S. S. (eds) *Site Specific Drug Therapy,* John Wiley, Chichester.
[7] Magin, R. L. & Weinskein, T. N. (1980). Delivery of drugs in temperature-sensitive liposomes. In: Gregoriadis, G., Senior, J. & Trouet, A. (eds) *Targeting of Drugs,* Plenum Press, New York.
[8] Julian, T. W. & Zentner, G. M. (1986). Ultrasonically mediated solute permeation through polymer barriers. *J. Pharm. Pharmacol.* **38** 871.
[9] Hsieh, D. S. T. & Langer, R. (1983). Zero-order drug delivery systems with magnetic control. In: Roseman, T. J. & Mansdorf, S. Z. (eds) *Controlled Release Delivery Systems,* Marcel Dekker, New York, Chapter 7.

[10] Yates, F. E. (1972). In Urquhart, J. & Yates, F. E. (eds) *Temporal Aspects of Therapeutics,* Plenum Press, New York, p. 125.

[11] Vaughan, A. T. M., Bradwell, A. R., Dykes, P. W. & Anderson, P. (1986). Illusions of tumour killing using radio-labelled antibodies. *Lancet* **i** 1492.

[12] Willmott, N., Cummings, J., Stuart, J. F. B. & Florence, A. T. (1985). Adriamycin-loaded albumin microspheres: preparation, *in vivo* distribution and release in the rat. *Biopharm. Drug Dispos.* **6** 91.

[13] Kovach, J. S., Buck, M., Tsukamoto, T., Odegaard, A. & Leiber, M. M. (1985). Regional targeting of Bisantrene by directed intravascular precipitation. *Cancer Chemother. Pharmacol.* **15** 192.

[14] Davis, S. S. & Illum, L. (1986). Colloidal delivery systems—opportunities and challenges. In: Tomlinson, E. & Davis, S. S. (eds) *Site Specific Drug Therapy,* John Wiley, Chichester, p. 93.

[15] Rogerson, A., Cummings, J. & Florence, A. T. (1987) Adriamycin-loaded niosomes: drug entrapment, stability and release. *J. Microencapsulation,* in press.

[16] Azmin, M. N., Florence, A. T., Jandjani-Vila, R. M., Stuart, J. F. B., vanlerberghe, G. & Whittaker, J. S. (1985). The effect of nonionic surfactant vesicles (niosomes) entrapment on the absorption and distribution of methotrexate in mice. *J. Pharm. Pharmacol.* **37** 237–242.

[17] Azmin, M. N., Florence, A. T., Handjani-Vila, R. M., Stuart, J. F. B., vanlerberghe, G. & Whittaker, J. S. (1986). The effect of niosomes and polysorbate 80 on the metabolism and excretion of methotrexate in the mouse. *J. Microencapsulation* **3** 95.

[18] Ryman, B. E. (1983). Liposomes: possible potential in drug delivery. In: Roseman, T. J. & Mansdorf, S. Z. (eds) *Controlled Release Delivery Systems,* Marcel Dekker, New York.

[19] Poste, G. & Fidler, I. J. (1981). Stimulation of macrophage-mediated destruction of lung metastases by administration of immunomodulators encapsulated in liposomes. In: Nicolau, G. & Paraf, A. (eds) *Liposomes, Drugs and Immunocompetent Cell Functions,* Academic Press, London.

[20] Drake, C. F. & Allen, W. M. (1985). The use of controlled-release glass for the controlled delivery of bioactive materials. *Biochem. Soc. Trans.* **13** Pt. 2, 516–520.

[21] Gröning, R. & Heun, G. (1984). Oral dosage forms with controlled gastrointestinal transit. *Drug. Dev. Ind. Pharm.* **10** 527.

[22] Tyle, P. (1986). Iontophoretic devices for drug delivery. *Pharm. Res.* **3** 318–326.

[23] Ostro, M. J. (ed.) (1983). *Liposomes,* Marcel Dekker, New York.

Index

absorbable, 224
absorbed, 225, 239
absorption, 155, 224, 226, 227, 228, 232, 234, 235, 239
  enhancers, 175, 176
  of peptides and proteins, 175
  windows, 165, 169
acrylic polymers, 185
active ester, 85
adhesion, 182, 183
administered, 231
  nasally, 224
administering, 224, 239
administration, 226, 232, 234, 235, 239
Adriamycin, 69, 83, 85
alkaloid, 85
allergic skin reactions, 219
Alzet™ pump, 125
amino sugar, 85
amphotericin B, 69, 71
ampicillin, 70
amylopectin, 71
animal, 225, 232
  models, 225
antibodies, 24, 81, 82, 83, 84, 85, 86, 87, 88, 89, 90
  conjugate, 86, 87, 88, 89, 90
  conjugation, 85
antibody coupling, 85
anticancer drugs, 82, 88
anticancer drug targeting, 83
anti-CEA, 88
anti-CEA antibody, 87
anti-CEA monoclonals, 84
anti-CEA monoclonal, 11.285.14, 85, 86
antiferritin, 90
antigen, 82, 83, 84, 85, 86, 87, 90
antigenic heterogeneity, 84
antineoplastic drugs, 73
[14]C-antipyrine, AP), 129
antiserum, 82
antitoxin, 36
antitumour, 90
antitumour antibodies, 82

antiviral, 45
arthritis, 76
asiafetuin, 68
autoimmune disease, 89
azide, 85
Azone, 207, 214

bacteria, 37
basement membrane, 69
betamethasone 17-benzoate, 207
binding sites, 204
bioadhesion, 161
bioadhesive polymers, 180
bioavailability of topical steroids, 207
biodegradable carrier, 108
biodegradable formulations, 108
biodegradable hydrogels, 108
biodegradable polymers for controlled release, 106
biodistribution, 89
bioerodible systems, 256
bleomycin, 129
Brunner's glands, 181
brush border, 183
buoyancy, 152

cancer, 40, 83, 89, 90
  cell, 90
candidiasis, 71
Carbopol 934P, 193, 195
carboxylate groups, 183
carboxyl concentration, 186
carboxymethyl cellulose, 184
carcino-embryonic antigen (CEA), 84
carcinoma, 84
cardiotoxicity, 73
carrier, 33, 35, 36, 37, 40, 41, 44, 45, 46, 50, 52, 54, 84, 95, 96, 97, 100
catecholamine, 224, 235, 240
CEA, 84, 86, 87, 89
  (Colo 320 DM), 87
cells, 86, 87, 88
M-cells, 175
cellulosics, 186

central nervous system (CNS), 24, 25, 26
chemical derivative formation, 247
chemical interaction, 187
chemical potential, 206, 207
chimaeras, 90
chimaeric, 90, 91
    antibody, 90
chlorambucil, 82, 83, 85
chloroquine, 68
cholesterol, 67
cholesteryl- [^{14}C] oleate, 75
circadian, 134
cis-aconityl, 85
clearance, 86, 89
clinical, 88, 89
clonidine, 205, 216, 218
CNS, 24, 25, 26
colloids, 35, 38, 39, 42, 46, 47, 51
colloidal, 33, 35, 42, 46, 50, 53
    carrier, 37, 39
    particle endothelia, 51
    particles, 37, 48, 50, 51
colon, 89, 152, 154, 161, 165
    adenocarcinoma, 72
colorectal cancer, 89
colorectal carcinoma, 84
conjugates, 82, 84, 85, 86, 87, 89, 90, 96, 97, 100, 102
conjugated drug, 86
conjugation, 85, 88, 89
controlled release, 164
copolymers, 48, 99
copolymerized, 99
correlation *in vitro*, 173
correlation *in vivo*, 173
cortisol palmitate, 76
coupling, 84, 85, 86, 90
    daunomycin, 85
cross-reactivity, 84
cryptococcosis, 71
cytosine arabinoside, 69, 83, 86
cytotoxic, 32, 39, 44, 71
cytotoxicity, 86

daunomycin, 83, 85
deconvolution, 165
    of pharmacokinetic data, 173
decylmethylsulphoxide, 214
degradation of poly (lactide-co-glycolide), 111
degradation studies on poly (d,1-lactide-co-glycolide), 109
delivery of drugs to the colon, 175
delivery rate, 19, 23
density, 170
depot sites, 205
detoxify, 32
devices, 12, 13, 16, 18, 19, 21, 22, 23
diazotisation, 85
diffusional systems, 252
dimensional change, 152
dimethylformamide, 207
dimethylisosorbide, 207

dimethylsulphoxide, 211
dimyristoylphosphatidycholine, 68
dipalmitoyl phosphatidylglycerol (DPPG), 74
dissolution, 159, 160
distearoyl phosphatidylcholine (DSPC), 74
dogs, 225, 239, 240
^{14}C-dopamine hydrochloride (DA), 130
dosage forms, 164
doxorubicin (DXR), 73
drug-antibody conjugate, 85, 86, 87, 88, 90
drug-antibody targeting, 85
drug-carrier, 83
drug delivery, 12, 14, 15, 19, 21, 23, 28
drug delivery device, 16
drug delivery system, 66
drug-monoclonal conjugates, 89
drug pulse, 162
drug release studies, 173
drug scheduling, 120
drug targeting, 83, 89, 90
duration of drug action, 157

11.285.14, 8
egg phosphatidylcholine (PC), 74
elasticity, 182
electrostatic, 184
ELISA, 84
emulsions, 247
endocytosis, 95, 96, 97
endothelia, 40, 41, 49, 50, 51, 52, 83
endothelial, 38, 39, 40, 42, 49, 50, 51, 52
    cells, 68
endotheliu, 36, 38, 52
enzymes, 95, 96, 100, 204
    inhibitors, 2–4
enzymic, 100, 102
epithelia, 37
epithelial, 36
epithelium, 36
ergosterol, 71
exercise tachycardia, 259
extravascular, 33, 34, 45, 50, 53
eye, 12, 35, 36

F(ab')$_2$ fragments, 69
fenestrations, 68
fentanyl, 216
Fick's law, 252
first-pass effect, 259
first pass phenomenon, 205
floating tablets, 170
fluid, 75
5-fluorouracil, 214
formulation, 237, 239
fungal, 44
fungally, 44

galactose-receptors, 68
gamma scintigraphy, 165
gastric emptying, 16, 18
gastric retention, 181
gastrointestinal motility, 152

gastrointestinal tract, 164
gastrointestinal transit of foods, 171
gastroscopy, 165
gelatin, 184
gel state, 67
gene cloning, 90
GI transit, 180, 195
glycocalyx, 184
glycoproteins, 84, 182
goblet cells, 181
Guar gum, 185
gum tragacanth, 184

hairless mouse skin, 212
hepatocytes, 68
high density lipoproteins (HDL), 68
histoplasmosis, 71
homo- and co-polymers of lactic and glycolic
    acid, 107
homopolymers, 99
hormone-responsive animal and human
    mammary and prostate tumours, 113
housekeeper wave, 167
human skin, 200
hybridoma, 83, 90
hydration, 213
hydrocortisone, 210
hydrogel, 153, 158
hydrophobic interactions, 184
hydrophilic matrices, 245
hydrophobic matrix, 257
hydrophobic polymer, 183
hydroethylcellulose, 185
hyoscine (scopolamine), 216
hyoscine, 217
hypersensitivity, 89

IgM immunocytoma, 74
ileocaecal sphincter, 171
imaging, 83, 84, 88
immunisation, 82, 90
immunoconjugate, 84, 86
    targeting, 83, 86
immunocytochemistry, 83, 84
immunofluorescence, 83
immunogen, 84
immunoglobulin, 81, 85, 90
immunomodulators, 71
immunotargeting, 83
immunotherapy, 76
immunotoxin, 90, 91
implants, 15, 16, 22, 23, 28, 120
implantable, 21
implant technology, 28
injection-infusion comparison protocol, 126
γ-interferon, 71
interstitial, 37, 39
interstitially, 38
interstitial particle, 38
interstitium, 37
intestinal motility, 161
intranasal, 224, 228, 234, 235, 239, 240, 241

absorption, 225
administration, 224, 225, 227, 231, 232, 235,
    237, 239
drug delivery systems, 224
sustained release formulation, 224, 237, 239,
    241
intranasally, 224, 240
intratumour, 39
[^{3}H] inulin, 75
ion pairs, 247
iontophoresis, 220
irritable bowel, 175
isosorbide dinitrate, 217

Karya gum, 185
keratin fibrils, 211
Kupffer, 36, 42, 43, 46
    cells, 67

(d, 1-lactide-co-glycolide), 109
lactosylceramide, 68
lag times, 206
Lamellae, 249
LDL, 52
Legionella pneumophila, 71
Leishmaniasis, 70
liposomal, 35, 36, 44, 46
liposomes, 33, 35, 37, 38, 39, 43, 44, 45, 46, 47,
    48, 49, 50, 53, 54, 55, 66, 247
    particles, 35, 38, 44, 50, 51
liquid-crystalline phase, 67
Listeria monocytogenes, 70
liver parenchymal cells, 68
liver sinusoids, 68
localisation, 88, 89
localise, 89
LS174T, 87
lungs, 35, 36, 41, 42, 47
luteinising hormone releasing hormone, 106
lymph, 35, 37, 38, 39
lymphatic, 37, 38, 39, 54
    carriers, 39
    endothelial, 9
lymph node metastases, 76
lymphocytes, 37
lymphoid, 37
lymphoidal, 37
lymphokines, 71
lymphoma, 83
lymphoscintigraphy, 38
lymphotropic, 38
lysine, 85
lysosomal, 45, 67, 102
    endocytosis, 67
    enzymes, 96, 97, 100, 101, 102
lysosomally, 45, 100, 102
lysosomes, 45, 54, 95, 96, 97, 100, 102

macromolecular, 37, 55, 97
    drugs, 107
macromolecules, 36, 37, 38, 39, 42, 48, 51, 54, 85,
    95, 96, 97, 98, 100

macrophage, 35, 42, 43, 44, 45, 46, 47, 67
matrix system, 216
mechanisms of transport, 108
meglumine antimoniate, 70
melanoma, 83
β16-melanoma, 72
melphalan, 83
metabolic, 205
metabolism, 204
metastatic, 71
methotrexate, 82, 83
    conjugate, 89
methoxerate-monoclonal conjugate, 89
methylcellulose (MeC), 185
N-methylpyrrolidone, 207
mice, 86, 87, 88
microparticles, 36
microvilli, 184
microviscosity, 183
migrating myoelectric complex (MMC), 167
mini-osmotic pumps, 122
modulating the intensity of drug action, 154
monoclonals, 82, 83, 84, 85, 86, 87, 88, 90
    11.285.14, 85
    antibodies, 69, 82, 83, 84, 89, 90
    anti-CEA, 86, 87
monolithic, 35, 52, 216
    particles, 48, 51
mononitrate, 217
motility of the gastrointestinal tract, 167
MPS, 41, 42, 44, 45, 46, 47, 48, 51, 53, 54
mucin-mucin interaction, 183
mucoadhesives, 181
mucoadhesive bond, 182
mucoadhesive materials, 170
mucosal adhesives, 152, 155
mucosal surface, 181
mucus, 181, 182
    cells, 181
    layer, 181
mucus-mucosa interaction, 182
myramyl dipeptide (MDP), 71
myristic acid, 155

nanoparticles, 33, 34, 36, 37, 47
nasal, 27, 28, 36, 37, 225, 226, 228, 229, 234, 235
    absorption, 224, 225, 226, 227, 229, 231, 232,
        234, 235, 237, 239
    administration, 225, 226, 227, 228, 229, 232,
        235, 237, 239, 240
nasally, 234
nasopalatine, 225
nitroglycerin, 204, 216, 217
non-colloidal, 33
nose, 235
nostrils, 226

ocular, 12, 13, 36
    inserts, 249
oestradoil, 210, 216
ointments, 246
oleic acid, 207, 214

oligopeptide, 95, 99, 100, 101, 102
onocogene, 90
ophthalmic systems, 244
opsonins, 42, 43, 46
opsonisation, 43, 47, 48
opsonised, 43, 45
optimal site, 235
optimisation of percutaneous absorption, 206
orabase, 184
orahesive, 184
oral, 15, 16, 19, 21, 26, 27
    controlled release, 180
    delivery rate, 18
    dosage forms, 164
orally, 26
oral mucosa, 196
osmotic pumps, 120, 174
osmotic systems, 254
osteogenic sarcoma, 84
osteogenic sarcoma target cell 791T, 86
overview, 11

parenteral, 39, 55
particles, 33, 34, 35, 36, 37, 38, 39, 40, 41, 42, 43,
    45, 46, 47, 48, 49, 50, 51, 52, 53, 54, 55
particulates, 33, 34, 36, 37, 45, 50, 51, 52
    carriers, 33, 34, 35, 36, 37, 44, 45, 49, 51, 53,
        55
    macromolecules, 51
partition coefficient, 202, 210
pathological conditions, 171
patterned administration, 120
peak blood levels, 154
pectin, 184
peel strength, 187
pellets, 168
penetration enhancers, 204, 206, 207
peptide, 21, 22, 25, 26, 27, 28, 224, 225, 231, 234
    drugs, 220
percutaneous absorption, 220
phagocyte, 41, 42, 45, 46, 97, 98
phagocytic, 35, 36, 42, 43, 45, 47, 50
phagocytose, 38, 43, 44
phagocytosing, 36, 46, 48
phagocytosis, 36, 39, 42, 43, 45, 46, 47, 48, 96, 97
pharmacokinetic profiles, 165
phosphatidylcholine, 67
phosphatidylserine, 67, 74
phospholipids, 67
physiological factors, 167
    on the gastrointestinal transit of
        pharmaceutical systems, 170
pinocytic, 96, 100
pinocytosis, 95, 96, 97, 98, 99, 102
platinum, 83
polycarbophil, 155, 195, 196
polyclonal, 82, 83, 88
    antibodies, 81, 82, 83
    antobody vindesine, 89
polyethylene glycol (PEG), 185
poly(ethylene oxide) (PEO), 186
polyHPMA, 96, 99, 100, 101, 102

polyisobutylene, 219
poly (d,1-lactide), 109
polymers, 23, 95, 97, 98, 99, 100, 101, 102
polymeric carrier, 8
polymer mucin interaction, 183
polypeptides, 106
    hormones, 107
preservatives, 259
pro-drug, 24, 25, 27, 247
propylene glycol, 207, 214
proteins, 26, 28, 211, 224, 225, 231, 234
pulsatile, 21, 23
2-pyrrolidone, 207

quaternary ammonium compound, 224, 226, 228
quaternary ammonium drugs, 229

rabbit antibodies, 83
radiocolloids, 35
radioimmunoimaging, 88
radiommunolocalisation, 84
radiolabelling, 88
radiolocalisation, 88
radiological (X-ray) studies, 165
radionuclides, 166
rats, 225, 226, 228, 232, 235
rate-controlled drug release, 251
rate-controlling membrane, 203
rate-limiting membrane, 216
rate of absorption, 154
C-reactive protein, 72
receptor, 205
recombinant DNA, 90, 91
rectal, 28
release studies with Zoladex™, 113
RES, 42
reserve length concept, 164
reservoir, 204
respiratory distress syndrome, 76
retene, 185
reticuloendothelial system (RES), 67
rhythm, 134
ricin, 91

791T/36, 84, 89
scintigraphy, 89
secondary bonding, 185
sensitisation reactions, 205
single units, 168
sisomycin, 71
site-specific, 33, 34, 41, 45, 54
    carriers, 34
    delivery, 120
sodium alginate, 185
sodium carboxymethyl cellulose (SCMC), 184
^{3}H-sodium methotrexate (MTX), 130
sodium-5-methoxysalicylate, 155
sodium salicylate, 155
solid, 75
solubility, 154, 157
soluble, 95
    gels, 246

macromolecules, 96, 97
    polymer, 95
stearylamine, 67
steroid esters, 204
stratum corneum, 204
subendothelial, 38, 49
surfactants, 211
suspensions, 247
sustained release, 69, 107, 224
    biodegradable delivery systems for peptide
        drugs, 108
    formulation, 237

targets, 11, 12, 23, 24, 25, 82, 84, 87, 89, 90, 95,
    97, 100
targetable, 97, 100, 101
target antigen, 86, 87, 90
target cells, 86
target cytotoxicity, 86
targeted, 100, 102
    administration, 131
    delivery, 120
targeting, 23, 24, 25, 81, 84, 97, 100, 102
    of drugs in the gastrointestinal tract, 152
    with the gastrointestinal tract, 175
technology, 12, 16, 21, 22, 26, 28
tensile strength, 187
testosterone, 216
theory for penetration enhancer activity, 208
therapeutic index, 87
thermodynamic control, 207
timolol, 216
tissue surface, 183
total transit, 173
toxic, 53
toxicity, 33, 36, 44, 53, 84, 87, 88, 89
toxicology, 120
trachoma, 260
tragacanth, 185
transdermal, 14, 15, 16, 21, 22
    delivery devices, 200
    drug delivery, 200
    drug delivery systems, 216
transdermally, 14
Transderm system, 216
transition temperature (T_c), 67
transit of dosage forms in the small intestine, 170
transit times, 180
transport mechanisms, 201
treatment of ulcerative colitis, 175
tumour, 38, 39, 41, 42, 45, 47, 50, 83, 85, 86, 87,
    88, 89, 90
    cells, 82
    endothelia, 50, 51
    targets, 83
    xenograft (MAWI), 86, 87, 88
tyroxines, 85

valproic acid (VPA), 126
vasoconstrictor assay, 207
VDS, 86, 87, 88
    monoclonal, 87

vinca, 84, 86
  alkaloid, 85, 86
vindesine, 84, 86, 87, 88, 89, 90
  antibody conjugate, 88, 89
  anti-CEA, 87
  monoclonal antibody conjugates, 85
  monoclonal conjugate, 86
viral, 45, 46

virally, 45
virus, 45, 46

xenografts, 84

zero order, 120
Zoladex™, 106